Imaging of the Small Bowel and Colorectum

Editor

JUDY YEE

RADIOLOGIC CLINICS OF NORTH AMERICA

www.radiologic.theclinics.com

Consulting Editor
FRANK H. MILLER

September 2018 • Volume 56 • Number 5

ELSEVIER

1600 John F. Kennedy Boulevard • Suite 1800 • Philadelphia, Pennsylvania, 19103-2899

http://www.theclinics.com

RADIOLOGIC CLINICS OF NORTH AMERICA Volume 56, Number 5
September 2018 ISSN 0033-8389, ISBN 13: 978-0-323-61410-8

Editor: John Vassallo (j.vassallo@elsevier.com)
Developmental Editor: Donald Mumford

Radiologic Clinics of North America (ISSN 0033-8389) is published bimonthly by Elsevier Inc., 360 Park Avenue South, New York, NY 10010-1710. Months of issue are January, March, May, July, September, and November. Periodicals postage paid at New York, NY and additional mailing offices. Subscription prices are USD 493 per year for US individuals, USD 889 per year for US institutions, USD 100 per year for US students and residents, USD 573 per year for Canadian individuals, USD 1136 per year for Canadian institutions, USD 680 per year for international individuals, USD 1136 per year for international institutions, and USD 315 per year for Canadian and international students/residents. To receive student and resident rate, orders must be accompanied by name of affiliated institution, date of term and the signature of program/residency coordinatior on institution letterhead. Orders will be billed at individual rate until proof of status is received. Foreign air speed delivery is included in all *Clinics* subscription prices. All prices are subject to change without notice. **POSTMASTER:** Send address changes to *Radiologic Clinics of North America*, Elsevier Health Sciences Division, Subscription Customer Service, 3251 Riverport Lane, Maryland Heights, MO63043. **Customer Service: Telephone: 1-800-654-2452** (U.S. and Canada); **1-314-447-8871** (outside U.S. and Canada). **Fax: 1-314-447-8029. E-mail: journalscustomerservice-usa@ elsevier.com (for print support); journalsonlinesupport-usa@elsevier.com (for online support)**.

Reprints. For copies of 100 or more of articles in this publication, please contact the Commercial Reprints Department, Elsevier Inc., 360 Park Avenue South, New York, New York 10010-1710. Tel.: +1-212-633-3874; Fax: +1-212-633-3820; E-mail: reprints@elsevier.com.

Radiologic Clinics of North America also published in Greek Paschalidis Medical Publications, Athens, Greece.

Radiologic Clinics of North America is covered in *MEDLINE/PubMed (Index Medicus), EMBASE/Excerpta Medica, Current Contents/Life Sciences, Current Contents/Clinical Medicine, RSNA Index to Imaging Literature, BIOSIS, Science Citation Index,* and *ISI/BIOMED.*

Contributors

CONSULTING EDITOR

FRANK H. MILLER, MD, FACR
Lee F. Rogers MD Professor of Medical
Education, Chief, Body Imaging Section and
Fellowship Program, Medical Director, MRI,
Department of Radiology, Northwestern Memorial
Hospital, Northwestern University, Feinberg
School of Medicine, Chicago, Illinois, USA

EDITOR

JUDY YEE, MD, FACR
Professor and University Chair, Department of
Radiology, Montefiore Medical Center, Albert
Einstein College of Medicine, New York, New
York, USA

AUTHORS

MAHMOUD AL-HAWARY, MD
Associate Professor, Department of Radiology,
Medical School, Director, GI Radiology
Service, Abdominal Radiology Division,
Michigan Medicine, University of Michigan,
Ann Arbor, Michigan, USA

MARK E. BAKER, MD
Professor of Radiology, Cleveland Clinic Lerner
College of Medicine of Case Western Reserve
University, Staff, Abdominal Imaging Section,
Imaging Institute, Cleveland Clinic, Cleveland,
Ohio, USA

DAVID BRUINING, MD
Associate Professor of Medicine, Mayo Clinic
School of Medicine, Consultant, Division of
Gastroenterology and Hepatology,
Department of Internal Medicine, Mayo Clinic,
Rochester, Minnesota, USA

ONOFRIO CATALANO, MD, PhD
Assistant Professor, Department of Radiology,
Division of Abdominal Imaging, Medical
Director of PET/MR, A. Martinos Center for
Biomedical Imaging, Massachusetts General
Hospital, Harvard Medical School, Boston,
Massachusetts, USA

KEVIN J. CHANG, MD
Department of Radiology, Newton-Wellesley
Hospital, Adjunct Associate Professor of
Diagnostic Imaging, The Warren Alpert Medical
School of Brown University, Newton,
Massachusetts, USA

JAY COLEMAN, MD
Department of Radiology, University of Texas
Southwestern Medical Center, Dallas, Texas,
USA

LAURA EISENMENGER, MD
Departments of Radiology and Biomedical
Imaging, University of California, San
Francisco, San Francisco, California,
USA

JEFF L. FIDLER, MD
Professor, Department of Radiology, Mayo
Clinic, Rochester, Minnesota, USA

JOEL G. FLETCHER, MD
Professor, Department of Radiology, Mayo
Clinic School of Medicine, Consultant,
Department of Radiology, Mayo Clinic,
Rochester, Minnesota, USA

MARC J. GOLLUB, MD, FACR
Department of Radiology, Memorial Sloan
Kettering Cancer Center, New York, New York,
USA

LIJUN GUO, MD
Post-doctoral Fellow, Joint Department of
Medical Imaging, University Health Network,
Toronto, Ontario, Canada

MUKESH G. HARISINGHANI, MD
Professor of Harvard Medical School,
Director of Abdominal MRI, Section Editor
for GU Imaging and American Journal
of Roentgenology, Department of Abdominal
Imaging, Massachusetts General
Hospital, Boston, Massachusetts,
USA

NATALLY HORVAT, MD
Department of Radiology, Memorial Sloan
Kettering Cancer Center, New York,
New York, USA; Department of Radiology,
Hospital Sírio-Libanês, São Paulo, São Paulo,
Brazil

EUGENE HUO, MD
Department of Radiology, San Francisco VA
Medical Center, San Francisco, California,
USA

KARTIK S. JHAVERI, MD
Director of Abdominal MRI, CME Director of
Medical Imaging, Joint Department of Medical
Imaging, University Health Network, Mount
Sinai Hospital, Women's College Hospital,
Associate Professor, University of Toronto,
Toronto, Ontario, Canada

GAURAV KHATRI, MD
Associate Professor, Department of Radiology,
University of Texas Southwestern Medical
Center, Dallas, Texas, USA

AOIFE KILCOYNE, MD
Instructor, Department of Radiology, Division
of Abdominal Imaging, Massachusetts General
Hospital, Harvard Medical School, Boston,
Massachusetts, USA

DAVID H. KIM, MD
Professor, Department of Radiology, University
of Wisconsin-Madison School of Medicine
and Public Health, Madison, Wisconsin,
USA

AMY B. KOLBE, MD
Department of Radiology, Mayo Clinic,
Rochester, Minnesota, USA

JOHN R. LEYENDECKER, MD
Professor, Department of Radiology, University
of Texas Southwestern Medical Center, Dallas,
Texas, USA

UMAR MAHMOOD, MD, PhD
Professor, Massachusetts General Hospital,
Director of Precision Medicine, A. Martinos
Center for Biomedical Imaging, Harvard
Medical School, Charlestown, Massachusetts,
USA

COURTNEY C. MORENO, MD
Associate Professor, Department of Radiology
and Imaging Sciences, Emory University
School of Medicine, Atlanta, Georgia,
USA

TREVOR C. MORRISON, MD
Assistant Professor of Radiology, Boston
University Medical Center, Boston,
Massachusetts, USA

MARKUS M. OBMANN, MD
Research Specialist, Department of Radiology,
University of California, San Francisco,
San Francisco, California, USA

MICHAEL A. OHLIGER, MD, PhD
Associate Professor, Department of
Radiology, University of California,
San Francisco, San Francisco, California,
USA

IVA PETKOVSKA, MD
Department of Radiology, Memorial Sloan
Kettering Cancer Center, New York, New York,
USA

PERRY J. PICKHARDT, MD
Professor, Department of Radiology, University
of Wisconsin-Madison School of Medicine and
Public Health, Madison, Wisconsin,
USA

BRUCE ROSEN, MD, PhD
Professor, Director, Martinos Center for
Biomedical Imaging, Harvard Medical School,
Professor of Health Sciences, Massachusetts
Institute of Technology, Charlestown,
Massachusetts, USA

SHANNON P. SHEEDY, MD
Department of Radiology, Mayo Clinic, Rochester, Minnesota, USA

ALBERTO SIGNORE, MD, PhD
Professor, Nuclear Medicine Unit, Department of Medical-Surgical Sciences and of Translational Medicine, Faculty of Medicine and Psychology, Sapienza University, Rome, Italy

JORGE A. SOTO, MD, PhD
Professor of Radiology, Boston University Medical Center, Boston, Massachusetts, USA

JAAP STOKER, MD, PhD
Department of Radiology and Nuclear Medicine, Academic Medical Center, University of Amsterdam, Amsterdam, The Netherlands

YUXIN SUN, MS
Senior Research Assistant, Department of Radiology, University of California, San Francisco, San Francisco, California, USA

SENG THIPPHAVONG, MD
Abdominal Radiologist, Joint Department of Medical Imaging, University Health Network, Mount Sinai Hospital, Women's College Hospital, Associate Professor, University of Toronto, Toronto, Ontario, Canada

MARIJE P. VAN DER PAARDT, MD, PhD
Resident, Department of Radiology, Albert Schweitzer Ziekenhuis, Dordrecht, The Netherlands; Department of Radiology and Nuclear Medicine, Academic Medical Center, University of Amsterdam, Amsterdam, The Netherlands

ZHEN J. WANG, MD
Associate Professor, Department of Radiology, University of California, San Francisco, San Francisco, California, USA

STEFANIE WEINSTEIN, MD
Department of Radiology, San Francisco VA Medical Center, San Francisco, California, USA

MICHAEL WELLS, MD
Assistant Professor, Department of Radiology, Mayo Clinic, Rochester, Minnesota, USA

ANTONIO C. WESTPHALEN, MD, PhD
Professor, Department of Radiology, University of California, San Francisco, San Francisco, California, USA

JUDY YEE, MD, FACR
Professor and University Chair, Department of Radiology, Montefiore Medical Center, Albert Einstein College of Medicine, New York, New York, USA

BENJAMIN M. YEH, MD
Professor, Department of Radiology, University of California, San Francisco, San Francisco, California, USA

Contents

Preface: Innovations in Bowel Imaging   xiii

Judy Yee

Computed Tomography Enterography   649

Shannon P. Sheedy, Amy B. Kolbe, Joel G. Fletcher, and Jeff L. Fidler

Computed tomography enterography (CTE) is a noninvasive imaging modality with superb spatial and temporal resolution, specifically tailored to evaluate the small bowel. It has several advantages over other radiologic and optical imaging modalities, all of which serve as complementary investigations to one another. This article describes the CTE technique, including dose reduction techniques, special considerations for the pediatric population, and common technical and interpretive pitfalls, and reviews some of the more common small bowel entities seen with CTE.

Magnetic Resonance Enterography for Inflammatory and Noninflammatory Conditions of the Small Bowel   671

Gaurav Khatri, Jay Coleman, and John R. Leyendecker

Magnetic resonance enterography (MRE) is an effective noninvasive tool for the evaluation of inflammatory and noninflammatory conditions of the small bowel. MRE allows for repeated evaluation of patients with Crohn's disease without exposure to ionizing radiation and can be used to assess disease status and direct management. MRE also allows the evaluation of neoplastic and other nonneoplastic conditions of the small bowel. Adequate patient preparation and acquisition techniques are required for optimal image quality.

Interdisciplinary Updates in Crohn's Disease Reporting Nomenclature and Cross-Sectional Disease Monitoring   691

Mark E. Baker, Joel G. Fletcher, Mahmoud Al-Hawary, and David Bruining

Computed tomography enterography and magnetic resonance enterography are essential in the evaluation and treatment of patients with Crohn's disease. As such, examination reporting must use standardized nomenclature for effective communication. This report documents an interdisciplinary consensus of the Society of Abdominal Radiology, the Society of Pediatric Radiology, and the American Gastroenterology Association on the computed tomography enterography/magnetic resonance enterography imaging findings and imaging-based morphologic phenotypes.

Low-Dose Computed Tomography Colonography Technique   709

Kevin J. Chang and Judy Yee

Significant anxiety has been expressed by some over the radiation risks associated with computed tomography (CT), particularly when it applies to a screening examination such as CT colonography. These theoretic risks are far outweighed by the significant benefits colorectal cancer screening offers. Regardless of how significant the theoretic risk of CT radiation is in the older population, the ALARA principle maintains that radiation dose should be reduced to As Low As Reasonably Achievable. This article discusses various strategies that may be used to reduce radiation dose and mitigate any increase in image noise that may occur.

Computed Tomography Colonography: Pearls and Pitfalls   719

David H. Kim, Courtney C. Moreno, and Perry J. Pickhardt

This article serves as a practical reference to optimize the performance of computed tomography colonography in the detection of colorectal neoplasia. A specific protocol in use at 2 US university programs and defined interpretation strategies are described. With this framework in place, various clinical pearls as well as pitfalls to avoid are a major focus of this article.

Current Status of Magnetic Resonance Colonography for Screening and Diagnosis of Colorectal Cancer   737

Marije P. van der Paardt and Jaap Stoker

Magnetic resonance colonography with its high tissue contrast and without the use of ionizing radiation was designed as a minimally invasive screening tool for colorectal cancer and its precursors. Nonetheless, heterogeneous data on diagnostic performance and patient burden have hindered its use in screening. This article provides an overview on the status and potential of magnetic resonance colonography in the setting of detection and screening of colorectal cancer and its precursors.

MR Imaging of Rectal Cancer   751

Natally Horvat, Iva Petkovska, and Marc J. Gollub

This article reviews current concepts in the management of patients with rectal cancer, including the most common surgical techniques, anatomic landmarks with MR imaging correlation, and the role of each imaging modality in local staging, focusing on MR imaging technique and its importance in primary staging, restaging, and local recurrence.

MR Imaging of Perianal Fistulas   775

Kartik S. Jhaveri, Seng Thipphavong, Lijun Guo, and Mukesh G. Harisinghani

In this article, the authors begin with an introduction of the perianal region anatomy, then review the definition, etiology, epidemiology, and 2 major classification systems of perianal fistulas. The role of MR imaging for the assessment of perianal fistulas is mainly discussed. Finally, the medical and surgical treatment principles are reviewed.

Imaging Workup of Acute and Occult Lower Gastrointestinal Bleeding   791

Trevor C. Morrison, Michael Wells, Jeff L. Fidler, and Jorge A. Soto

Lower gastrointestinal bleeding is defined as occurring distal to the ligament of Treitz and presents as hematochezia, melena, or with anemia and positive fecal occult blood test. Imaging plays a pivotal role in the localization and treatment of lower gastrointestinal bleeds. Imaging tests in the workup of acute lower gastrointestinal bleeding include computed tomography (CT) angiography, nuclear medicine scintigraphy, and conventional catheter angiography. Catheter angiography can also be used to deliver treatment. Imaging tests in the workup of occult lower gastrointestinal bleeding include CT enterography and nuclear medicine Meckel scan.

Dual-Energy Computed Tomography Scans of the Bowel: Benefits, Pitfalls, and Future Directions   805

Benjamin M. Yeh, Markus M. Obmann, Antonio C. Westphalen, Michael A. Ohliger, Judy Yee, Yuxin Sun, and Zhen J. Wang

Current computed tomography bowel imaging is challenging given the variable distension, content, and location of the bowel; the different appearance of tumors within and adjacent to bowel; and peristaltic artifacts. Published data remain sparse. Derangements in enhancement may be highlighted, image artifacts reduced, and radiation dose from multiphase scans minimized. This modality is suited for bowel tumor detection and characterization and imaging gastrointestinal bleeding, bowel inflammation, and ischemia. Experimental results on computed tomography colonography and novel bowel contrast material offer hope for major improvements in bowel interrogation. It is likely to become increasingly valuable for bowel-related disease diagnosis and monitoring.

Lower Gastrointestinal Tract Applications of PET/Computed Tomography
and PET/MR Imaging   821

Onofrio Catalano, Aoife Kilcoyne, Alberto Signore, Umar Mahmood, and Bruce Rosen

This article discusses the role of PET/CT and PET/MR imaging in the evaluation of inflammatory and malignant disorders of the lower gastrointestinal tract, including a review of the current literature and a discussion of new and emerging research.

Imaging of the Postoperative Colon   835

Eugene Huo, Laura Eisenmenger, and Stefanie Weinstein

Recognition of postoperative complications is important for the immediate diagnosis and treatment needed for appropriate patient care. Identification of postoperative complications from colon surgery requires knowledge of not only the type of procedure but also the expected normal postoperative appearance. This article discusses and reviews the expected anatomic changes after colorectal surgery and the appearance of the most common postoperative complications.

PROGRAM OBJECTIVE
The objective of the *Radiologic Clinics of North America* is to keep practicing radiologists and radiology residents up to date with current clinical practice in radiology by providing timely articles reviewing the state of the art in patient care.

TARGET AUDIENCE
Practicing radiologists, radiology residents, and other healthcare professionals who provide patient care utilizing radiologic findings.

LEARNING OBJECTIVES
Upon completion of this activity, participants will be able to:
1. Review magnetic resonance imaging of rectal cancer.
2. Discuss MR enterography for Inflammatory and Non-Inflammatory Conditions of the Small Bowel.
3. Recognize the benefits and pitfalls of dual energy CT of the Bowel and CT colonography.

ACCREDITATION
The Elsevier Office of Continuing Medical Education (EOCME) is accredited by the Accreditation Council for Continuing Medical Education (ACCME) to provide continuing medical education for physicians.

The EOCME designates this enduring material for a maximum of 15 *AMA PRA Category 1 Credit*(s)™. Physicians should claim only the credit commensurate with the extent of their participation in the activity.

All other healthcare professionals requesting continuing education credit for this enduring material will be issued a certificate of participation.

DISCLOSURE OF CONFLICTS OF INTEREST
The EOCME assesses conflict of interest with its instructors, faculty, planners, and other individuals who are in a position to control the content of CME activities. All relevant conflicts of interest that are identified are thoroughly vetted by EOCME for fair balance, scientific objectivity, and patient care recommendations. EOCME is committed to providing its learners with CME activities that promote improvements or quality in healthcare and not a specific proprietary business or a commercial interest.

The planning committee, staff, authors and editors listed below have identified no financial relationships or relationships to products or devices they or their spouse/life partner have with commercial interest related to the content of this activity:
Mahmoud Al-Hawary, MD; David Bruining, MD; Onofrio Catalano, MD, PhD; Kevin J. Chang, MD; Jay Coleman, MD; Laura Eisenmenger, MD; Jeff L. Fidler, MD; Joel G. Fletcher, MD; Marc J. Gollub, MD, FACR; Lijun Guo, MD; Mukesh G. Harisinghani, MD; Natally Horvat, MD; Eugene Huo, MD; Kartik S. Jhaveri, MD; Alison Kemp; Gaurav Khatri, MD; Aoife Kilcoyne, MD; Amy B. Kolbe, MD; Pradeep Kuttysankaran; John R. Leyendecker, MD; Umar Mahmood, MD, PhD; Frank H. Miller, MD, FACR; Courtney C. Moreno, MD; Trevor C. Morrison, MD; Markus M. Obmann, MD; Michael A. Ohliger, MD, PhD; Iva Petkovska, MD; Bruce Rosen, MD, PhD; Shannon P. Sheedy, MD; Alberto Signore, MD, PhD; Jorge A. Soto, MD, PhD; Yuxin Sun, MS; Seng Thipphavong, MD; Marije P. van der Paardt, MD, PhD; John Vassallo; Zhen J. Wang, MD; Stefanie Weinstein, MD; Michael Wells, MD; Antonio C. Westphalen, MD, PhD.

The planning committee, staff, authors and editors listed below have identified financial relationships or relationships to products or devices they or their spouse/life partner have with commercial interest related to the content of this CME activity:
Mark E. Baker, MD: receives research support from Siemens Medical Solutions USA
Joel G. Fletcher, MD: receives research support from Siemens Medical Solutions USA, and is a consultant for Medtronic
David H. Kim, MD: is co-founder of VirtuoCTC LLC; and owns stock in Elucent Medical and Cellectar Biosciences, Inc.
Perry J. Pickhardt, MD: is co-founder of VirtuoCTC LLC; a consultant for Bracco and Check-Cap; and owns stock in Elucent Medical, Cellectar Biosciences, and SHINE Medical Technologies
Jaap Stoker, MD, PhD: is a consultant for Robarts Clincial Trials, Inc.
Judy Yee, MD, FACR: receives research support from EchoPixel, Inc. and Koninklijke Philips N.V.
Benjamin M. Yeh, MD: receives research support from Koninklijke Philips N.V. and Guerbet LLC; and is a speaker and receives research support for General Electric Company

UNAPPROVED/OFF-LABEL USE DISCLOSURE
The EOCME requires CME faculty to disclose to the participants:
1. When products or procedures being discussed are off-label, unlabelled, experimental, and/or investigational (not US Food and Drug Administration [FDA] approved); and
2. Any limitations on the information presented, such as data that are preliminary or that represent ongoing research, interim analyses, and/or unsupported opinions. Faculty may discuss information about pharmaceutical agents that is outside of FDA-approved labelling. This information is intended solely for CME and is not intended to promote off-label use of these medications. If you have any questions, contact the medical affairs department of the manufacturer for the most recent prescribing information.

TO ENROLL

To enroll in the *Radiologic Clinics of North America* Continuing Medical Education program, call customer service at 1-800-654-2452 or sign up online at http://www.theclinics.com/home/cme. The CME program is available to subscribers for an additional annual fee of USD 327.60.

METHOD OF PARTICIPATION

In order to claim credit, participants must complete the following:

1. Complete enrolment as indicated above.
2. Read the activity.
3. Complete the CME Test and Evaluation. Participants must achieve a score of 70% on the test. All CME Tests and Evaluations must be completed online.

CME INQUIRIES/SPECIAL NEEDS

For all CME inquiries or special needs, please contact elsevierCME@elsevier.com.

RADIOLOGIC CLINICS OF NORTH AMERICA

FORTHCOMING ISSUES

November 2018
Imaging of the Pelvis and Lower Extremity
Laura Bancroft and Kurt Scherer, *Editors*

January 2019
Cardiovascular CT
Suhny Abbara and Prabhakar Rajiah, *Editors*

March 2019
The Spine
Lubdha M. Shah, *Editor*

RECENT ISSUES

July 2018
Multi-Energy CT: The New Frontier in Imaging
Savvas Nicolaou and Mohammed F. Mohammed, *Editors*

May 2018
Imaging of Lung Cancer: Update on Staging and Therapy
Jeremy J. Erasmus and Mylene T. Truong, *Editors*

March 2018
MR Imaging of the Prostate
Aytekin Oto, *Editor*

RELATED SERIES

Magnetic Resonance Imaging Clinics
Neuroimaging Clinics
PET Clinics

THE CLINICS ARE AVAILABLE ONLINE!
Access your subscription at:
www.theclinics.com

Preface
Innovations in Bowel Imaging

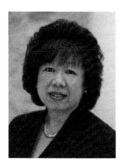

Judy Yee, MD, FACR
Editor

In this issue, a series of timely and important topics related to imaging of the small bowel and colorectum are presented by a renowned panel of experts. You will find each article an important reference that will be helpful to return to when interpreting and reporting diseases of the small bowel and the colorectum.

It is imperative that imaging techniques for evaluation of the bowel remain up-to-date concurrent with important technological advances, particularly in CT and MR. CT enterography is an established test used to evaluate and characterize small bowel inflammatory processes and masses and to identify causes of small bowel bleeding. Radiation dose reduction strategies are provided, including reducing tube current through the use of automatic exposure control, reducing tube potential, and the use of iterative reconstruction. MR enterography (MRE) avoids exposure to ionizing radiation, which is relevant to patients with Crohn disease who often require scans at repeat intervals. MRE techniques optimizing patient preparation and scan acquisition, including cine imaging, are provided. Of importance is the multidisciplinary development of reporting nomenclature that radiologists should use to describe the imaging findings of Crohn disease.

Advances in CT colonography (CTC) technique for colorectal cancer (CRC) screening include a large drop in radiation dose to levels lower than 3 mSv, addressing a concern of the US Preventive Services Task Force (USPSTF) and the Centers for Medicare and Medicaid Services. The USPSTF has included CTC under its "A" rating for CRC screening. Strategies to reduce CTC radiation dose include reducing tube current, reducing tube voltage, using automatic dose modulation, and incorporating iterative reconstruction. A presentation of interpretive pearls and pitfalls accumulated by experts over many years is provided to assist both novice and experienced CTC readers. Although MR colonography is not currently suitable for CRC screening and additional performance studies are needed, there is still interest in its development as a screening test given the avoidance of ionizing radiation. The difference in accuracy of the "bright lumen" versus the "dark lumen" technique needs additional evaluation.

Rectal MR imaging plays a central role in the pretreatment and posttreatment assessment of rectal carcinoma. Expertise in rectal MR imaging using the newest techniques is important as the incidence of rectal carcinoma continues to increase dramatically in young patients under the age of 50. Optimization of MR technique allows accurate primary staging, restaging, and determining local recurrence of rectal carcinoma. MR imaging using external phased array coils is the imaging technique of choice for detection of perianal fistula, determining the relation to the anal sphincter complex and any complications.

Imaging plays an essential role in the localization and treatment of lower gastrointestinal bleeds. Imaging tests in the workup of acute lower gastrointestinal bleeding include CT angiography, nuclear medicine scintigraphy, and catheter angiography. CT enterography and nuclear medicine Meckel scan are valuable in the workup of occult lower gastrointestinal bleeding.

Radiol Clin N Am 56 (2018) xiii–xiv
https://doi.org/10.1016/j.rcl.2018.06.014
0033-8389/18/© 2018 Published by Elsevier Inc.

Exciting new imaging modalities have the potential to improve bowel evaluation. Dual-energy CT (DECT) shows promise to improve the sensitivity, specificity, and reader confidence for the detection and characterization of tumor, gastrointestinal bleeding, and bowel inflammation and ischemia. The use of DECT for CTC and novel bowel contrast material offer additional areas of possible improved bowel evaluation. PET/CT is an established technique in the staging and assessment of bowel malignancies and is being assessed for evaluation of Crohn disease. PET/MR may have a role in the long-term evaluation of patients with inflammatory bowel disease. The surgical management of bowel disease can be complex, and the differentiation between expected postoperative findings from unexpected complications on imaging is critical.

I extend my sincerest gratitude to the authors who participated in this issue, which I am very proud to present to the readership. I thank the Elsevier staff for their assistance from inception to the end of this project. In particular, I am grateful to John Vassallo, Associate Publisher, and Donald Mumford, Developmental Editor. I would like to recognize the faculty at Montefiore Medical Center and the Albert Einstein College of Medicine, who inspire me every day. Finally, I thank my husband, David Leong, and my daughter, Taylor, for their support during every project I undertake.

Judy Yee, MD, FACR
Department of Radiology
Montefiore Medical Center
Albert Einstein College of Medicine
111 East 210th Street
New York, NY 10467, USA

E-mail address:
jyee@montefiore.org

Computed Tomography Enterography

Shannon P. Sheedy, MD*, Amy B. Kolbe, MD, Joel G. Fletcher, MD, Jeff L. Fidler, MD

KEYWORDS

• Computed tomography (CT) • Enterography • CTE • Small bowel

KEY POINTS

• Computed tomography enterography (CTE) has several advantages over other radiologic and optical imaging modalities and is ideally suited for imaging of the small bowel.
• Ingestion of a large volume of neutral oral contrast material combined with imaging during peak small bowel enhancement increases conspicuity of small bowel abnormalities.
• A major limitation of CTE is the need for ionizing radiation; radiologists should use the latest available dose reduction techniques for CTE, particularly for young patients and for those with chronic inflammatory bowel disease who often require repeated imaging.
• CTE excels at detection and surveillance of small bowel inflammatory processes, evaluation of suspected small bowel bleeding, and detection and characterization of small bowel masses.

INTRODUCTION

Superb spatial and temporal resolution of multidetector row computed tomography (CT) has made CT the first-line imaging modality for many abdominopelvic indications. CT enterography (CTE) is a modification of the standard abdominopelvic CT and is tailored specifically to evaluate the small bowel (SB). Patients are required to ingest a large volume of (usually neutral) oral contrast material to optimally distend the SB. Following rapid injection of intravenous (IV) contrast material, thin-section image acquisition during the peak bowel wall enhancement allows for increased conspicuity of abnormally enhancing processes of the SB.

CTE has many advantages over other SB radiologic and optical imaging techniques, including widespread availability, lack of need for sedation, reproducible high-quality images, the ability to visualize the entire thickness and length of SB, and the ability to also assess extraenteric structures in high resolution. Therefore, CTE is well suited for evaluation of SB in many scenarios (**Box 1**).

In this review, the authors describe their protocol for performing CTE and potential modifications depending on the clinical scenario as well as opportunities for dose reduction. The authors

---

Box 1
Common clinical indications for computed tomography enterography

• Detection/surveillance of inflammatory SB conditions and complications (eg, CD and CeD)
• Unexplained diarrhea
• Evaluate suspected SB bleeding
• Detect/characterize SB masses
• Detect low-grade SB obstruction
• Combined high-quality evaluation of other organs and SB

Disclosure Statement: The authors have no funding or conflicts of interest to disclose.
Department of Radiology, Mayo Clinic, 200 First Street Southwest, Rochester, MN 55905, USA
* Corresponding author.
E-mail address: Sheedy.Shannon@mayo.edu

Radiol Clin N Am 56 (2018) 649–670
https://doi.org/10.1016/j.rcl.2018.04.002

discuss and provide illustrative examples of technical limitations of CTE and of common interpretive pitfalls. Last, they describe several of the more common CT enterographic findings encountered in their practice, including Crohn disease (CD), celiac disease (CeD), SB tumors, vascular lesions, and nonsteroidal anti-inflammatory drug (NSAID) enteropathy.

TECHNIQUE
Oral Contrast

Adequate SB distension is necessary to maximize detection of SB abnormalities and requires ingestion of a large volume of oral contrast material over a relatively short period of time (45–60 minutes) (Table 1). Neutral contrast agents, VoLumen (Bracco Diagnostics, Inc, Monroe Township, NJ, USA) and Breeza (Beekley Medical, Bristol, CT, USA), have attenuation values near or just above water attenuation and are the preferred agents for most CTE examinations because they provide superior conspicuity of hyperenhancing SB abnormalities.

Side effects of both of these agents include loose stools, diarrhea, and cramping. Water can be administered to patients who are unable or unwilling to drink the above agents. Although water does not incur additional cost to the examination, it is more rapidly absorbed from the SB; therefore, distal SB distension may be suboptimal.

Some abnormalities may be obscured by neutral contrast agents especially in poorly distended bowel. New oral contrast agents that are able to provide biphasic characteristics using dual-energy techniques are being developed. For more information on dual-energy technique, please see Benjamin M. Yeh and colleagues' article, "Dual Energy CT of the Bowel: Benefits, Pitfalls, and Future Directions," in this issue.

Intravenous Contrast and Scan Timing

IV contrast should be used unless there are contraindications because it helps demonstrate areas of hyperenhancement that can be seen with inflammation and masses. CTE can be performed as a single-phase or multiphase examination (mpCTE). Table 1 provides a summary of the technique used in the authors' institution. Single-phase CTE is more commonly performed and is used for most indications. Iodinated contrast is administered at a rapid rate, and imaging can be performed during the enteric phase when there is peak SB wall enhancement[1] or during the portal venous phase when the liver is more enhanced.

In the evaluation of patients with occult gastrointestinal (GI) bleeding, mpCTE can be helpful for improving the detection and characterization of lesions causing SB bleeding. The authors perform an mpCTE using a bolus triggering threshold of 150 HU for the arterial phase, an enteric phase at 50 seconds, and delayed phase at 90 seconds.[2] Some sites prefer to obtain unenhanced images to help differentiate pathologic condition from high-attenuation ingested material (Fig. 1) and only perform 2 phases with IV contrast to reduce the overall radiation exposure. If dual-energy technology is available, virtual noncontrast (VNC) images can be generated without the need for additional radiation. More information regarding multiphase technique for GI bleeding can be found in Trevor C. Morrison and colleagues' article, "Imaging Workup of Acute and Occult Lower Gastrointestinal Bleeding," in this issue.

Computed Tomographic Parameters and Dose Reduction Strategies

The Society of Abdominal Radiology, the American College of Radiology, and the Society of Pediatric Radiology have established technical parameters for the performance of CTE in CD.[3,4] As CTE examinations generate thin (2–4 mm) multiplanar images, the examination should be performed on 16-slice and higher multidetector CT systems.[3] Multiphasic imaging is used in patients with acute and overt SB bleeding and with suspected SB bleeding; however, currently there is no clear consensus on the technical requirements in these settings.[5] The field-of-view should be adapted to fit the patient, with some practices reducing the scan range to image only the SB to minimize radiation dose and exclude the lung bases and breast tissue.[6] Every CTE should image the anal sphincter complex owing to the potential for unsuspected perianal CD.[7] For older CT systems, the detector configuration should be chosen so that image acquisition can be performed in a single breath-hold with the minimal possible configuration chosen so as to maintain z-axis spatial resolution on coronal and sagittal images.

Radiation dose should be minimized to perform the diagnostic task, and CT enterography examinations should additionally be adapted to patient size, with volume CT Dose Index (CTDI$_{vol}$) generally between 5 and 15 mGy.[3] Radiation dose can be reduced by reducing the scan coverage, lowering the tube potential, reducing tube current, and using automatic exposure control (AEC), and tolerating more noise in CT images. "Low kV" scanning is the term used for CT imaging performed with a tube potential of less than 120 kV, with the potential for low kV scanning depending

Table 1
Computed tomography enterography protocol

Parameter	Technique	Notes
Patient preparation	Avoid solid foods (clear liquids only) for 4 h	
CT scanner specifications	16-slice and higher multidetector CT system	
Oral contrast		Patient compliance crucial for success of CTE; supervision and encouragement during drinking phase recommended
Neutral contrast agent	1350 mL neutral contrast agent (450 mL increments every 15 min over 45 min) 500 mL water consumed during the last 15 min just before examination	Maximize contrast between lumen and enhancing SB wall and/or hyperenhancing bowel abnormalities
Positive contrast agent	Same as above, no water Can use water-soluble or CT barium agents	Potential uses: polyposis syndromes or other isoenhancing masses; known serosal disease, establish fistula patency; assessing bowel transit, patency of complex postoperative anatomy, patients with iodine allergy May obscure mural enhancement, intraluminal hemorrhage, vascular lesions, or detection of subtle mural disease
Agents with biphasic properties, new		Being developed for dual-energy scanning
Water alone		Usually inadequate distension due to rapid reabsorption
IV contrast (weight-based volume)	300 mg/mL iodinated contrast material through ≥18-gauge IV 4 mL/s rapid injection rate, followed by 30 mL saline flush	
Scan acquisition timing	Single phase: • Enteric phase (50-s scan delay)	Peak SB wall enhancement, allows maximum contrast between lumen and enhancing SB wall and/or hyperenhancing bowel abnormalities May prefer 60- to 70-s delay (portal venous) for improved hepatic enhancement
	Multiphasic (mpCTE): • Arterial phase (bolus trigger 150 HU threshold) • Enteric phase • Delay phase (90 s)	For suspected SB bleeding (Trevor C. Morrison and colleagues' article, "Imaging Workup of Acute and Occult Lower Gastrointestinal Bleeding," in this issue)
Image acquisition and reconstruction	0.6-mm collimation 2-mm slice thickness 1-mm reconstruction interval	
Reformations	2- to 3-mm coronal and sagittal multiplanar reformats coronal MIP	Coronal MIP help detect acute/chronic mesenteric venous occlusion; make engorged vasa recta more conspicuous; easier assessment of length of involvement

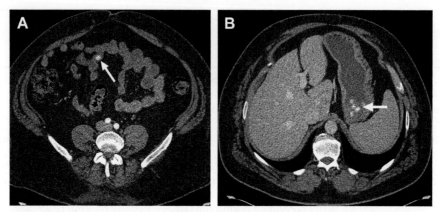

Fig. 1. Pill fragment simulating active GI bleeding. CTE (*A*) shows a high-density intraluminal focus in the distal SB in a patient with GI blood loss (*arrow*). This was a presumed pill fragment given the additional pills seen in the stomach (*B, arrow*) rather than a focus of contrast extravasation due to active bleeding. NC or VNC images can help differentiate between ingested material and SB abnormality if unclear.

on both the size of the patient and the CT system being used.[8] Lowering the tube potential increases iodine signal, increasing the conspicuity of inflamed bowel segments or enhancing SB masses. The subsequent increase in iodine contrast-to-noise ratio permits the radiation dose to be lowered substantially while still preserving the conspicuity and identification of inflamed bowel segments (**Fig. 2**).[6] Several investigators have shown that using low kV techniques in appropriately sized patients can reduce the radiation dose for routine CT enterography by 50% or more.[6,8,9] Lowering the tube potential requires an assessment of the patient size and the ability of

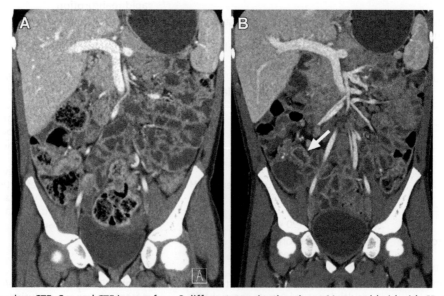

Fig. 2. Low-dose CTE. Coronal CTE images from 2 different examinations in an 11-year-old girl with CD. Initial CTE was performed with a tube potential of 100 kV and a lower strength of iterative reconstruction with a $CTDI_{vol}$ of 3.94 mGy; this examination was interpreted as negative (*A*). Because of continued clinical suspicion for CD, a repeat CTE was performed 1 year later using a lower tube potential (70 kV), lower AEC settings, and a stronger strength of iterative reconstruction, yielding a $CTDI_{vol}$ of 1.47 mGy, a 62% reduction in dose with effective dose corresponding to 0.9 mSv (*B*). The subsequent and lower dose CTE is of similar image quality and demonstrates mild mural thickening, stratification, and segmental hyperenhancment in the terminal ileum typical of active inflammatory CD (*B, arrow*).

the CT system to deliver the higher tube currents that will be required to avoid excessive image noise at the lower potential. This objective can be accomplished via the use of technique charts, which specify patient weights or lateral widths at which specific lower tube potentials can be used,[6,9] or by routine use of a vendor-supplied kV selection tool.[10] Tube current can be reduced using a lower fixed tube current (determined by a technique chart for patients of different sizes) or by using AEC, with several studies also showing that 2-fold dose reductions are possible by lowering tube current.[11,12]

Iterative reconstruction reduces noise in CT images by using an optimization-based framework that uses a system model that takes into account image noise and CT system characteristics.[13] It improves visual image quality, thereby facilitating the adoption of lower-dose CT images by changing the appearance of lower-dose CT images so that they have a high degree of fidelity to routine, standard-dose CT images.[11,14] Several studies have shown that for CD detection by low-dose CTE, iterative reconstruction improves image quality, but is not needed to preserve detection of inflamed bowel segments.[12,15] Image-based denoising techniques can also be used to reduce image noise and improve image quality of lower-dose CT images.[16] Both iterative reconstruction

and other denoising methods are often used in conjunction with low kV imaging at CTE to reduce radiation dose while increasing conspicuity of diseased bowel segments.[9,17] CT dose reduction strategies are reviewed in **Table 2**.

PEDIATRIC CONSIDERATIONS

CTE can be performed in most children to image the bowel and has the same advantages as for adults. MR enterography (MRE) may be warranted in children with known inflammatory bowel disease (IBD) who will require repeated imaging over their lifetime, but in many instances, CTE remains a superior option. The principles of ALARA (as low as reasonably achievable) should be followed; technical parameters and techniques to reduce radiation exposure should be implemented as discussed above.

Child Life specialists provide support and encouragement to anxious children.[18] They use developmental stage and age-appropriate techniques to introduce the child to the radiology equipment. Occasionally, a child will not tolerate the scan despite these measures. In such patients, sedation or anesthesia may be necessary.

The taste, texture, or volume of oral contrast material required for CTE may be poorly tolerated by some children, but the authors have found

Table 2	
Computed tomographic dose reduction strategies	
Ways to Reduce Radiation Dose	**Hardware/Software or Implementation Comment**
Reduce scan coverage	No hardware/software Cover bowel and anus only (no lung or breast tissue) Requires technologist training
Reduce tube current	Best accomplished through use of AEC system, which will deliver a reproducible level of image quality AEC paradigms vary by vendor, for some vendors a single AEC setting is used for each task; for others, a size-specific technique chart must be used Size-specific technique charts for tube current (mA) adapted to the diagnostic task are the alternative Tube current settings for CT enterography are generally the same or less than routine abdominopelvic CT
Reduce tube potential	Use a vendor-supplied kV selection tool, if available Size-specific technique charts must be adapted for each CT system due to different tube current limitations Low kV scanning used in conjunction with iterative reconstruction or other denoising strategy
Reduce image noise	Iterative reconstruction (expensive, purchased with each CT system) Image-based denoising (less expensive, can service multiple CT systems, but noise reduction more limited) Select a smoother reconstruction kernel Accommodate noisier images (requires radiologist acceptance across a practice)

that patients as young as 3 years old generally tolerate a weight-based algorithm of the Breeza flavored beverage. Occasionally, transnasogastric enteric tube administration is necessary. The paucity of mesenteric fat in many pediatric patients poses a challenge and can result in decreased conspicuity of SB abnormalities. In addition, one must tailor the differential diagnosis in pediatric patients, which may include entities not as often seen in adults such as Meckel diverticum, Henoch Schölein purpura, bowel wall hemorrhage, and lymphoid hyperplasia (**Fig. 3**).

IMAGE RECONSTRUCTION AND IMAGE REVIEW

Images should be reconstructed using 2- to 3-mm slice thickness in the coronal and sagittal plane. Coronal maximum intensity projection images (MIPs) may be helpful giving an overview of the bowel and vascular structures. Accurate detection of SB abnormalities requires a comprehensive and systematic evaluation of the GI tract. For example, tracking the lumen combined with zonal assessment on multiple projections may be needed because abnormalities may be most conspicuous

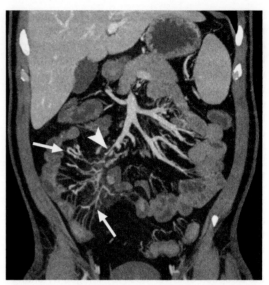

Fig. 4. Coronal MIP reconstruction shows chronic superior mesenteric vein (SMV) occlusion. A 45-year-old man with history of CD. Typical appearance of chronic SMV occlusion (*arrowhead*) with prominent peripheral dilatation (*arrows*) and mesenteric edema.

in one projection. After assessment of the bowel, the extraenteric structures, including the mesentery and mesenteric vasculature, must be evaluated (**Fig. 4**).

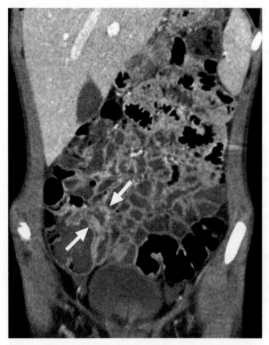

Fig. 3. Thickening of the terminal ileum (TI) due to lymphoid hyperplasia mimicking CD. A 5-year-old with distal TI thickening without mural hyperenhancement (*arrows*). Nodular mucosa was seen on ileocolonoscopy and histopathology showed lymphoid hyperplasia without granulomas.

Box 2
Inflammatory bowel disease imaging

Features of active CD on CTE (**Fig. 5**)

- Bowel wall thickening (>3 mm)
- Mural hyperenhancement (homogeneous or striated)
- Engorgement of the vasa recta ("comb sign")
- Perienteric inflammation or edema
- Reactive perienteric lymph nodes

Specificity for CD increases when mural disease:

- Is asymmetric or associated with pseudosacculations
- Is multisegmental with "skip" lesions (often of varying severity)
- Is associated with perienteric fibrofatty proliferation
- Involves the terminal ileum
- Demonstrates submucosal mural fat, indicating a chronic component of disease
- Has associated mural ulcers and/or penetrating disease
- Has associated penetrating disease

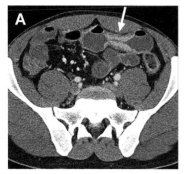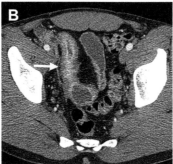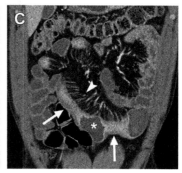

Fig. 5. Active inflammatory CD. Axial (*A, B*) and coronal (*C*) CTE images demonstrate multisegmental active SB CD with wall thickening, mural hyperenhancement, and luminal narrowing (*arrows*). Note the pseudosacculation from asymmetric inflammation (*asterisk, C*) and the "comb sign" (*arrowhead, C*).

COMMON SMALL BOWEL DISORDERS AT COMPUTED TOMOGRAPHY ENTEROGRAPHY
Inflammatory Bowel Disease

CTE exquisitely demonstrates active CD and in contradistinction to endoluminal imaging also permits detection of perienteric complications and extraintestinal manifestations of the disease. Radiologic response detected with CTE is associated with improved long-term clinical outcomes, and thus, CTE can be used not only to help diagnose CD but also to assess therapeutic response.[19,20] The findings of active CD are shown in **Box 2**.

Luminal narrowing in CD can be secondary to active inflammation and potentially reversible with medical therapy or may be more fixed due to a combination of inflammation and fibrosis and require surgery. The location and length of any stricture and presence/absence of superimposed active inflammation and obstruction (>3 cm diameter) should be documented.

Penetrating disease rarely occurs in the absence of stricture. CTE identifies clinically occult penetrating disease (**Figs. 6** and **7**), often resulting in a change in patient management.[21] Penetrating manifestations are detailed in **Box 3**.

The radiology report should detail the presence of extraintestinal manifestations of CD, including acute or chronic mesenteric venous or portal thrombosis (see **Fig. 4**), cholelithiasis, nephrolithiasis, primary sclerosing cholangitis, perianal disease, sacroiliitis, and avascular necrosis of femoral heads. Please see Mark E. Baker and colleagues' article, "Interdisciplinary Updates in

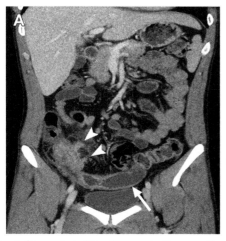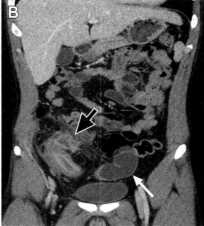

Fig. 6. Active inflammatory CD with penetrating manifestations. Coronal CTE images demonstrate active inflammation of the terminal ileum with luminal narrowing and mild upstream SB dilatation (*arrows*). One of the sinus tracts (*A, arrowheads*) communicates with a small perienteric abscess (*B, black arrow*). Penetrating disease is rarely, if ever, present in the absence of stricture.

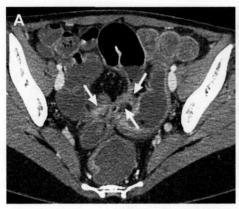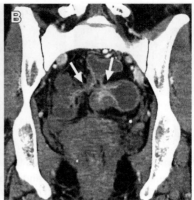

Fig. 7. Fistulizing CD. Axial (*A*) and coronal (*B*) CTE images show a complex fistula network involving multiple ileal loops (*arrows*). Multiple bowel segments tethered together by fistulas often results in an "asterisk" appearance.

Crohn's Disease Reporting Nomenclature, and Cross-sectional Disease Monitoring," in this issue for a more thorough discussion on CD.

CTE is tailored to evaluate the SB, and although the colon can be assessed when adequately distended, CTE is less sensitive than endoscopy for the evaluation of colitis. The colonic findings of ulcerative colitis (UC) and Crohn colitis intersect, with findings of wall thickening, hyperenhancement, mural stratification, IBD-related polyps, and dilatation of pericolonic vasculature seen with both entities. Terminal ileal (TI) inflammation can be seen in UC patients from backwash ileitis. Isolated involvement of the right hemicolon, discontinuous segmental involvement, involvement of the SB, and extraenteric complications, including perianal fistulizing disease, support the diagnosis of CD over UC. CTE is not typically performed to diagnose UC, but is performed in patients previously diagnosed with UC who subsequently have signs and symptoms of CD.

Box 3
Penetrating disease in Crohn disease on computed tomography enterography

- Sinus tract and fistula: simple or branching linear, enhancing tracts. Fistulas often cause tethering of bowel or adjacent organs, and complex fistulas may have an "asterisk" shape (see **Fig. 7**). Fluid or air is rarely identified within the tracts.

- Inflammatory mass:, ill-defined masslike extension of the transmural inflammation into the perienteric fat

- Abscess: ring-enhancing fluid collection with or without air (see **Fig. 6**)

Small Bowel Neoplasms

SB neoplasms account for a small percentage of all GI tumors.[22,23] Patients may present with nonspecific GI symptoms or may remain asymptomatic until complications of obstruction, perforation, or bleeding occur. With increasing usage of cross-sectional imaging, SB neoplasms are being detected as incidental findings more frequently. CTE can guide surgical or endoscopic management by providing accurate tumor localization and also enables assessment for locoregional and distant metastatic disease.

Neuroendocrine neoplasms

The incidence of NEN has recently surpassed that of adenocarcinoma.[24] Most SB NENs arise in the ileum from enterochromoffin cells in the bowel wall and produce serotonin. The World Health Organization proposed the term "carcinoid" to describe most GI neuroendocrine tumors in 1980; however, based on a more recently revised histology classification, that term has been discouraged. These tumors vary in their biologic behavior and in their ability to metastasize, and they are now classified as grade 1 to 2 NEN or as grade 3 small or large cell neuroendocrine carcinoma.[25] On CTE, SB NENs typically hyperenhance and can appear as a mural or intraluminal polypoid nodule, focal eccentric plaquelike thickening with serosal puckering and retraction (**Fig. 8**), or as a carpet-type lesion with segmental submucosal spread (mimicking CD). SB NEN is typically a slow-growing neoplasm, but as it progresses, it frequently infiltrates into the adjacent mesentery. The infiltrative tumor and nodal metastatic disease incite a desmoplastic response in the adjacent mesentery, often creating a "sunburst" appearance with tethering and angulation

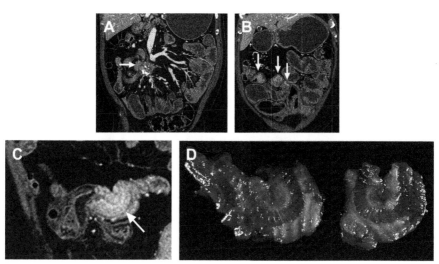

Fig. 8. Metastatic SB NEN. A 66-year-old man with diarrhea and unintentional weight loss. Coronal CTE images (*A*, *B*) demonstrate a partially calcified metastatic mesenteric mass with surrounding desmoplastic change (*arrow*, *A*). Note how the mass constricts and occludes the SMV. This was initially misdiagnosed as sclerosing mesenteritis; however, notice the multifocal hyperenhancing, SB NEN (*arrows*, *B*). Because of the relatively high rate of multicentric tumors, it is important to carefully assess the entire length of the SB. (*C*, *D*) CTE image and gross pathology from another patient demonstrate the characteristic plaquelike thickening of SB NEN with serosal puckering and retraction (*C*, *arrow*).

of the adjacent SB (see **Fig. 8**). Tumor and fibrosis encase mesenteric vessels (see **Fig. 8**), placing patients at risk for SB ischemia and rendering surgical excision particularly challenging or impossible. Metastases often hyperenhance similar to the primary tumor and can calcify (see **Fig. 8**). Large metastatic tumor burden in the liver may result in carcinoid syndrome. Similar plaquelike lesions may be seen with CD, serosal metastases, and bowel invasive endometriosis.

Adenocarcinoma

Although most small bowel adenocarcinomas (SBA) are sporadic, predisposing conditions, including polyposis syndromes, CeD, and CD, have been identified. For example, the increased relative risk of SBA in CD has been estimated in population-based studies to be between 17 and 41 compared with the non-Crohn general population.[26] Most adenocarcinomas develop in the proximal SB with the exception of CD patients in whom adenocarcinoma more often arises in the ileum.[27–29] Early adenocarcinomas are polypoid endoenteric masses or ulcerative plaquelike lesions, but as they progress, they tend to have an annular, constrictive growth pattern (**Fig. 9**). These biologically aggressive malignancies are solitary, typically

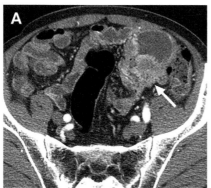
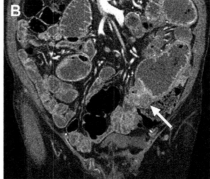

Fig. 9. SBA. Axial (*A*) and coronal (*B*) CTE images demonstrate an obstructive "apple-core" malignancy (*arrows*) with sharp shouldering margins and luminal narrowing.

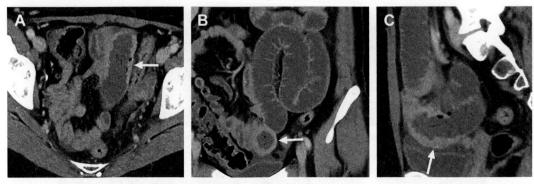

Fig. 10. Small intestinal lymphoma. Axial (*A*), coronal (*B*), and sagittal (*C*) CTE images demonstrate a mass in the distal jejunum with circumferential wall thickening and aneurysmal dilatation (*arrows*). Although SB lymphoma does not classically constrict the lumen and cause obstruction, upstream dilatation can occur and may be a result of damage of the myenteric plexus in the wall of the SB.

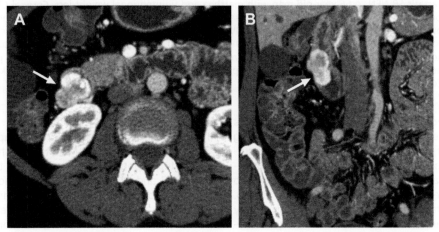

Fig. 11. Small bowel gastrointestinal tumor (GIST). A 63-year-old woman with iron deficiency anemia and normal upper and lower endoscopy. Axial (*A*) and coronal (*B*) mpCTE images demonstrate an endoexoenteric hyperenhancing mass in the second portion of the duodenum with a small focus of calcification (*arrows*).

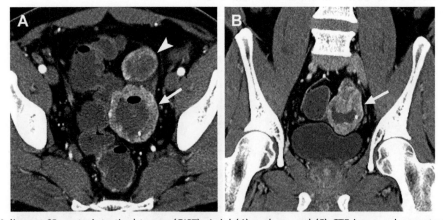

Fig. 12. Malignant SB gastrointestinal tumor (GIST). Axial (*A*) and coronal (*B*) CTE images demonstrate a large, centrally necrotic mass with eccentric focal calcification (*arrows, A, B*). See also the second similar-appearing mass without necrosis in the adjacent SB (*arrowhead, A*). Most GISTs are solitary; however, patients with neurofibromatosis 1 (NF1) or familial GIST syndrome may have multiple.

> **Box 4**
> **Imaging features of vascular lesions causing small bowel bleeding**
>
> Arterial lesions: hyperenhance during the arterial phase, often fading rapidly; high flow and can pose potential for life-threatening bleeding
>
> - AVM
>   - Nodular or masslike enhancement
>   - May have an enlarged feeding artery and/or an early and prominent draining veins
> - Dieulafoy
>   - Tortuous arteriole in the submucosal bowel wall, subject to erosion and bleeding
>   - At CTE, nodular focus of hyperenhancement in arterial phase only unless actively bleeding (Fig. 13), no prominent feeding artery or draining vein
>   - At endoscopy, seen as a small, red, pulsatile protrusion through the mucosa, but may be overlooked if not actively bleeding[35]
>
> Angioectasia (angiodysplasia)
>
> - Usually in the jejunum and often multifocal
> - On mpCTE, appear as nodular foci of enhancement or as bulbous, prominence of intramural veins, most conspicuous during the enterographic phase (Fig. 14); MIPs may make more apparent
> - At endoscopy, seen as patchy areas of erythema on the mucosal surface with scalloped or frondlike edges, may bleed on contact
>
> Venous lesions: progressive enhancement during the enteric and delayed phases, often undetectable on arterial phase images
>
> - Angiomas: slow progressive globular enhancement due to slow filling of blood-filled sinuses; venous phlebolith can help increase diagnostic confidence
> - Varices: serpiginous pattern of enhancement; usually develop as a result of prior venous thrombosis, previous surgery, or cirrhosis

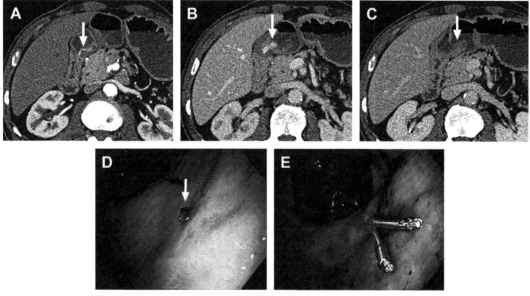

Fig. 13. Active bleeding from a Dieulafoy lesion. A 69-year-old man with suspected SB bleeding. mpCTE demonstrates a linear focus of active extravasation of contrast material in the gastric antrum on the arterial phase (*arrow, A*) with progressive accumulation during the enteric (*arrow, B*) and delayed (*arrow, C*) phases. Subsequent upper endoscopy showed an exposed visible vessel in the antrum (*arrow, D*) with fresh arterial-type bleeding attached to its surface, suggestive of a Dieulafoy lesion. The lesion was treated with epinephrine and hemoclips (*E*).

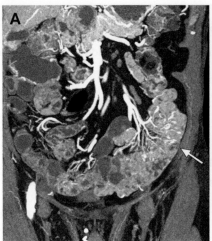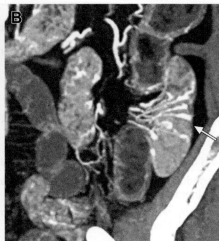

Fig. 14. Small bowel angioectasias. Coronal (*A*) and coronal MIP (*B*) CTE images demonstrate focal bulbous swelling of intramural veins of the jejunum (*arrows*). Small bowel angioectasias are a common cause of SB bleeding; however, they are often detected incidentally.

short, and frequently produce SB obstruction because of their radial growth pattern. Mucosal ulceration is typical, and large aggressive adenocarcinoma with marked central ulceration may mimic lymphoma. Adenocarcinomas tend to locally infiltrate into the surrounding mesenteric fat, and regional nodal metastases are common.

Box 5
Computed tomography enterography findings of celiac disease, nonspecific related to inflammation and/or malabsorption

Nonspecific findings related to inflammation and/or malabsorption

- Dilated, fluid-filled SB: most common finding, due to decreased absorption and increased fluid secretion

- SB wall and fold thickening: inflammation and/or edema

- Peptic ulcers/strictures: particularly susceptible to gastric, biliary, and pancreatic secretions due to villus atrophy

- Submucosal fat deposition: chronic inflammation in duodenum or jejunum[36] (Fig. 15)

- SB conformation (obliteration of interloop pelvic fat) and transient intussusception: due to dilated, hypotonic bowel[37–39]

- "Jejunoileal fold pattern reversal": most specific finding,[40,41] but may be absent in more than half of patients[42] (see Fig. 15)

Lymphoma

SB lymphoma may be primary or more commonly occurs as secondary involvement in systemic disease. The most common site of occurrence is the ileum. Non-Hodgkin B-cell lymphoma of mucosa-associated lymphoid tissue lymphoma is the most common subtype of primary SB lymphoma.[30] The CT imaging manifestations of lymphoma are protean. The most characteristic appearance is that of circumferential bowel wall thickening with aneurysmal dilatation of the lumen due to infiltration of the muscularis layer and destruction of the myenteric plexus[30] (Fig. 10). Other morphologies include endoentric polypoid mass or masses; diffuse, segmental, or multifocal wall thickening and nodularity; ulcerative mucosal lesion; and endoexoenteric mass with necrosis, cavitation, and rarely, fistula formation. Obstruction is less common with lymphoma than adenocarcinoma, and when present, may be related to hypomotility or disruption of the myenteric plexus rather than to luminal constriction[30] (see Fig. 10). Splenomegaly and/or bulky lymphadenopathy in the abdomen are other clues to the diagnosis.

Gastrointestinal stromal tumor

Gastrointestinal stromal tumor (GIST) is the most common mesenchymal tumor of the GI tract, but represents a small proportion of primary SB neoplasms.[28] When small, they are usually well circumscribed and may have an endoenteric, exoenteric, or endoexoenteric growth pattern (Fig. 11). Predominantly exoenteric GISTs are often large at the time of presentation, whereas smaller lesions that erode through the mucosa

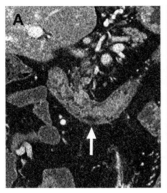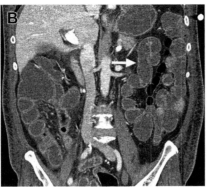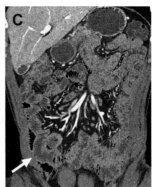

Fig. 15. CeD. Submucosal fat deposition in the duodenum (*arrow, A*) or jejunum should raise suspicion for possible CeD. Coronal CTE images from different patients with known CeD demonstrate fold pattern reversal with a decrease in the number of jejunal folds (*arrow, B*) and an isolated increase in the number of ileal folds (*arrow, C*). The fold pattern alterations are often best appreciated on coronal images.

Box 6
Computed tomography enterography of complications in celiac disease

- Cavitary mesenteric lymph node syndrome (CMLNS): multiple small or mildly enlarged mesenteric lymph nodes are typical in CeD, but CMLNS is a rare complication of severe disease presenting as abnormal, central low-density nodes[43,44]
- Splenic atrophy or hypofunction: may accompany CMLNS, both portend a poor prognosis
- Ulcerative jejunoileitis (UJ): marked wall thickening with mural edema or hyperenhancement and stratification, may see associated with mesenteric inflammation; considered premalignant because of risk of enteropathy-associated T-cell lymphoma (EATL)[45–47]
- EATL: rare aggressive primary intestinal T-cell lymphoma found almost exclusively in CeD patients; can be difficult to differentiate from UJ. More likely to occur in the jejunum compared with lymphoma in non-CeD patients (Fig. 16). Involvement of intra-abdominal lymph nodes, liver, and spleen may occur, but extra-abdominal involvement atypical
- Nonlymphomatous GI malignancies: increased risk in CeD patients, particularly SBA[48]

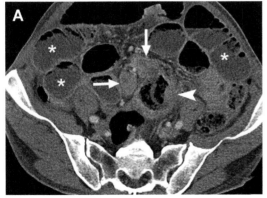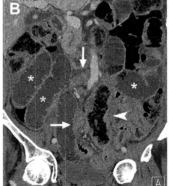

Fig. 16. EATL. A 62-year-old CeD patient, not adherent to a gluten-free diet. Axial (*A*) and coronal (*B*) CTE images demonstrate dilated, fluid-filled loops of SB (*asterisks*) upstream from an irregular annular mass in the distal jejunum (*arrowheads, A, B*). Notice the aneurysmal dilatation and the invasion into the mesenteric fat where there is also lymphadenopathy (*arrows, A, B*).

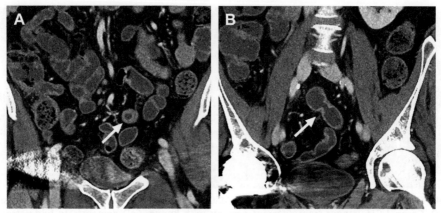

Fig. 17. NSAID-induced diaphragm disease. Enteric phase coronal mpCTE images demonstrate typical NSAID strictures in the midileum (*arrows*), one viewed en face (*A*) and the other longitudinally (*B*). These subtle strictures are more conspicuous when actively inflamed or when obstruction is present.

and result in GI bleeding may be discovered earlier; because the tumor is submucosal, this erosion can be mistaken at endoscopy for ulcers.[31] They enhance variably, usually avidly, and tend to enhance more heterogeneously as

they increase in size. Calcification is sometimes present. In the absence of obvious local invasion or metastatic disease, there are no reliable CT signs to determine malignancy. However, larger size, internal necrosis, and ulceration are

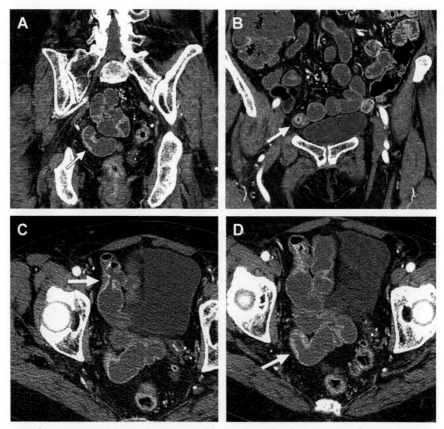

Fig. 18. CD mimicking NSAID strictures. An 84-year-old woman with a long history of CD presents with recurrent obstructive symptoms. Coronal (*A, B*) and axial (*C, D*) images from CTE demonstrate several short, symmetric, circumferential, strictures in the ileum with mild wall thickening and hyperenhancement (*arrows*) suggesting mild active inflammation. This was initially misinterpreted (no history) as suspected NSAID-related strictures.

Box 7

Pitfalls, limitations and tips: computed tomography enterography

Pitfalls or Limitations	Comments
Technical	
• Poor luminal distension	• Particularly in jejunum, normally appears thicker and enhances more intensely than the ileum
Incompletely distended bowel mistaken for abnormally thickened or hyperenhancing bowel and result in false positive diagnoses (**Fig. 19**) or can obscure subtle findings resulting in underdiagnosis (**Fig. 20**) (eg, early or subtle inflammation, nonobstructing strictures)	• Causes: inability to drink large volumes, rapid transit through SB, or excessive time delay between drinking and scan acquisition
	• Provide written instructions or drinking timetable for patients to follow; helpful to have personnel supervise/encourage patients
	• Review of multiplanar reformats aid in diagnostic sensitivity and confidence.
	• May need follow-up with MRE (multiple sequences allow evaluation during multiple time points) or CT enteroclysis (provides more complete SB distension than CTE and better spatial resolution than MRE); SB series may be helpful to evaluate poorly distended jejunum
• Isolated mucosal abnormalities	• Endoscopy and CTE are complementary; endoscopy excels at detecting mucosal abnormalities; CTE assesses full bowel wall thickness, entire length of SB (especially important in patients with TI skipping in CD), penetrating complications from CD, and extraenteric structures
Early or isolated abnormalities, such as apthous ulcer, may be missed at CTE	
• Need for ionizing radiation	• Especially relevant in young patients with CD; chronic and relapsing nature often necessitates multiple examinations
Imperative to use scanners capable of dose reduction techniques	• Can limit number of phases (eg, exclude the arterial phase in young patients with suspected SB bleeding because they less frequently have vascular causes of bleeding)
Dose reduction techniques can result in excessive noise and can obscure important anatomic detail or limit diagnostic ability	
• Inadequate radiation dose	• Dose reduction techniques should be used, but must be sufficient enough to permit visualization of mural thickness, enhancement pattern, and fold pattern
Efforts to maximally decrease radiation dose can result in excessive image noise that can obscure anatomic detail and contribute to missed diagnoses	• Consider limiting the dose reduction if evaluation of the solid organs is important
• Lack of therapeutic capability	• Although no therapeutic capabilities, CTE can guide subsequent surgery or endoscopic procedures
mpCTE performed for suspected SB bleeding sources, but if found, no therapeutic intervention is possible	
Interpretive	
• Small bowel contraction/spasm	• Closely evaluate for presence of hyperenhancement, associated mesenteric abnormalities
May mimic stricture or wall thickening (**Fig. 21**); or true stricture may be mistaken for contraction (**Fig. 22**)	• Evaluate segment on all phases and planes to assess for change or consider obtaining delay

(continued on next page)

Box 7
(continued)

Pitfalls or Limitations	Comments
• Poorly or isoenhancing abnormalities Hypoenhancing/isoenhancing abnormalities (some metastases, adenocarcinomas, lymphoma, polyps) may be poorly visualized with the use of neutral oral contrast material (**Fig. 23**) Low-density or cystic mesenteric abnormalities (**Figs. 24–26**)	• For some indications, may consider using positive oral contrast material (eg, serosal metastatic disease, SB polyposis syndromes) • Routine use of positive oral contrast material not recommended for CTE because of decreased conspicuity of hyperenhancing abnormalities (**Figs. 27 and 28**)
• Nonspecific findings of inflammation Many entities present with similar appearance of nonspecific wall thickening and/or hyperenhancement	• Patient clinical history is important as is knowledge of differentiating features of disease processes (eg, asymmetric inflammation, skip lesions, and penetrating disease for CD)
• Ingested opaque pills/opaque debris Can simulate enhancing masses, vascular lesions, or active bleeding (see **Fig. 1**)	• Ingested material may change in position with time due to peristalsis • Ingested material remains the same density on all phases of contrast enhancement and will not change shape over time • Noncontrast (NC) or VNC when dual-energy technique is used are helpful because the ingested material will be hyperdense on NC or VNC
• Minimal mesenteric fat Makes evaluation of bowel wall and of mesenteric abnormalities challenging	• Particularly challenging in pediatric patients • May consider positive enteric contrast in patients with very low body mass index

associated with high-grade and malignant tumors, and irregular or invasive tumor borders are associated with malignant tumors[32] (**Fig. 12**). Metastatic spread is usually to the liver and peritoneum, whereas nodal and extra-abdominal metastases are rare.

Suspected small bowel bleeding SB sources of GI blood loss are many, including inflammation, neoplasm, and vascular lesions. In general, vascular lesions can be categorized by mpCTE into arterial lesions, angioectasia (angiodysplasia), and venous lesions (**Box 4**).[33] Please refer to Trevor C. Morrison and colleagues' article, "Imaging Workup of Acute and Occult Lower Gastrointestinal Bleeding," in this issue for a more detailed discussion on the use of mpCTE in suspected SB bleeding.

Celiac disease CeD is an autoimmune disorder resulting in inflammation and damage to the SB mucosa in genetically susceptible individuals following ingestion of gluten. The intestinal

damage may cause any number of GI symptoms. Other patients may be asymptomatic or have symptoms related to chronic malabsorption of nutrients.

CTE is often normal in CeD patients, but may show nonspecific findings, many of which are from inflammation and/or a pattern of SB malabsorption (**Box 5**). CTE may be able to suggest the diagnosis in patients who present with atypical or nonspecific clinical signs and symptoms.

Given the high diagnostic accuracy of serologic testing and of SB biopsies, CTE is of limited value in the diagnosis of clinically suspected CeD, but is critical in patients who have a poor response to or suffer symptomatic recurrence despite a strict gluten-free diet, because these patients and patients with undiagnosed/untreated disease are most likely to experience complications (**Box 6**).

Nonsteroidal anti-inflammatory drug enteropathy Early injury from NSAID use results in superficial linear ulcerations, but as injury progresses, larger annular ulcers and strictures may develop

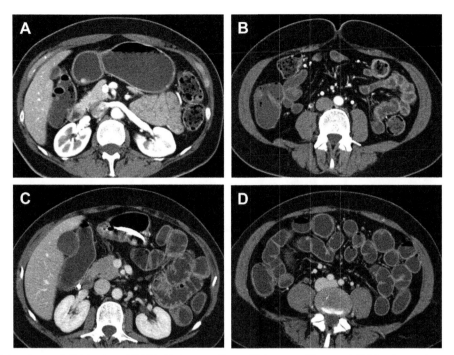

Fig. 19. Jejunal pseudothickening. CTE (*A, B*) shows collapsed jejunum with pseudothickening and pseudohyperenhancement suggesting jejunal CD. SB enteroclysis (*C, D*) provides better jejunal distension and normal appearance of the bowel wall.

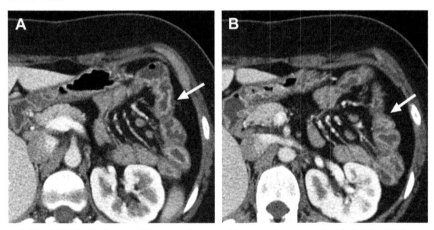

Fig. 20. Jejunal CD. CTE (*A, B*) shows diffuse subtle mural hyperenhancement related to CD (*arrows*). This was missed on previous scans because of incomplete distension.

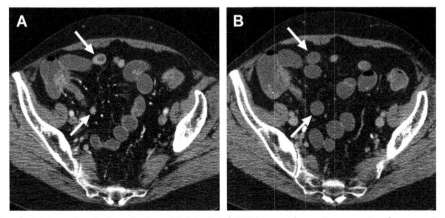

Fig. 21. Pseudostricture due to transient peristalsis. Axial CTE image shows 2 segments of apparent narrowing and wall thickening without upstream dilatation (*arrows, A*). Delayed acquisition shows these segments to open with normal appearance (*arrows, B*), consistent with transient peristalsis.

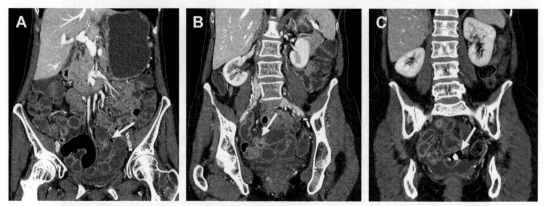

Fig. 22. Radiation-induced strictures of the SB. Coronal CTE images (*A, B*) show multiple strictures related to history of pelvic radiation therapy that were misattributed to contractions (*arrows*). Capsule endoscopy resulted in retention of the pill camera proximal to a stricture (*C, arrow*).

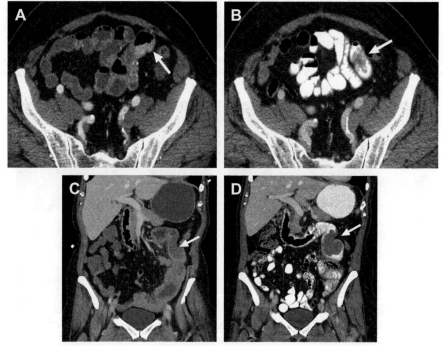

Fig. 23. Isodense neoplasms obscured by neutral contrast. Two patients with neoplasms of the SB, both missed on initial CT with neutral enteric contrast (*A, C*, axial, *arrows*). Coronal CTE images using positive enteric contrast (*B, D*) show the large hypoenhancing lesions in the SB (*arrows, B, D*), eventually proven to be ileal adenoma and jejunal adenocarcinoma, respectively.

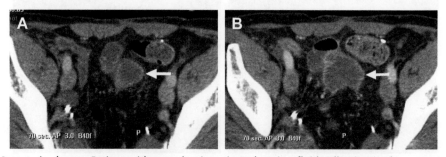

Fig. 24. Mesenteric abscess. Patient with an enlarging, rim-enhancing fluid collection in the mesentery. At the initial study (*A*), the collection (*arrow*) was attributed to fluid-filled loop of bowel. Follow-up study (*B*) shows increase in abscess size (*arrow*), which is now more apparent.

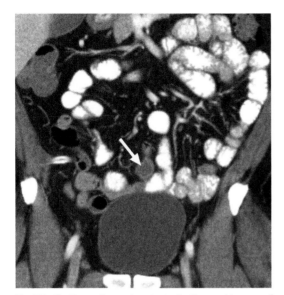

Fig. 25. Cystic peritoneal metastasis. Coronal image of a conventional abdominopelvic CT with positive oral contrast material. Small cystic peritoneal metastasis (*arrow*) is well seen adjacent to high-density enteric contrast and could be mistaken for a loop of fluid-filled bowel next to neutral enteric contrast.

and cause bleeding and/or obstruction. Multiple short segment (5- to 10-mm length) strictures (**Fig. 17**) or web-like diaphragms are the hallmark CTE finding. Multiphase imaging can help differentiate from contraction, and CT enteroclysis may increase sensitivity for detection, especially if not associated with partial SB obstruction. Multifocal short segment strictures can also be seen with chronic radiation-induced injury, CD (**Fig. 18**), and can be mistaken for adhesive disease, which typically has more tapered narrowing without wall thickening; clinical history is imperative. Although capsule endoscopy may be more sensitive for superficial erosions and ulcerations, its use is controversial in the setting of suspected NSAID enteropathy because of the risk of capsule retention.[34]

SUMMARY

CTE is a well-tolerated, accurate, and efficient modality used to assess pathologic condition arising from the SB. CTE benefits from widespread availability, rapid scan time, relatively lower cost compared with MR and optical modalities, and ability to evaluate extraenteric

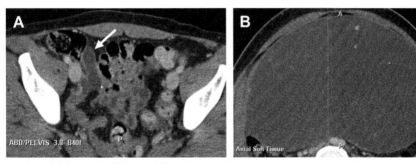

Fig. 26. Mucocele. Initial axial CTE image (*A*) with neutral contrast shows a mucocele of the appendix (*arrow*). This was mistaken for fluid-filled bowel. Examination 2 years later (*B*) shows pseudomyxoma peritonei from a mucocele that grew and perforated.

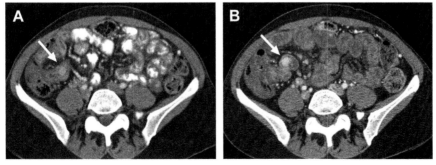

Fig. 27. Ileal carcinoid obscured by contrast. Axial CT image using positive enteric contrast (*A*) was interpreted as normal. Axial CTE image using neutral enteric contrast (*B*) well demonstrated a hyperenhancing carcinoid in the distal ileum (*arrow*). The mass was initially mistaken as contrast (*arrow, A*).

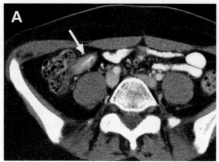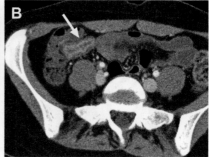

Fig. 28. CD obscured with positive oral contrast. Initial axial CT with positive contrast (*A*) was interpreted as negative in an adult with suspected CD. Because of persistent symptoms, CTE with neutral contrast (*B*) was done and better shows the hyperenhancement associated with active inflammation (*arrows*).

structures. Clinical scenarios well suited to CTE include detection and monitoring of inflammatory conditions and their complications, suspected SB bleeding, and detection and characterization SB masses. Proper technique is critical, including ingestion of a large volume of neutral oral contrast material and scanning during peak bowel wall enhancement. Radiologists should be familiar with dose reduction strategies, particularly for children and patients with chronic IBD requiring repeated studies. Familiarity with technical and interpretive pitfalls of CTE (**Box 7**) also improves diagnostic accuracy.

ACKNOWLEDGMENTS

The authors acknowledge the assistance of Sonia Watson, PhD, in editing the article.

REFERENCES

1. Schindera ST, Nelson RC, DeLong DM, et al. Multidetector row CT of the small bowel: peak enhancement temporal window–initial experience. Radiology 2007;243(2):438–44.
2. Huprich JE, Fletcher JG, Fidler JL, et al. Obscure GI bleeding: the role of multiphase CT enterography. Appl Radiol 2011;40(12):16–20.
3. Baker ME, Hara AK, Platt JF, et al. CT enterography for Crohn's disease: optimal technique and imaging issues. Abdom Imaging 2015;40(5):938–52.
4. Bruining DH, Zimmerman EM, Loftus EV Jr, et al. Consensus recommendations for evaluation, interpretation and utilization of computed tomography and magnetic resonance enterography in patients with small bowel Crohn's disease. Radiology 2018; 286(3):776–99.
5. Soto JA, Park SH, Fletcher JG, et al. Gastrointestinal hemorrhage: evaluation with MDCT. Abdom Imaging 2015;40(5):993–1009.
6. Del Gaizo AJ, Fletcher JG, Yu L, et al. Reducing radiation dose in CT enterography. Radiographics 2013;33(4):1109–24.
7. Sheedy SP, Bruining DH, Dozois EJ, et al. MR imaging of perianal Crohn disease. Radiology 2017; 282(3):628–45.
8. Guimaraes LS, Fletcher JG, Harmsen WS, et al. Appropriate patient selection at abdominal dual-energy CT using 80 kV: relationship between patient size, image noise, and image quality. Radiology 2010;257(3):732–42.
9. Kaza RK, Platt JF, Al-Hawary MM, et al. CT enterography at 80 kVp with adaptive statistical iterative reconstruction versus at 120 kVp with standard reconstruction: image quality, diagnostic adequacy, and dose reduction. AJR Am J Roentgenol 2012; 198(5):1084–92.
10. Yu L, Fletcher JG, Grant KL, et al. Automatic selection of tube potential for radiation dose reduction in vascular and contrast-enhanced abdominopelvic CT. AJR Am J Roentgenol 2013; 201(2):W297–306.
11. Kambadakone AR, Chaudhary NA, Desai GS, et al. Low-dose MDCT and CT enterography of patients with Crohn disease: feasibility of adaptive statistical iterative reconstruction. AJR Am J Roentgenol 2011; 196(6):W743–52.
12. Lee SJ, Park SH, Kim AY, et al. A prospective comparison of standard-dose CT enterography and 50% reduced-dose CT enterography with and without noise reduction for evaluating Crohn disease. AJR Am J Roentgenol 2011;197(1):50–7.
13. Ehman EC, Yu L, Manduca A, et al. Methods for clinical evaluation of noise reduction techniques in abdominopelvic CT. Radiographics 2014;34(4): 849–62.
14. Sagara Y, Hara AK, Pavlicek W, et al. Comparison of low-dose CT with adaptive statistical iterative reconstruction and routine-dose CT with filtered back projection in 53 patients. AJR Am J Roentgenol 2010; 195(3):713–9.

15. Gandhi NS, Baker ME, Goenka AH, et al. Diagnostic accuracy of CT enterography for active inflammatory terminal ileal Crohn disease: comparison of full-dose and half-dose images reconstructed with FBP and half-dose images with SAFIRE. Radiology 2016; 280(2):436–45.

16. Fletcher JG, Hara AK, Fidler JL, et al. Observer performance for adaptive, image-based denoising and filtered back projection compared to scanner-based iterative reconstruction for lower dose CT enterography. Abdom Imaging 2015; 40(5):1050–9.

17. Guimaraes LS, Fletcher JG, Yu L, et al. Feasibility of dose reduction using novel denoising techniques for low kV (80 kV) CT enterography: optimization and validation. Acad Radiol 2010;17(10): 1203–10.

18. Khan JJ, Donnelly LF, Koch BL, et al. A program to decrease the need for pediatric sedation for CT and MRI. Appl Radiol 2007; 36(4):30–3.

19. Bruining DH, Loftus EV Jr, Ehman EC, et al. Computed tomography enterography detects intestinal wall changes and effects of treatment in patients with Crohn's disease. Clin Gastroenterol Hepatol 2011;9(8):679–83.e1.

20. Deepak P, Fletcher JG, Fidler JL, et al. Radiological response is associated with better long-term outcomes and is a potential treatment target in patients with small bowel Crohn's disease. Am J Gastroenterol 2016;111(7):997–1006.

21. Booya F, Akram S, Fletcher JG, et al. CT enterography and fistulizing Crohn's disease: clinical benefit and radiographic findings. Abdom Imaging 2009; 34(4):467–75.

22. Buckley JA, Fishman EK. CT evaluation of small bowel neoplasms: spectrum of disease. Radiographics 1998;18(2):379–92.

23. Sailer J, Zacherl J, Schima W. MDCT of small bowel tumours. Cancer Imaging 2007;7:224–33.

24. Bilimoria KY, Bentrem DJ, Wayne JD, et al. Small bowel cancer in the United States: changes in epidemiology, treatment, and survival over the last 20 years. Ann Surg 2009;249(1): 63–71.

25. Rindi G, Arnold R, Bosman FT, et al. Nomenclature and classification of neuroendocrine neoplasms of the digestive system. In: Bosman TF, Carneiro F, Hruban RH, et al, editors. WHO Classification of Tumours of the Digestive System. 4th edition. Lyon (France): International Agency for Research on cancer (IARC); 2010. p. 13.

26. Aparicio T, Zaanan A, Svrcek M, et al. Small bowel adenocarcinoma: epidemiology, risk factors, diagnosis and treatment. Dig Liver Dis 2014;46(2): 97–104.

27. Weber NK, Fletcher JG, Fidler JL, et al. Clinical characteristics and imaging features of small bowel adenocarcinomas in Crohn's disease. Abdom Imaging 2015;40(5):1060–7.

28. McLaughlin PD, Maher MM. Primary malignant diseases of the small intestine. AJR Am J Roentgenol 2013;201(1):W9–14.

29. Miller TL, Skucas J, Gudex D, et al. Bowel cancer characteristics in patients with regional enteritis. Gastrointest Radiol 1987;12(1):45–52.

30. Ghai S, Pattison J, Ghai S, et al. Primary gastrointestinal lymphoma: spectrum of imaging findings with pathologic correlation. Radiographics 2007;27(5): 1371–88.

31. Levy AD, Sobin LH. From the archives of the AFIP: gastrointestinal carcinoids: imaging features with clinicopathologic comparison. Radiographics 2007; 27(1):237–57.

32. Vasconcelos RN, Dolan SG, Barlow JM, et al. Impact of CT enterography on the diagnosis of small bowel gastrointestinal stromal tumors. Abdom Radiol (NY) 2017;42(5):1365–73.

33. Huprich JE, Barlow JM, Hansel SL, et al. Multiphase CT enterography evaluation of small-bowel vascular lesions. AJR Am J Roentgenol 2013;201(1):65–72.

34. Cheifetz AS, Lewis BS. Capsule endoscopy retention: is it a complication? J Clin Gastroenterol 2006;40(8):688–91.

35. Yano T, Yamamoto H, Sunada K, et al. Endoscopic classification of vascular lesions of the small intestine (with videos). Gastrointest Endosc 2008;67(1): 169–72.

36. Scholz FJ, Behr SC, Scheirey CD. Intramural fat in the duodenum and proximal small intestine in patients with celiac disease. AJR Am J Roentgenol 2007;189(4):786–90.

37. Cohen MD, Lintott DJ. Transient small bowel intussusception in adult coeliac disease. Clin Radiol 1978;29(5):529–34.

38. Gonda TA, Khan SU, Cheng J, et al. Association of intussusception and celiac disease in adults. Dig Dis Sci 2010;55(10):2899–903.

39. Scholz FJ, Afnan J, Behr SC. CT findings in adult celiac disease. Radiographics 2011;31(4):977–92.

40. Herlinger H, Maglinte DD. Jejunal fold separation in adult celiac disease: relevance of enteroclysis. Radiology 1986;158(3):605–11.

41. Rubesin SE, Herlinger H, Saul SH, et al. Adult celiac disease and its complications. Radiographics 1989; 9(6):1045–66.

42. Barlow JM, Johnson CD, Stephens DH. Celiac disease: how common is jejunoileal fold pattern reversal found at small-bowel follow-through? AJR Am J Roentgenol 1996;166(3):575–7.

43. Freeman HJ. Mesenteric lymph node cavitation syndrome. World J Gastroenterol 2010;16(24): 2991–3.

44. Reddy D, Salomon C, Demos TC, et al. Mesenteric lymph node cavitation in celiac disease. AJR Am J Roentgenol 2002;178(1):247.
45. Buckley O, Brien JO, Ward E, et al. The imaging of coeliac disease and its complications. Eur J Radiol 2008;65(3):483–90.
46. Lohan DG, Alhajeri AN, Cronin CG, et al. MR enterography of small-bowel lymphoma: potential for suggestion of histologic subtype and the presence of underlying celiac disease. AJR Am J Roentgenol 2008;190(2):287–93.
47. Van Weyenberg SJ, Meijerink MR, Jacobs MA, et al. MR enteroclysis in refractory celiac disease: proposal and validation of a severity scoring system. Radiology 2011;259(1):151–61.
48. Freeman HJ. Malignancy in adult celiac disease. World J Gastroenterol 2009;15(13):1581–3.

Magnetic Resonance Enterography for Inflammatory and Noninflammatory Conditions of the Small Bowel

Gaurav Khatri, MD, Jay Coleman, MD, John R. Leyendecker, MD*

KEYWORDS

• MR enterography • Crohn's disease • Small bowel

KEY POINTS

- Magnetic resonance enterography (MRE) is an effective noninvasive means to assess disease activity in Crohn disease (CD) patients on a recurrent basis without exposure to ionizing radiation.
- Elements of successful MRE technique typically include patient preparation, good bowel distention with biphasic enteric contrast, use of anti-peristaltic agents, administration of a gadolinium-based contrast agent, and acquisition of cine images.
- CD findings on MRE correlate with disease status and can be used to guide management and assess response to therapy.
- MRE can depict findings of active inflammatory CD, fibrostenotic CD, penetrating CD, quiescent or inactive CD, as well as enteric and extraenteric complications.
- Cine images acquired as part of MRE protocol assist in differentiating luminal narrowing secondary to active inflammation from luminal narrowing due to fibrostenotic disease.

INTRODUCTION

Over the last several years, cross-sectional imaging has replaced fluoroscopic techniques for the evaluation of select inflammatory and noninflammatory conditions of the small and large bowel. Computed tomography (CT) and magnetic resonance (MR) enterography are routinely performed for assessment of inflammatory bowel disease (IBD), small bowel neoplasms, bowel obstructions, infection, or for systemic conditions, such as celiac disease or systemic sclerosis. These cross-sectional techniques allow for direct visualization of the bowel wall and better detection for extraenteric complications.[1] Visualization in multiple planes allows for easier separation and tracking of bowel segments and associated abnormalities.

MR and CT enterography have similar diagnostic accuracy for detection of findings of active small bowel Crohn disease (CD)[1–3]; however, magnetic resonance enterography (MRE) may be superior in terms of stricture detection.[2] MRE costs more and takes longer to perform than computed tomography enterography (CTE). Other

Disclosure Statement: The authors have no pertinent commercial or financial disclosures, or sources of external funding.
Department of Radiology, University of Texas Southwestern Medical Center, 5323 Harry Hines Boulevard, Dallas, TX 75390, USA
* Corresponding author.
E-mail address: John.Leyendecker@utsouthwestern.edu

Radiol Clin N Am 56 (2018) 671–689
https://doi.org/10.1016/j.rcl.2018.04.003
0033-8389/18/© 2018 Elsevier Inc. All rights reserved.

limitations of MRE include variable image quality related to patient and technical factors; however, MRE avoids exposure to ionizing radiation and iodinated contrast. The lack of exposure to ionizing radiation is particularly advantageous in young CD patients who require multiple examinations over time to evaluate disease status. Gadolinium-based contrast agents (GBCAs) used for MR imaging are not nephrotoxic at approved doses, but caution should be used when administering GBCAs to patients with renal insufficiency. MR imaging also offers superior soft tissue contrast resolution, which assists in detecting abnormal enhancement, edema, and mural fibrosis. The lack of exposure to ionizing radiation during MRE allows for multiple acquisitions at various time points and phases of contrast enhancement. Dynamic cine imaging provides functional information about motility and helps differentiate transient narrowing of bowel segments from persistent strictures. Newer MR imaging techniques also offer higher spatial resolution, allowing for subtle details such as linear ulcers to be detected. Utilization of proper, efficient technique and interpretive expertise allows one to leverage these advantages of MRE to improve diagnosis and management of small bowel disease. In this article, the authors review optimal MRE technique, demonstrate its application to various disease processes afflicting the small bowel, discuss pearls and pitfalls that may be encountered during image acquisition and interpretation, and discuss reporting strategies.

TECHNIQUE
Patient Preparation

Optimal MRE technique requires patient preparation before image acquisition. Appropriately timed administration of a sufficient volume of oral contrast material facilitates adequate distention of the bowel. Oral contrast agents used for MRE can be categorized as positive contrast agents, negative contrast agents, or biphasic agents. Positive contrast agents result in high intraluminal signal intensity (SI) on both T1-weighted (T1w) and T2-weighted (T2w) images and include paramagnetic substances, such as dilute gadolinium solutions, or manganese-containing liquids, including low concentrations of blueberry juice.[4,5] Positive enteric agents depict bowel wall thickening well; however, the high SI luminal contents obscure mucosal enhancement on postcontrast T1w images. Negative contrast agents such as superparamagnetic iron oxide solution or air induce low SI in bowel lumen on both T1w and T2w sequences[5]

and allow for visualization of bowel wall edema and perienteric inflammatory changes on T2w images, and mucosal enhancement on T1w postcontrast images, although susceptibility artifact can degrade bowel wall visualization on gradient echo– and echo planar–based diffusion-weighted sequences and obscure low SI intraluminal lesions.[6] The most commonly used MRE contrast agents are biphasic, exhibiting high SI on T2w images (allowing for detection of wall thickening, endoluminal abnormalities, and transmural ulcers) and low SI on T1w images (enhancing detection of mucosal enhancement and hypervascular endoluminal masses).[6] Examples of biphasic contrast agents include water, polyethylene glycol (PEG), mannitol, and sorbitol-containing 0.1% barium sulfate (SCBS) solution. Because of their osmotic properties, PEG and SCBS solution provide better bowel distention than water. Water fails to provide adequate distal bowel distention but is better tolerated with a lower incidence of side effects and does not incur additional cost.[7] At the authors' institution, patients are asked to remain fasting before the examination and to ingest 900 mL of SCBS solution starting 45 minutes before the examination. They are instructed to ingest the oral contrast at a steady pace to obtain uniform distention throughout the small bowel. Immediately before supine positioning on the MR table, patients ingest one 16-ounce cup of water to distend the stomach and duodenum. Multichannel phased-array torso coils are used to cover the abdomen and pelvis. Images from initial sequences are assessed to ensure adequate small bowel distention before further image acquisition. The authors administer additional oral contrast or water if needed for adequate bowel distention as discussed in the pearls and pitfalls section.

Imaging Protocol

The standard MRE protocol at the authors' institution as published previously (Table 1)[8] includes thick-slab (40 mm) 2-dimensional (2D) heavily T2w single-shot fast spin echo (SSFSE) sequences with fat suppression (FS) and balanced fast field echo (BFFE) sequences. Each of these sequences is acquired in the coronal plane from anterior to posterior repeatedly over 2.5 minutes. The images are sorted by slice location and viewed as cine-loops, thus allowing for visualization of bowel wall and change in luminal content over time. An important technical consideration after completion of these cine-type sequences is the administration of an

Table 1
Sample magnetic resonance enterography protocol

Sequence	Imaging Plane	Field of View (mm)	Number of Slices	Slice Thickness (mm)	Repetition Time (ms)	Time to Echo (ms)	Flip Angle (°)	Matrix
2D CINE FS T2w SSFSE	Coronal	400	5	40	2180	593	180	384 × 307
2D CINE BFFE[a]	Coronal	400	28	6	3.98	1.99	70	256 × 154
2D BFFE	Coronal	400	32	5	4.37	2.19	70	320 × 192
2D BFFE (upper abd)	Axial	360	40	6	3.67	1.47	70	256 × 166
2D BFFE (lower abd/pelvis)	Axial	360	40	6	3.67	1.47	70	256 × 166
2D T2w SSFSE	Coronal	450	49	5	1480	115	150	320 × 288
2D T2w FS SSFSE	Coronal	400	49	5	1480	115	150	320 × 288
3D T1w FS 3D GRE pre- and post (×2)	Coronal	450	60	4	4.16	1.41	10	288 × 173
3D T1w FS GRE Post (upper abd)	Axial	380	60	4	4.06	1.52	10	320 × 192
3D T1w FS GRE Post (lower abd/pelvis)	Axial	380	60	4	4.06	1.52	10	320 × 192

Abbreviation: abd, abdomen.
[a] Radiologist checks for luminal distension after 2D cine BFFE and determines need for additional oral contrast.

antiperistaltic agent to minimize bowel wall motion on the remainder of the examination. A one-time dose of 1 mg intramuscular glucagon is administered after completion of the cine sequences at the authors' institution. Alternatively, patients with known hypersensitivity or contraindications to glucagon, such as insulin-dependent or poorly controlled diabetes, known pheochromocytoma, insulinoma, or glucagonoma, or certain cardiac diseases[9] can be administered 0.250 mg sublingual hyoscyamine sulfate. Although MRE has been shown to perform well even in the absence of antiperistaltic agents,[10,11] subjective image quality is typically lower without antiperistaltic agents, and their routine use is recommended.[12]

After administration of the antiperistaltic agent, T2w SSFSE sequences, without and with FS, and high-resolution BFFE sequences are acquired in the coronal plane. The field-of-view for all the coronal acquisitions should extend from the stomach down to the rectum.

Axial BFFE images are then acquired in 2 separate breath-holds, one for the upper abdomen and a second through the lower abdomen and pelvis. The T2w SSFSE sequences provide high contrast between the bowel lumen and bowel wall when used in conjunction with positive or biphasic contrast agents and allow identification of bowel wall thickening. FS highlights submucosal edema within the thickened wall as well as surrounding mesenteric inflammation. BFFE sequences are relatively motion insensitive. They are acquired at an out-of-phase echo time and hence demonstrate an India ink artifact at the interface of the bowel wall and adjacent perienteric fat, and also within the bowel wall itself when submucosal fat is present. Mesenteric findings such as lymph nodes are also well delineated on BFFE images because of surrounding India ink artifact.

Finally, 3-dimensional (3D) T1w gradient recall echo (GRE) images with FS are obtained before and after the administration of a single dose of gadolinium-based contrast at 2 mL/s. The authors advocate the use of macrocyclic gadolinium-based contrast agents in order to minimize risk of nephrogenic systemic fibrosis in these patients who may receive multiple doses during their lifetimes. Postcontrast images are acquired in the coronal plane during the early enteric phase of contrast and then again after a 40-second delay. Subsequently, axial postcontrast 3D T1w FS GRE images are obtained in 2 separate breath-holds, one through the upper abdomen and the second through the lower abdomen and pelvis. Subtraction images are created to increase sensitivity for areas of bowel wall hyperenhancement and fistulas. Standard sequence parameters are provided in **Table 1**.

Additional Sequences and Techniques

Additional optional sequences and techniques that can be performed include diffusion-weighted imaging (DWI), high temporal resolution dynamic contrast-enhanced (DCE)-MR imaging to measure perfusion and other pharmacokinetic parameters, and magnetization transfer imaging (MTI). DWI measures the microscopic motion of intracellular and extracellular water molecules within tissue. It can detect subtle areas of inflammation or abscess formation. Studies show lower apparent diffusion coefficient (ADC) values in inflamed bowel segments than in noninflamed segments. ADC values correlate with CD clinical measures of disease activity, such as the Harvey-Bradshaw Index (HBI).[13–15] Oto and colleagues[15] reported 95% sensitivity and 82% specificity of DWI for detection of active inflammation in the small bowel. DWI is also able to detect inflammation in the colon without oral preparation[16] and is a reliable tool for evaluation of both ileal and colonic CD.[17] It may be most useful in patients with contraindications to GBCAs. Perfusion DCE MR imaging and MTI are currently under investigation and have not been widely adopted for routine clinical use. Although initial studies demonstrated correlation between peak enhancement in the bowel wall during DCE imaging and the Crohn Disease Activity Index (CDAI),[18] some more recent studies have shown only weak correlation between enhancement measures and disease activity scores.[19,20] Perfusion parameters such as K_{trans} can be combined with ADC values from DWI to provide quantitative measures of bowel inflammation.[14] MTI provides quantification of magnetization transfer between hydrogen protons in tissue and in doing so provides an indirect measure of concentrations of macromolecules, such as collagen within the tissue. It has shown potential in humans for identification of fibrotic scarring in bowel segments.[21]

APPLICATIONS
Crohn Disease

CD is an idiopathic inflammatory condition that can affect any portion of the gastrointestinal tract but with a predilection to involve small bowel. Because of its relapsing and remitting nature, propensity to affect young patients, nonspecific symptoms, and high rate of extraintestinal complications, CD remains the most common indication for performance of MRE. For known CD patients presenting with symptoms, MRE assists in assessing disease status, detecting complications, such as fistulas, strictures, and abscesses (**Fig. 1**), determining appropriate therapy, and monitoring treatment response without exposure to ionizing radiation. Traditional management of CD has focused on symptom control and relies on clinical indices of inflammation such as the HBI and the CDAI as measurable endpoints.[22,23] Unfortunately, clinical indices are limited in their ability to assess the full extent and severity of bowel inflammation, and mitigation of symptoms does not necessarily reflect resolution of inflammation.[24–26] Unresolved inflammation is thought to result in cumulative bowel damage and fibrosis, potentially requiring eventual surgical intervention. More recently, mucosal healing has been suggested as an appropriate endpoint for medical therapy.[27] Although endoscopy remains the gold standard for assessment of mucosal healing and disease activity, a few newer imaging-based indices attempt to quantify disease status and severity noninvasively. Most MR imaging–based disease activity indices incorporate measures of wall thickness and degree of wall enhancement after

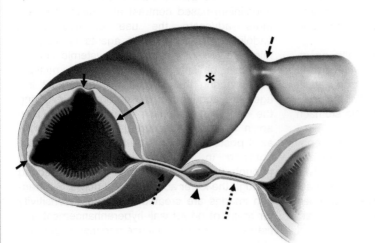

Fig. 1. Enteric complications of CD. Coexistence of findings of active disease such as mucosal inflammation (*long solid arrow*) and ulcerations (*short arrows*) with enteric complications such as stricture formation (*dashed arrow*) with upstream bowel dilatation (*asterisks*) and of sequelae of penetrating disease, including fistula (*dotted arrows*) and abscess (*arrowhead*).

contrast administration. Other common parameters include presence or absence of luminal stenosis, mucosal irregularity/ulceration, mural edema (resulting in target sign), engorgement of the vasa recta (comb sign), and regional lymphadenopathy, whereas less commonly used parameters include hyperintensity on DWI, subjective or semiquantitative evaluation of bowel motility, presence of penetrating lesions, and fibrofatty proliferation.[28] The Magnetic Resonance Index of Activity (MaRIA) was developed using ileocolonoscopy and the Crohn disease endoscopic index of severity (CDEIS) as reference standards and is based on bowel wall thickness, relative contrast enhancement, and the presence or absence of bowel wall edema and mucosal ulceration on MR imaging. MaRIA has been shown to correlate well with CDEIS[29,30] and is useful in assessing response to medical therapy.[31] A more recent study, however, found that the MaRIA score was not predictive of disease course.[32] Other MRE indices have been developed including the Clermont index, which modifies the MaRIA with addition of DWI,[33] and the London MR imaging index for CD activity, which is based on wall thickness and mural T2w SI.[34] These indices have similar high diagnostic accuracy for assessment of disease activity in CD.[35]

CD can be categorized as active inflammatory CD with or without luminal narrowing, fibrostenotic CD, penetrating CD, mixed stenotic and active inflammatory CD, or quiescent or inactive CD. CD patients often progress along a spectrum from active inflammation to fibrostenotic disease, with or without penetrating disease, and many patients manifest a mixture of inflammation and fibrosis histologically. MRE findings associated with these categories of CD are discussed.

Active Inflammatory Crohn Disease

There are several imaging findings that contribute to a determination of active disease. Bowel wall thickening (>3 mm) and increased contrast enhancement on MRE are associated with inflammatory activity in CD patients and can be used to predict disease severity and differentiate active disease from bowel segments in remission.[29,30,36] Other studies have shown weak to moderate correlation between wall thickening and enhancement and disease activity.[37] Mucosal hyperenhancement, along with submucosal edema, results in a stratified appearance of the bowel wall (Fig. 2), which correlates with active disease, whereas homogeneous enhancement of the bowel wall favors inactive or quiescent disease.[38,39] Bowel wall thickening with high SI on T2w images

can result from either submucosal edema or submucosal fat deposition, and T2w images with FS allow differentiation (see Fig. 2). Wall thickening with submucosal edema is associated with acute inflammation[39] and correlates with disease activity on CDEIS,[29,30] whereas submucosal fat deposition is a sequela of chronic disease. As mentioned previously, bowel inflammation also increases SI in the bowel wall on DWI and lowers mural ADC values compared with noninflamed bowel segments.[13–15] Inflamed bowel segments may be noncontiguous, resulting in skip lesions in the gastrointestinal tract, a hallmark of CD (Fig. 3).

Mucosal ulceration is a hallmark of active inflammatory CD on endoscopy. Although superficial ulcers are difficult to detect on MR imaging, deep or transmural ulcerations appear as linear or saccular protrusions into the bowel wall on high-resolution images. Using a high-resolution, thin-section T2w acquisition increases sensitivity for superficial and deep ulceration.[40] Bowel mucosa between transmural ulcerations appears irregular and polypoid in appearance, resulting in formation of pseudo-polyps.[41] Chronic ulceration results in asymmetric fibrosis and shortening of the mesenteric border of the bowel wall with associated pseudo-saccule formation on the antimesenteric border[41] (Fig. 4).

In addition to changes within the small bowel mucosa and submucosa, changes in the associated mesentery, particularly edema, correlate with active inflammation.[42] Engorgement of the vasa recta, often called the "comb sign" (see Fig. 2; Fig. 5),[43] also correlates with biologic activity of disease.[44] These additional findings improve confidence in a diagnosis of active inflammatory CD. Mesenteric lymphadenopathy is a common finding in the setting of active inflammatory CD, and one study has demonstrated higher enhancement relative to adjacent vessels in the setting of active CD compared with lymph nodes in patients with predominately fibrostenotic CD[45] (see Fig. 5).

Luminal Narrowing and Fibrostenotic Crohn Disease

CD patients often manifest focal luminal narrowing on MRE. In the absence of extraenteric mass effect, luminal narrowing typically results from either mural inflammation or submucosal fibrosis or both. Submucosal edema due to inflammation manifests as high SI on T2w images that persists with FS (see Fig. 2), whereas fibrosis appears low in SI with similar technique (Fig. 6). Upstream bowel dilatation implies some degree of obstruction, but partial obstruction does not necessarily require surgery, particularly when accompanied by

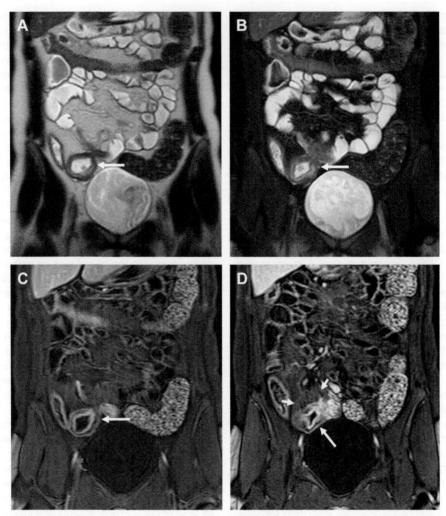

Fig. 2. A 26-year-old woman with CD. Coronal (Cor) T2w SSFSE image demonstrates bowel wall thickening with submucosal high SI in right lower quadrant (*arrow* in *A*), which could be due to edema or fat. Submucosal high SI persists on Cor T2w SSFSE image with FS (*arrow* in *B*) consistent with submucosal edema rather than fat. On Cor T1w 3D FS GRE images, the edematous loop demonstrates stratified enhancement with mucosal hyperenhancement due to active inflammation (*long arrows* in *C, D*) along with engorgement of adjacent vasa recta resulting in the comb sign (*short arrows* in *D*).

imaging findings of active inflammation that might respond to medical treatment. Although stratified or layered enhancement in the bowel wall generally denotes active inflammatory CD, it can also be present when active mucosal inflammation coexists with fibrostenotic disease. In fact, fibrosis and active inflammation frequently coexist at sites of luminal narrowing in patients with small bowel CD[39] (see **Fig. 6**; **Fig. 7**). Cine T2w or BFFE sequences can help differentiate between luminal narrowing secondary to fibrosis, which appears fixed with loss of normal peristalsis (see **Fig. 7**) and luminal narrowing due to active inflammation alone, which does not persist on repeated acquisition (**Fig. 8**). In patients with fibrotic strictures, the degree of bowel dilatation upstream on MRE is a significant predictor of success of surgical management with strictureplasty versus bowel resection.[46]

Penetrating Crohn Disease

Unchecked transmural ulceration progresses to penetrating disease in the form of sinus tract or fistula formation. Of patients with penetrating disease, 93% to 96% have associated strictures on surgical specimens.[47,48] Most fistulas and sinus tracts occur proximal to the associated stricture, whereas a few occur within the stricture itself[47,48] (see **Figs. 6** and **7**). The association between

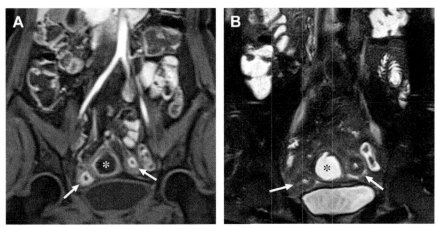

Fig. 3. A 47-year-old woman with CD. Cor T1w FS 3D GRE image demonstrates stratified enhancement in pelvic ileal loops (*arrows* in *A*), which are separated by a more central dilated loop (*asterisks* in *A, B*). Findings are typical of skip lesions in CD. Cor T2w FS image demonstrates perienteric edema and some areas of high SI in the thickened wall due to submucosal edema suggesting active disease (*arrows* in *B*). Dark SI in the wall on T2 FS image may be due to underlying fibrosis or submucosal fat.

strictures and fistulas is important, because most fistulas will not heal as long as the stricture persists. Fistulas often form between loops of small bowel (enteroenteric) or between small bowel and colon (enterocolic), may extend to the abdominal wall, may be confined to the mesentery, and less commonly may be between small bowel and bladder or gynecologic structures.[47] Perianal fistulas are common, requiring additional targeted high-resolution sequences for adequate evaluation. MRE has high sensitivity and specificity for detection of fistulas,[40,42,49] which appear as enhancing tubular tracts between loops of bowel or extending to other organs with associated bowel angulation and tethering due to adhesion formation. Fistulas are often best demonstrated on FS T1w images after GBCA administration due to enhancing granulation tissue in the wall of the tract[50] (see **Fig. 6**; **Fig. 9**). Surrounding inflammation and hyperemia may be present on T2w images. When large enough, fistulas or sinus tracts contain enteric contrast or gas. Fistulas may be complex, involving multiple bowel loops, and multiplanar reformations may be necessary to show their true extent (see **Fig. 9**).

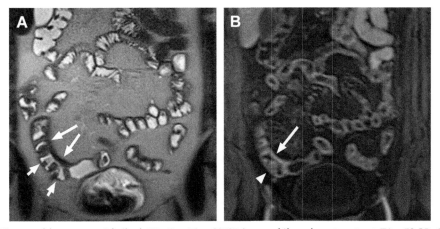

Fig. 4. A 43-year-old woman with ileal CD. Cor T2w SSFSE image (*A*) and postcontrast T1w FS 3D GRE image demonstrate wall thickening with low SI consistent with fibrosis along the mesenteric border of the distal ileum in the right lower quadrant (*long arrows*) and pseudo-sacculations along the antimesenteric border (*short arrows* in *A*). There is no significant surrounding active inflammatory change. Pseudo-polyp seen in the bowel lumen on postcontrast image (*arrowhead* in *B*).

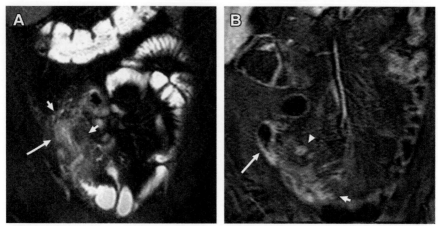

Fig. 5. A 37-year-old woman with history of CD and acute right-sided pain. Cor FS T2w SSFSE image demonstrates wall thickening of an ileal segment in the right lower quadrant with high SI in the wall consistent with submucosal edema suggesting active inflammation (*long arrow* in *A*). Surrounding perienteric stranding (*short arrows* in *A*) is reactive. Cor postcontrast 3D T1w FS GRE image demonstrates wall thickening and hyperenhancement (*long arrow* in *B*) with engorgement of the adjacent vasa recta consistent with the "comb sign" (*short arrow* in *B*). Reactive hypervascular mesenteric lymph nodes are seen in the adjacent mesentery (*arrowhead* in *B*).

Penetrating disease may result in formation of abscesses, for which MRE has high sensitivity.[42,46,49] These perienteric organized fluid collections typically develop within the mesentery adjacent to sites of inflammation and demonstrate a thick enhancing wall with surrounding inflammatory changes (see **Fig. 8**). Gas within an abscess can demonstrate evidence of susceptibility artifact. Abscesses are often very bright on DWI and low SI on ADC maps, helping to distinguish them from adjacent bowel loops.[51] Identification of an abscess alters medical management, because certain therapies, such as steroids or tumor

necrosis factor-alpha inhibitors, are contraindicated in the setting of abscess. Furthermore, accessible abscesses can be managed by percutaneous drainage, which may obviate emergent surgical intervention.[46]

Quiescent or Inactive Crohn Disease

Inactive CD can demonstrate mild wall thickening with homogeneous enhancement of the small bowel wall.[38] The bowel wall lacks the mural edema typical of active inflammation on T2w images, although may contain intramural fat

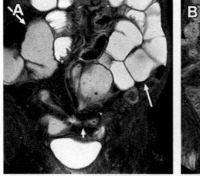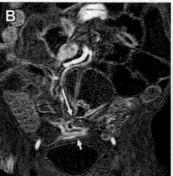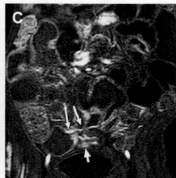

Fig. 6. A 62-year-old woman with ileocolonic fistulizing CD with persistent abdominal bloating/distention. Cor FS T2 SSFSE image demonstrates a short segment of luminal narrowing that is hypointense (*short arrow* in *A*) that could be due to fibrosis or submucosal fat. There is bowel dilatation in the upper abdomen indicating at least partial obstruction (*long arrows* in *A*) upstream to the luminal narrowing. Postcontrast T1w 3D FS GRE images demonstrate a corresponding fixed stricture (*short arrows* in *B, C*). Superimposed mucosal hyperenhancement and stratified enhancement are present at the stricture. There are associated enteroenteric fistulas (*long arrows* in *B, C*) arising at and proximal to the stricture with involvement of multiple bowel loops, which appear tethered centrally.

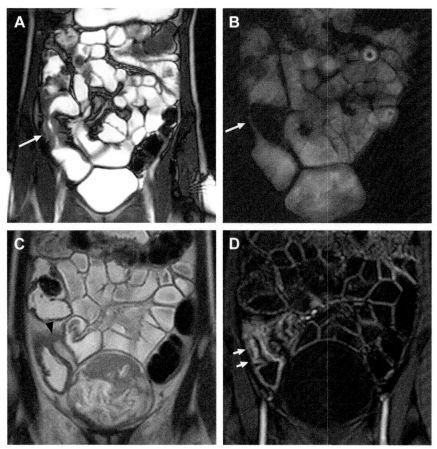

Fig. 7. A 31-year-old woman with history of CD. Cor cine BFFE image (*A*) and thick slab T2w FS SSFSE image (*B*) through the same location at 2 different time points demonstrate persistent luminal narrowing of a right lower quadrant loop (*arrows*) indicating fixed stricture. Coronal T2w SSFSE image shows a sinus tract (*arrowhead* in *C*) arising from the proximal portion of the stenotic segment. Cor postcontrast T1w FS 3D GRE image demonstrates hyperenhancement of the stenotic segment (*arrows* in *D*).

deposition (discussed under "Pitfalls"). There may also be proliferation of the associated mesenteric fat, the so-called creeping fat sign.

Other Complications of Crohn Disease

Besides stricture and fistula formation, which can result in bowel obstruction or abscesses, patients with CD have higher risk for small bowel adenocarcinoma and lymphoma.[52,53] Early small bowel adenocarcinoma may be difficult to differentiate from nonmalignant stricture on imaging. The presence of a focal or circumferential mass with intraluminal/extraluminal growth, and heterogeneous SI on T2w images with moderate heterogeneous enhancement is worrisome for adenocarcinoma.[54,55] Associated lymphadenopathy may be present. Appearance of small bowel adenocarcinoma and lymphoma is discussed further under "Small Bowel Neoplasms."

Other extraenteric conditions associated with CD can be seen incidentally on MRE, such as sclerosing cholangitis, renal calculi, and sacroiliitis.

Small Bowel Neoplasms

MRE has been proposed as a noninvasive tool for detection of small bowel polyps in patients with polyposis syndromes, including Peutz-Jeghers syndrome, Cowden disease, juvenile polyposis, and Gardner syndrome. In patients with Peutz-Jeghers syndrome, small bowel manifestations include multiple hamartomatous polyps throughout the bowel. Patients have an increased risk of small bowel, colorectal, and other gastrointestinal and nongastrointestinal malignancies.[56,57] Large polyps may result in obstruction and gastrointestinal bleeding, and the American College of Gastroenterology guidelines recommend surveillance with colonoscopy,

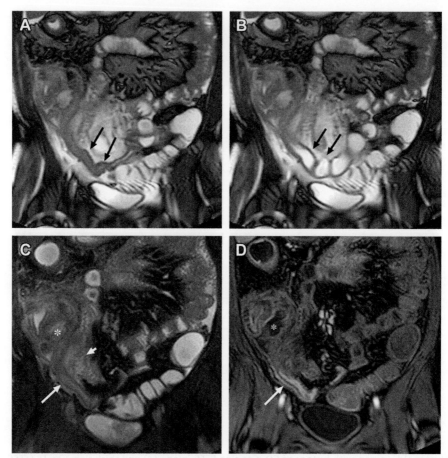

Fig. 8. A 35-year-old man with history of ileal CD, abdominal distention, pain, and clinical concern for stricture. Coronal cine BFFE images through the same location at 2 different time points are shown. At the first time point, there is a thick-walled ileal loop in the right lower quadrant with luminal narrowing (*arrows* in *A*). This loop demonstrates normal luminal distention at the second time point (*arrows* in *B*), excluding a fixed stricture. Cor T2w FS image (*C*) and postcontrast T1w FS 3D GRE image (*D*) demonstrate wall edema and enhancement of the terminal ileum (*long arrows*), inflammatory changes in the adjacent mesentery (*short arrow* in *C*), and an abscess (*asterisks*) that was secondary to perforated appendicitis in setting of CD.

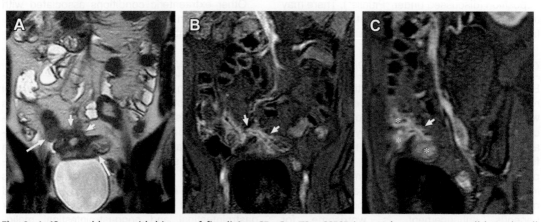

Fig. 9. A 42-year-old man with history of fistulizing CD. Cor T2w SSFSE image demonstrates small bowel wall thickening (*long arrows* in *A*) with an enteroenteric fistula (*short arrows* in *A*). Cor postcontrast T1w FS 3D GRE image demonstrates hyperenhancement of the fistulous tract (*short arrows* in *B*). Sagittal oblique reformation of the postcontrast T1w FS 3D GRE image (*C*) demonstrates the complex nature of the fistula (*short arrow* in *C*) involving at least 3 bowel loops (*asterisks* in *C*).

esophagogastroduodenoscopy, and capsule endoscopy (CE) every 3 years.[57] A few studies have assessed the performance of MRE for detection of small bowel polyps. Caspari and colleagues[58] demonstrated similar performance of MRE and CE for detection of large polyps greater than 15 mm, whereas polyps smaller than 5 mm were seen only on CE. Maccioni and colleagues[59] demonstrated high concordance (93%) between MRE and pushed-double-balloon enteroscopy, laparoscopic endoscopy, or surgery for detection of polyps greater than 15 mm; however, concordance for smaller polyps was 73%. They suggested that MRE may offer an effective alternative to CE for surveillance in these patients on a more frequent yearly basis. To the authors' knowledge, the appropriate time interval for surveillance by MRE has not been systematically studied or reported. Gupta and colleagues[60] demonstrated similar performance of MRE and CE for detection of polyps larger than 10 mm. Polyps present as round or oval filling defects within the bowel lumen, are hypointense relative to positive or biphasic contrast on T2w and BFFE images, and are best visualized when the bowel lumen is well distended with oral contrast (Fig. 10). Gas within the bowel can obscure or mimic polyps. Addition of prone imaging to traditional supine acquisition displaces the gas within the lumen and can result in higher detection rate of small polyps.[59] Polyps can be differentiated from intraluminal contents and gas bubbles by their persistent location and appearance on multiple sequences and the presence of enhancement (see Fig. 10). Biphasic enteric contrast material allows visualization of enhancing polyps on 3D postcontrast T1w FS images against a background of low SI bowel lumen. SSFSE T2w sequences are particularly susceptible to intraluminal filling defects due to flow artifacts, debris, or gas. Filling defects seen on these sequences should thus always be confirmed on other sequences and planes.

Carcinoid tumors, a subset of neuroendocrine tumors (NETs), commonly arise in the gastrointestinal system, and the jejunum and ileum are relatively common locations for these tumors, particularly in Caucasian patients and male patients.[61] Carcinoid tumors may be asymptomatic or cause nonspecific symptoms. Of patients with carcinoid tumor, 10% to 15% develop carcinoid syndrome, typically in the setting of hepatic metastases from an intestinal primary.[62] Primary carcinoid tumors and associated metastatic mesenteric masses are typically isointense relative to muscle on T1w images and isointense to mildly hyperintense on T2w images, often demonstrating a radiating, spiculated appearance because of surrounding desmoplastic reaction. They may present as intraluminal filling defects that are hypointense relative to positive or biphasic oral contrast in the lumen on T2w or BFFE images. They typically enhance avidly after GBCA administration.[55] Associated hyperenhancing lymphadenopathy may be present in the adjacent mesentery (Fig. 11). Dohan and colleagues[63] evaluated the sensitivity of MRE for detection of NETs of the small bowel and found a per lesion sensitivity of 74%. All the NETs in that study were seen in the ileum in keeping with the most common location for small bowel carcinoid. In 16 of 19 patients, NETs were seen as well-demarcated intraluminal masses with marked enhancement, whereas in 2 patients, NETs presented as focal thickening of

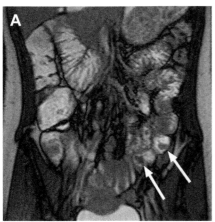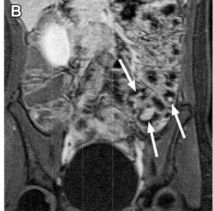

Fig. 10. A 26-year-old woman with history of Peutz-Jeghers syndrome. Coronal BFFE (A) and postcontrast T1w FS 3D GRE (B) images show multiple endoluminal masses with enhancement consistent with hamartomatous polyps (arrows).

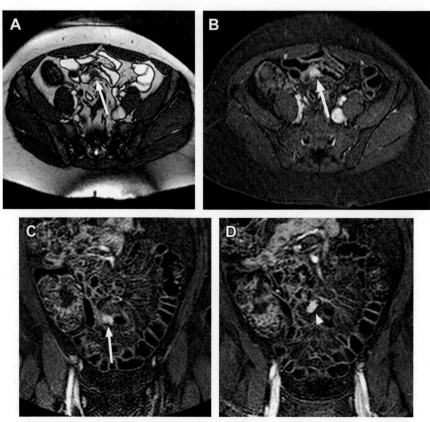

Fig. 11. A 35-year-old woman with intermittent small bowel obstruction and pain. Axial BFFE (*A*) and axial (*B*) and coronal (*C, D*) postcontrast T1w FS 3D GRE images demonstrate an intraluminal filling defect with low SI on BFFE and hyperenhancement (*arrows* in *A–C*). An associated hypervascular mesenteric lymph node (*arrowhead* in *D*) was also noted. Lesion was resected. Pathology confirmed well-differentiated NET.

the mesenteric margin of the ileum with marked enhancement. 3D postcontrast T1w FS GRE images provided the best visualization of NETs in this study. Common associated findings included mesenteric stranding, mesenteric mass with or without vascular encasement, and enhancing mesenteric lymph nodes.

Among symptomatic tumors of the small bowel, up to 70% may be malignant.[55] Some factors concerning for malignancy include mesenteric infiltration, fixed, nonpedunculated lesions, bulky or fungating masses, and concurrent enlarged mesenteric lymph nodes.[55] The most common primary malignancy of the small bowel is adenocarcinoma, accounting for up to 42% of small bowel malignancies in some case series, arising most commonly in the duodenum.[64] MR findings include a focal eccentric or circumferential mass with intraluminal or extraluminal growth pattern, heterogeneous SI on T2w images, heterogeneous moderate enhancement, and associated luminal narrowing.[54,55] Stratified enhancement, more indicative of inflammation, is typically absent in

the setting of malignancy. A prospective study of 75 patients with 37 pathologically confirmed small bowel tumors in 26 patients demonstrated a 70% per lesion sensitivity of MRE. Positive predictive value (PPV) on a per lesion basis was 93%, whereas sensitivity and PPV on a per patient basis were 96% and 93%, respectively. Injection of gadolinium-based contrast increased sensitivity compared with evaluation of noncontrast images. Of lesions in the study, 76% were located in the ileum, and most were malignant neoplasms, including carcinoid tumors, metastases, gastrointestinal stromal tumors, lymphomas, and adenocarcinomas.[65] The addition of DWI to unenhanced MRE examinations may help improve sensitivity for small bowel neoplasms, particularly for less experienced readers.[66]

Unlike adenocarcinoma, small bowel lymphoma has a predilection for the distal small bowel. Lymphoma presents with varied imaging characteristics, including long smooth or irregular continuous segment of bowel wall thickening with or without aneurysmal dilatation, polypoid endophytic lesions, and large exophytic fungating masses.[55,67,68] Lesions usually appear homogeneous and intermediate in SI on T1w images and isointense to slightly hyperintense compared with muscle on T2w images. Enhancement is typically mild to moderate in intensity. Lymphoma typically demonstrates very high SI on DWI and low SI on ADC maps. Associated mesenteric lymphadenopathy may be present.

Other Applications

Although not a common indication for MRE, atypical enteric infection (eg, from mycobacterial, fungal, or parasitic causes) may be discovered during the evaluation of a patient's nonspecific symptoms. Typically, findings are nonspecific and include wall thickening, mural hyperenhancement, and lymphadenopathy. Atypical infections commonly affect the ileocecal region. Small bowel findings include areas of focal moderate mural thickening and stricture formation, or more segmental and mild wall thickening without luminal narrowing or upstream bowel dilatation.

MRE may be able to detect other conditions with gastrointestinal manifestations, such as celiac disease and systemic sclerosis. Celiac disease causes an enteropathy due to gluten sensitivity. MRE may not demonstrate significant bowel fold abnormalities or may demonstrate loss of folds isolated to the duodenum, jejunization of the ileum, and reversal of fold pattern in the jejunum and ileum. These findings have been shown to correlate with clinical disease severity.[69] Systemic sclerosis causes dysmotility due to fibrosis of the circular smooth muscle in the wall of the GI tract.[70] The GI tract is the second most commonly involved site after the skin, although the esophagus and anorectum are more commonly involved than small bowel.[71] Small bowel findings include dilatation of the proximal bowel, particularly the duodenum and jejunum, with associated sacculations and close regular spacing of the valvulae conniventes (**Fig. 12**). Prolonged transit time may result in a pseudo-obstruction; however, this is better appreciated with real-time fluoroscopic evaluation than with MR imaging.[70,72]

Other less common indications of MRE include evaluation of bowel ischemia or vasculitis, and radiation- or chemotherapy-related bowel inflammation.[73] Finally, MRE is comparable to CE for detection of the cause of obscure gastrointestinal bleeding in the pediatric population, with overall sensitivity and specificity of 86% and 100%, respectively.[74] There are few published data on the utility of MRE for detection of obscure gastrointestinal bleeding in adults.

PEARLS AND PITFALLS

MRE can be performed on either 1.5T or 3T magnets. Higher field strength imaging at 3T has the advantage of higher signal-to-noise ratio,[75,76] which can be used to generate images with higher spatial resolution or decreased scan time. Imaging at 3T does have certain limitations, including higher energy deposition and specific absorption rate in the patient.[76] Increased B1 inhomogeneity and standing wave artifacts may further limit use of 3T for MRE particularly in obese patients or when a large amount of ascites is present.[75,76] Imaging on 1.5T magnets may also be preferred in patients whereby there is concern for hardware that is either not conditional at 3T or due to the potential for larger susceptibility artifacts at 3T.[75,76]

Patient preparation is of utmost importance for adequate MRE technique. Patients should be instructed to remain fasting for at least 6 hours before arrival to the radiology department in order to decrease likelihood of gastric and bowel filling defects, which may be mistaken for pathologic

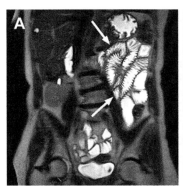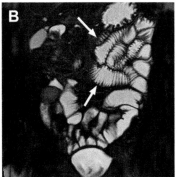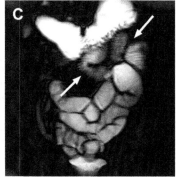

Fig. 12. A 61-year-old woman with weight loss and history of systemic sclerosis. Cor T2w SSFSE (*A*), FS T2w SSFSE (*B*), and thick slab FS T2w SSFSE cine (*C*) images demonstrate diffusely dilated bowel with thickened closely spaced folds involving the jejunum (*arrows*).

lesions. Traditional CTE techniques involve ingestion of 3 bottles of oral contrast (450 mL each bottle). In order to improve patient comfort and compliance, the authors instruct patients to drink 2 bottles of oral contrast. In lieu of the third bottle, patients drink a large cup of water immediately before scanning in order to distend the stomach and proximal small bowel. Patients are coached to drink the oral contrast at a steady pace over 45 to 60 minutes to facilitate uniform bowel distention. The authors advocate checking the examination after acquisition of the initial BFFE images to ensure adequate bowel distention to the level of the terminal ileum. In rare cases of suboptimal distention, imaging is delayed, and additional oral contrast is given. In cases of intractable nausea or vomiting, patients may not be able to tolerate the oral contrast, resulting in inadequate bowel distention, thus limiting evaluation of mild mucosal inflammation. In other cases, collapsed bowel loops may give the appearance of mucosal hyperenhancement, resulting in false positive findings. In patients with bowel obstruction, oral contrast administration is less critical because of the presence of bowel distention from the obstruction.

Timing of administration of the antiperistaltic agent is crucial. In order to adequately demonstrate bowel motility, the cine images should be acquired before onset of action of the antiperistaltic agent. If glucagon is used intramuscularly, it should be administered immediately after acquisition of the cine images, because maximum plasma concentration is attained at approximately 13 minutes.[77] If sublingual hyoscyamine sulfate is used, it may be given at the beginning of the study because of its more latent time of peak effect (30 minutes to 1 hour). Suspension of peristalsis is most helpful to decrease bowel motion artifact on the 3D T1w FS images and to minimize luminal collapse related to peristalsis. Some investigators report administering the antiperistaltic agent in 2 doses, with the second dose given intravenously immediately before the acquisition of precontrast and postcontrast 3D T1w FS images.[78]

During interpretation of MRE images, a common pitfall is the expected early and perceived higher degree of enhancement of jejunum relative to the ileum. This pattern of enhancement is a normal finding when seen affecting the jejunum uniformly and should not be interpreted as active inflammation. Collapsed bowel loops also appear to hyperenhance due to apposition of the mucosal surfaces and may be mistaken for segments with active mucosal inflammation. Conversely, subtle areas of mucosal inflammation may be difficult to perceive in the absence of bowel distention. The presence of luminal contents with the bowel that are hyperintense on precontrast T1w images can also obscure or mimic hyperenhancement of the mucosa. Subtraction images may be particularly helpful in this setting in order to provide a dark background for visualization of hyperenhancement of the bowel wall, provided images are appropriately registered. Adequate antiperistaltic effect not only decreases motion artifact but also decreases the likelihood of misregistration of bowel wall between precontrast and postcontrast images.

Another potential pitfall is the tendency to categorize areas of luminal narrowing as strictly either active inflammation or stricture. Radiologists must keep in mind that active inflammation and stricturing disease are not mutually exclusive and frequently coexist. Many small bowel strictures diagnosed with MRE have components of active inflammation and submucosal fibrosis. Although stratified enhancement is generally thought of as an indication of active disease, it can also be seen in strictures either due to mucosal apposition or due to superimposed active disease. Bowel wall SI on T2w images plays an important role in distinguishing inflammation from fibrosis in the setting of mural thickening. T2w images should be obtained before administration of GBCAs to avoid the T2-shortening effects of gadolinium that might suppress the high SI of mural edema in the presence of avid enhancement. In addition, submucosal fat can mimic edema on non-FS T2w images and fibrosis on FS T2w images, however is typically seen well as India ink artifact within the bowel wall on BFFE images (Fig. 13). An additional pitfall when evaluating bowel on T2w images pertains to intraluminal filling defects. T2w SSFSE images often demonstrate the appearance of filling defects in the center of the bowel lumen due to flow artifact. These artifacts can be correctly characterized due to lack of persistence on subsequent acquisitions or in other planes. BFFE sequences are less susceptible to flow artifact and do not confirm these filling defects within the lumen.

Finally, in cases of suspected perianal disease, additional targeted high-resolution images of the perineum are recommended, because the perianal area may not be appropriately evaluated on larger field-of-view images of the abdomen and pelvis.

REPORTING MAGNETIC RESONANCE ENTEROGRAPHY: WHAT THE CLINICIAN WANTS TO KNOW

For CD, MRE helps assess disease status and guide further management. In patients with acute symptoms, the authors recommend reporting the

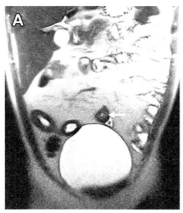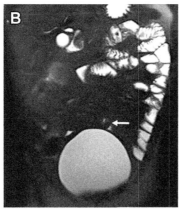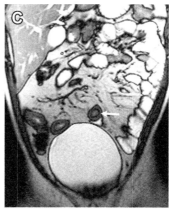

Fig. 13. A 34-year-old man with history of CD. Small bowel loops in the central and lower abdomen demonstrate predominant low SI with subtle areas of slightly higher SI in the submucosa on Cor T2 SSFSE image (*arrow* in *A*). On Cor T2 FS SSFSE image, the wall is diffusely hypointense and fibrosis cannot be differentiated from submucosal fat (*arrow* in *B*). Cor BFFE image demonstrates India ink artifact in the wall consistent with submucosal fat deposition (*arrow* in *C*).

Table 2
Key elements of magnetic resonance enterography reporting template for Crohn disease

History	Provide Patient History	
Technique	Report type and volume of oral and IV contrast; other medications and dose; sequences performed	
Comparison	Date of comparison study if available	
Findings (intestinal)	Disease location	Stomach
		Small bowel (duodenum, jejunum, ileum)
		Colon
	Enhancement pattern	Stratified vs homogeneous
	Bowel wall thickening	Site, location, length of involved segment(s)
	Stricture/luminal narrowing	Luminal narrowing without or with upstream bowel dilatation
		Fixed stricture vs inflammatory narrowing
		Stricture with concomitant active inflammation
	Penetrating disease	Sinus tract vs fistula
		Relationship to stricture
	Mesenteric findings	Stranding
		Vasa recta engorgement
		Fluid collections: location, drainable vs not
		Fibrofatty proliferation
		Lymphadenopathy
	Bowel masses	Endophytic vs exophytic
Findings (extraintestinal)	Describe extraintestinal findings	
Impression	Active inflammatory small bowel Crohn disease (SBCD)	With or without luminal narrowing
	Mixed stenotic and active inflammatory SBCD	
	Penetrating CD (add to either active inflammatory or mixed disease)	
	Quiescent or inactive SBCD	
	Fibrostenotic SBCD	

Adapted from Baker ME, Hara AK, Platt JF, et al. CT enterography for Crohn's disease: optimal technique and imaging issues. Abdom Imaging 2015;40(5):949; with permission.

presence and location of active inflammation along with the length of bowel segments involved. Skip lesions should be documented. Also important for management are the presence and location of strictures, the presence or absence of active inflammation within each strictured segment of bowel, and the presence or absence of upstream dilatation. Fistulae or sinus tracts and their relationship to strictures should be noted, because penetrating disease upstream to a stricture tends to be refractory to medical therapy as long as the stricture remains. Complications such as bowel obstruction and abscesses also have significant management implications and are important to report. Bowel obstruction often requires surgical evaluation, particularly if the obstruction is severe and little active inflammation is present. Patients with abscess might not qualify for certain medical therapies but might benefit from percutaneous drainage.

The Society of Abdominal Radiology (SAR) disease focus panel on CD has proposed a template for reporting findings in patients with CD.[79] Use of structured reporting templates allows for more uniform and standardized interpretation and has been shown to increase documentation of findings such as strictures, fistulas, fluid collections, and perianal disease.[80] Key elements from the reporting template proposed by the SAR are shown in **Table 2**.

SUMMARY

MRE is an effective noninvasive tool for imaging evaluation of CD as well as other conditions of the small bowel. Imaging findings of CD on MRE correlate with disease status, and MRE assists in guiding management and monitoring treatment response. MRE offers patients the opportunity to remain on extended periods of imaging surveillance without the risks of ionizing radiation. A typical MRE protocol includes biphasic enteric contrast for adequate bowel distention, antiperistaltic agents, use of cine sequences, and intravenous administration of gadolinium-based contrast. Use of structured reports can standardize interpretation and provide value to the referring physicians.

REFERENCES

1. Lee SS, Kim AY, Yang SK, et al. Crohn disease of the small bowel: comparison of CT enterography, MR enterography, and small-bowel follow-through as diagnostic techniques. Radiology 2009;251(3):751–61.
2. Fiorino G, Bonifacio C, Peyrin-Biroulet L, et al. Prospective comparison of computed tomography enterography and magnetic resonance enterography for assessment of disease activity and complications in ileocolonic Crohn's disease. Inflamm Bowel Dis 2011;17(5):1073–80.
3. Liu W, Liu J, Xiao W, et al. A diagnostic accuracy meta-analysis of CT and MRI for the evaluation of small bowel Crohn disease. Acad Radiol 2017;24(10):1216–25.
4. Hiraishi K, Narabayashi I, Fujita O, et al. Blueberry juice: preliminary evaluation as an oral contrast agent in gastrointestinal MR imaging. Radiology 1995;194(1):119–23.
5. Laghi A, Paolantonio P, Iafrate F, et al. Oral contrast agents for magnetic resonance imaging of the bowel. Top Magn Reson Imaging 2002;13(6):389–96.
6. Masselli G, Gualdi G. MR imaging of the small bowel. Radiology 2012;264(2):333–48.
7. Young BM, Fletcher JG, Booya F, et al. Head-to-head comparison of oral contrast agents for cross-sectional enterography: small bowel distention, timing, and side effects. J Comput Assist Tomogr 2008;32(1):32–8.
8. Gupta MK, Khatri G, Bailey A, et al. Endoluminal contrast for abdomen and pelvis magnetic resonance imaging. Abdom Radiol (NY) 2016;41(7):1378–98.
9. Administration USFD. Glucagon for injection prescribing information. 2015. Available at: https://www.accessdata.fda.gov/drugsatfda_docs/label/2015/201849s002lbl.pdf. Accessed November 10, 2017.
10. Grand DJ, Beland MD, Machan JT, et al. Detection of Crohn's disease: comparison of CT and MR enterography without anti-peristaltic agents performed on the same day. Eur J Radiol 2012;81(8):1735–41.
11. Grand DJ, Kampalath V, Harris A, et al. MR enterography correlates highly with colonoscopy and histology for both distal ileal and colonic Crohn's disease in 310 patients. Eur J Radiol 2012;81(5):e763–9.
12. Grand DJ, Guglielmo FF, Al-Hawary MM. MR enterography in Crohn's disease: current consensus on optimal imaging technique and future advances from the SAR Crohn's disease-focused panel. Abdom Imaging 2015;40(5):953–64.
13. Stanescu-Siegmund N, Nimsch Y, Wunderlich AP, et al. Quantification of inflammatory activity in patients with Crohn's disease using diffusion weighted imaging (DWI) in MR enteroclysis and MR enterography. Acta Radiol 2017;58(3):264–71.
14. Oto A, Kayhan A, Williams JT, et al. Active Crohn's disease in the small bowel: evaluation by diffusion weighted imaging and quantitative dynamic contrast enhanced MR imaging. J Magn Reson Imaging 2011;33(3):615–24.
15. Oto A, Zhu F, Kulkarni K, et al. Evaluation of diffusion-weighted MR imaging for detection of

bowel inflammation in patients with Crohn's disease. Acad Radiol 2009;16(5):597–603.

16. Oussalah A, Laurent V, Bruot O, et al. Diffusion-weighted magnetic resonance without bowel preparation for detecting colonic inflammation in inflammatory bowel disease. Gut 2010;59(8):1056–65.

17. Hordonneau C, Buisson A, Scanzi J, et al. Diffusion-weighted magnetic resonance Imaging in ileocolonic Crohn's disease: validation of quantitative index of activity. Am J Gastroenterol 2014;109(1):89–98.

18. Pupillo VA, Di Cesare E, Frieri G, et al. Assessment of inflammatory activity in Crohn's disease by means of dynamic contrast-enhanced MRI. Radiol Med 2007;112(6):798–809.

19. Ziech ML, Lavini C, Caan MW, et al. Dynamic contrast-enhanced MRI in patients with luminal Crohn's disease. Eur J Radiol 2012;81(11):3019–27.

20. Taylor SA, Punwani S, Rodriguez-Justo M, et al. Mural Crohn disease: correlation of dynamic contrast-enhanced MR imaging findings with angiogenesis and inflammation at histologic examination–pilot study. Radiology 2009;251(2):369–79.

21. Pazahr S, Blume I, Frei P, et al. Magnetization transfer for the assessment of bowel fibrosis in patients with Crohn's disease: initial experience. MAGMA 2013;26(3):291–301.

22. Harvey RF, Bradshaw JM. A simple index of Crohn's-disease activity. Lancet 1980;1(8167):514.

23. Best WR, Becktel JM, Singleton JW, et al. Development of a Crohn's disease activity index. National Cooperative Crohn's Disease Study. Gastroenterology 1976;70(3):439–44.

24. Gomes P, du Boulay C, Smith CL, et al. Relationship between disease activity indices and colonoscopic findings in patients with colonic inflammatory bowel disease. Gut 1986;27(1):92–5.

25. Jorgensen LG, Fredholm L, Hyltoft Petersen P, et al. How accurate are clinical activity indices for scoring of disease activity in inflammatory bowel disease (IBD)? Clin Chem Lab Med 2005;43(4):403–11.

26. Baars JE, Nuij VJ, Oldenburg B, et al. Majority of patients with inflammatory bowel disease in clinical remission have mucosal inflammation. Inflamm Bowel Dis 2012;18(9):1634–40.

27. Lichtenstein GR, Hanauer SB, Sandborn WJ. Management of Crohn's disease in adults. Am J Gastroenterol 2009;104(2):465–83 [quiz: 464, 484].

28. Rimola J, Ordas I, Rodriguez S, et al. Imaging indexes of activity and severity for Crohn's disease: current status and future trends. Abdom Imaging 2012;37(6):958–66.

29. Rimola J, Rodriguez S, Garcia-Bosch O, et al. Magnetic resonance for assessment of disease activity and severity in ileocolonic Crohn's disease. Gut 2009;58(8):1113–20.

30. Rimola J, Ordas I, Rodriguez S, et al. Magnetic resonance imaging for evaluation of Crohn's disease: validation of parameters of severity and quantitative index of activity. Inflamm Bowel Dis 2011;17(8):1759–68.

31. Ordas I, Rimola J, Rodriguez S, et al. Accuracy of magnetic resonance enterography in assessing response to therapy and mucosal healing in patients with Crohn's disease. Gastroenterology 2014;146(2): 374–82.e1.

32. Fiorino G, Morin M, Bonovas S, et al. Prevalence of bowel damage assessed by cross-sectional imaging in early Crohn's disease and its impact on disease outcome. J Crohns Colitis 2017;11(3):274–80.

33. Buisson A, Joubert A, Montoriol PF, et al. Diffusion-weighted magnetic resonance imaging for detecting and assessing ileal inflammation in Crohn's disease. Aliment Pharmacol Ther 2013;37(5):537–45.

34. Steward MJ, Punwani S, Proctor I, et al. Non-perforating small bowel Crohn's disease assessed by MRI enterography: derivation and histopathological validation of an MR-based activity index. Eur J Radiol 2012;81(9):2080–8.

35. Rimola J, Alvarez-Cofino A, Perez-Jeldres T, et al. Comparison of three magnetic resonance enterography indices for grading activity in Crohn's disease. J Gastroenterol 2017;52(5):585–93.

36. Sempere GA, Martinez Sanjuan V, Medina Chulia E, et al. MRI evaluation of inflammatory activity in Crohn's disease. AJR Am J Roentgenol 2005; 184(6):1829–35.

37. Florie J, Wasser MN, Arts-Cieslik K, et al. Dynamic contrast-enhanced MRI of the bowel wall for assessment of disease activity in Crohn's disease. AJR Am J Roentgenol 2006;186(5):1384–92.

38. Del Vescovo R, Sansoni I, Caviglia R, et al. Dynamic contrast enhanced magnetic resonance imaging of the terminal ileum: differentiation of activity of Crohn's disease. Abdom Imaging 2008;33(4):417–24.

39. Punwani S, Rodriguez-Justo M, Bainbridge A, et al. Mural inflammation in Crohn disease: location-matched histologic validation of MR imaging features. Radiology 2009;252(3):712–20.

40. Sinha R, Murphy P, Sanders S, et al. Diagnostic accuracy of high-resolution MR enterography in Crohn's disease: comparison with surgical and pathological specimen. Clin Radiol 2013;68(9):917–27.

41. Sinha R, Rajiah P, Murphy P, et al. Utility of high-resolution MR imaging in demonstrating transmural pathologic changes in Crohn disease. Radiographics 2009;29(6):1847–67.

42. Maccioni F, Bruni A, Viscido A, et al. MR imaging in patients with Crohn disease: value of T2- versus T1-weighted gadolinium-enhanced MR sequences with use of an oral superparamagnetic contrast agent. Radiology 2006;238(2):517–30.

43. Meyers MA, McGuire PV. Spiral CT demonstration of hypervascularity in Crohn disease: "vascular jejunization of the ileum" or the "comb sign". Abdom Imaging 1995;20(4):327–32.

44. Malago R, Manfredi R, Benini L, et al. Assessment of Crohn's disease activity in the small bowel with MR-enteroclysis: clinico-radiological correlations. Abdom Imaging 2008;33(6):669–75.

45. Gourtsoyianni S, Papanikolaou N, Amanakis E, et al. Crohn's disease lymphadenopathy: MR imaging findings. Eur J Radiol 2009;69(3):425–8.

46. Pozza A, Scarpa M, Lacognata C, et al. Magnetic resonance enterography for Crohn's disease: what the surgeon can take home. J Gastrointest Surg 2011;15(10):1689–98.

47. Oberhuber G, Stangl PC, Vogelsang H, et al. Significant association of strictures and internal fistula formation in Crohn's disease. Virchows Arch 2000; 437(3):293–7.

48. Kelly JK, Preshaw RM. Origin of fistulas in Crohn's disease. J Clin Gastroenterol 1989;11(2):193–6.

49. Rieber A, Aschoff A, Nussle K, et al. MRI in the diagnosis of small bowel disease: use of positive and negative oral contrast media in combination with enteroclysis. Eur Radiol 2000;10(9):1377–82.

50. Herrmann KA, Michaely HJ, Zech CJ, et al. Internal fistulas in Crohn disease: magnetic resonance enteroclysis. Abdom Imaging 2006;31(6):675–87.

51. Oto A, Schmid-Tannwald C, Agrawal G, et al. Diffusion-weighted MR imaging of abdominopelvic abscesses. Emerg Radiol 2011;18(6):515–24.

52. Beaugerie L, Itzkowitz SH. Cancers complicating inflammatory bowel disease. N Engl J Med 2015; 372(15):1441–52.

53. Chang M, Chang L, Chang HM, et al. Intestinal and extraintestinal cancers associated with inflammatory bowel disease. Clin Colorectal Cancer 2018;17(1): e29–37.

54. Semelka RC, John G, Kelekis NL, et al. Small bowel neoplastic disease: demonstration by MRI. J Magn Reson Imaging 1996;6(6):855–60.

55. Masselli G, Gualdi G. Evaluation of small bowel tumors: MR enteroclysis. Abdom Imaging 2010; 35(1):23–30.

56. Hearle N, Schumacher V, Menko FH, et al. Frequency and spectrum of cancers in the Peutz-Jeghers syndrome. Clin Cancer Res 2006;12(10): 3209–15.

57. Syngal S, Brand RE, Church JM, et al. ACG clinical guideline: genetic testing and management of hereditary gastrointestinal cancer syndromes. Am J Gastroenterol 2015;110(2):223–62 [quiz: 263].

58. Caspari R, von Falkenhausen M, Krautmacher C, et al. Comparison of capsule endoscopy and magnetic resonance imaging for the detection of polyps of the small intestine in patients with familial adenomatous polyposis or with Peutz-Jeghers' syndrome. Endoscopy 2004;36(12):1054–9.

59. Maccioni F, Al Ansari N, Mazzamurro F, et al. Surveillance of patients affected by Peutz-Jeghers syndrome: diagnostic value of MR enterography in prone and supine position. Abdom Imaging 2012; 37(2):279–87.

60. Gupta A, Postgate AJ, Burling D, et al. A prospective study of MR enterography versus capsule endoscopy for the surveillance of adult patients with Peutz-Jeghers syndrome. AJR Am J Roentgenol 2010;195(1):108–16.

61. Yao JC, Hassan M, Phan A, et al. One hundred years after "carcinoid": epidemiology of and prognostic factors for neuroendocrine tumors in 35,825 cases in the United States. J Clin Oncol 2008;26(18):3063–72.

62. Ganeshan D, Bhosale P, Yang T, et al. Imaging features of carcinoid tumors of the gastrointestinal tract. AJR Am J Roentgenol 2013;201(4):773–86.

63. Dohan A, El Fattach H, Barat M, et al. Neuroendocrine tumors of the small bowel: evaluation with MR-enterography. Clin Imaging 2016;40(3): 541–7.

64. Neugut AI, Jacobson JS, Suh S, et al. The epidemiology of cancer of the small bowel. Cancer Epidemiol Biomarkers Prev 1998;7(3):243–51.

65. Amzallag-Bellenger E, Soyer P, Barbe C, et al. Prospective evaluation of magnetic resonance enterography for the detection of mesenteric small bowel tumours. Eur Radiol 2013;23(7):1901–10.

66. Amzallag-Bellenger E, Soyer P, Barbe C, et al. Diffusion-weighted imaging for the detection of mesenteric small bowel tumours with magnetic resonance–enterography. Eur Radiol 2014;24(11): 2916–26.

67. Lohan DG, Alhajeri AN, Cronin CG, et al. MR enterography of small-bowel lymphoma: potential for suggestion of histologic subtype and the presence of underlying celiac disease. AJR Am J Roentgenol 2008;190(2):287–93.

68. Chou CK, Chen LT, Sheu RS, et al. MRI manifestations of gastrointestinal lymphoma. Abdom Imaging 1994;19(6):495–500.

69. Tomei E, Diacinti D, Stagnitti A, et al. MR enterography: relationship between intestinal fold pattern and the clinical presentation of adult celiac disease. J Magn Reson Imaging 2012;36(1):183–7.

70. Rohrmann CA Jr, Ricci MT, Krishnamurthy S, et al. Radiologic and histologic differentiation of neuromuscular disorders of the gastrointestinal tract: visceral myopathies, visceral neuropathies, and progressive systemic sclerosis. AJR Am J Roentgenol 1984;143(5):933–41.

71. Sjogren RW. Gastrointestinal motility disorders in scleroderma. Arthritis Rheum 1994;37(9):1265–82.

72. Madani G, Katz RD, Haddock JA, et al. The role of radiology in the management of systemic sclerosis. Clin Radiol 2008;63(9):959–67.

73. Amzallag-Bellenger E, Oudjit A, Ruiz A, et al. Effectiveness of MR enterography for the assessment of small-bowel diseases beyond Crohn disease. Radiographics 2012;32(5):1423–44.

74. Casciani E, Nardo GD, Chin S, et al. MR enterography in paediatric patients with obscure gastrointestinal bleeding. Eur J Radiol 2017;93:209–16.

75. Merkle EM, Dale BM. Abdominal MRI at 3.0 T: the basics revisited. Am J Roentgenol 2006;186(6): 1524–32.

76. Barth MM, Smith MP, Pedrosa I, et al. Body MR imaging at 3.0 T: understanding the opportunities and challenges. Radiographics 2007;27(5):1445–62 [discussion: 1462–4].

77. Eli Lilly and Company. Information for the physician. Glucagon for injection. 2012.

78. Fidler JL, Guimaraes L, Einstein DM. MR imaging of the small bowel. Radiographics 2009;29(6): 1811–25.

79. Baker ME, Hara AK, Platt JF, et al. CT enterography for Crohn's disease: optimal technique and imaging issues. Abdom Imaging 2015;40(5):938–52.

80. Wildman-Tobriner B, Allen BC, Davis JT, et al. Structured reporting of magnetic resonance enterography for pediatric Crohn's disease: effect on key feature reporting and subjective assessment of disease by referring physicians. Curr Probl Diagn Radiol 2017;46(2):110–4.

Interdisciplinary Updates in Crohn's Disease Reporting Nomenclature, and Cross-Sectional Disease Monitoring

Mark E. Baker, MD[a],*, Joel G. Fletcher, MD[b],
Mahmoud Al-Hawary, MD[c], David Bruining, MD[d]

KEYWORDS

• Crohn's disease • Reporting nomenclature • Imaging-based morphologic phenotypes

KEY POINTS

• There is now interdisciplinary consensus on terms and nomenclature used for effective communication in describing small bowel Crohn's disease at computed tomography and magnetic resonance enterography.
• An imaging-based morphologic construct that focuses on the role of enteric inflammation can be used to describe active inflammatory Crohn's disease and its stricturing and penetrating complications.
• Active inflammatory Crohn's disease can be diagnosed when imaging findings of inflammation are asymmetric and preferentially involve the mesenteric border, or when mural hyperenhancement and wall thickening are present in a patient with known Crohn's disease.
• Disease monitoring with computed tomography and magnetic resonance enterography can define response to treatment, which predicts long-term outcomes.

Over the last decade, computed tomography enterography (CTE) and magnetic resonance enterography (MRE) have become essential methods of guiding the clinical management of patients with Crohn's disease.[1–6] Multiple investigations have shown that biologic inflammatory activity in Crohn's disease is unrelated to patient signs and symptoms, and penetrating and stricturing complications can be present in asymptomatic patients.[7,8] Cross-sectional enterography is important at the time of diagnosis and in monitoring patients with small bowel inflammation, because up to 50% of patients with small bowel Crohn's disease will have active small bowel inflammation on CTE or MRE, despite a negative endoscopy.[4,9,10]

Disclosure Statement: M.E. Baker has a grant from Siemens Healthineers in the form of salary support, hardware, and software for investigating computed tomography exposure reduction; J.G. Fletcher has a grant from Siemens Healthineers and consults with Medtronic; M. Al-Hawary has no disclosures; D. Bruining has no disclosures.

[a] Abdominal Imaging Section, Imaging Institute, Cleveland Clinic, 9500 Euclid Avenue - L10, Cleveland, OH 44195, USA; [b] Department of Radiology, Mayo Clinic, 200 First Street Southwest, Rochester, MN 55905, USA; [c] Department of Radiology, Michigan Medicine, University of Michigan, 1500 East Medical Center Drive, Ann Arbor, MI 489109, USA; [d] Division of Gastroenterology and Hepatology, Department of Internal Medicine, Mayo Clinic, 200 First Street Southwest, Rochester, MN 55905, USA
* Corresponding author.
E-mail address: bakerm@ccf.org

Members of the Society of Abdominal Radiology Crohn's Disease-focused Panel have met yearly with gastroenterologists from the American Gastroenterological Association to discuss common issues.[11,12] Based on what has been observed with both CTE and MRE, it was apparent that distinct, imaging-based morphologic phenotypes seen in clinical practice are incompletely described using the Montreal and Paris classifications,[13,14] and that there are also distinct dynamic transitions between phenotypes, largely driven by progression and remission of enteric inflammation.

Over the years, the nomenclature used to describe these phenotypes has evolved with input from members of the group as well as adult and pediatric gastroenterologists and colorectal surgeons. The Society of Abdominal Radiology, the American Gastroenterological Association Institute Governing Council, and the Society for Pediatric Radiology Board have now approved the terms, in addition to recommendations for the use of CTE and MRE.[15] The purpose of this work is to review these consensus recommendations, terms, and interpretation of specific imaging findings at CTE and MRE in small bowel Crohn's disease, along with recommendations for reporting to maximize clinical benefit to the patient and referring gastroenterologist, and how to conceptualize implications for patient care in disease monitoring paradigms.

LIMITATIONS OF CURRENT CLASSIFICATION SYSTEMS

For years, physicians caring for patients with Crohn's disease have used a phenotypic classification that parses the disease state into discreet groups. These are (1) nonstricturing, nonpenetrating disease (active inflammatory), (2) stricturing disease, and (3) penetrating disease, with perianal disease added to any of these 3 phenotypes.[13,14] These classifications fail to recognize that Crohn's disease is dynamic and can wax and wane, but is often progressive. Second, strictures in Crohn's patients commonly have both radiographic and pathologic findings of active inflammation.[16,17] Third, penetrating disease is almost always associated with strictures with active inflammation.[18–21] In any particular patient, each of these processes may coexist in different anatomic locations and change over time.

Baker and associates[11] proposed that imaging portrayed distinct patterns of transition between morphologic phenotypes that paralleled observations in the pathologic literature. Imaging-based phenotypes (and the transitions between them), emphasize the coexisting and preeminent role of enteric inflammation in gut destruction and enteric

complications, and are linked to specific anatomic locations. For example, in many cases, there is a progression from wall thickening with active inflammation, to luminal narrowing, to stricture formation, and eventual development of penetrating disease. Analogous patterns proceeding in the opposite direction of this pathway are seen as inflammation moves toward transmural healing with appropriate medical therapy. A standardized method of interpreting the meaning of imaging findings coupled with the use of these imaging-based phenotypes will assist in describing Crohn's disease burden and response to medical or surgical therapy.

STANDARD NOMENCLATURE FOR DESCRIBING THE IMAGING FINDINGS OF CROHN'S DISEASE

The following describes the agreed upon terms that should be used to describe the imaging findings of Crohn's disease, the patterns of enteric involvement, as well as the morphologic phenotypes, based on the recommendations of this interdisciplinary group.

MURAL FINDINGS OF ACTIVE INFLAMMATION

Mural findings of active inflammation can be separated into segmental mural hyperenhancement, wall thickening, intramural edema, stricture formation, ulceration, sacculations, and diminished motility[22–28] (Box 1). Most investigations have shown that mural hyperenhancement is a good indicator of active inflammation.[29,30] In Crohn's disease, segmental hyperenhancement is generally patchy or asymmetric. Although different patterns of bowel wall enhancement are observed (eg, stratified or homogeneous), no meaning should be inferred from the enhancement pattern in the enteric or portal phase of enhancement. In contradistinction, a recent investigation suggested that delayed homogeneous enhancement is related to the degree of fibrosis.[31] The use of the term mucosal hyperenhancement should not be used, because the mucosa is often totally absent in regions of severe inflammation.

Wall thickening in Crohn's disease can be seen even in cases without active inflammation.[22,23] Early in the disease, wall thickening is often asymmetric, affecting the mesenteric border preferentially. With disease progression, thickening often becomes symmetric. Wall thickening can be mild (3–5 mm) or moderate (>5–9 mm). Whenever the wall is greater than 9 mm, one should consider a complicating carcinoma or neuroendocrine tumor, especially when there is a poorly marginated,

Box 1
Terms for imaging findings of active inflammation that should be used as descriptors in the body of the report

Segmental mural hyperenhancement

   Asymmetric

   Stratified (bilaminar or trilaminar)

   Homogeneous, symmetric

Wall thickening

   Mild (3–5 mm)

   Moderate (5–9 mm)

   Severe (≥10 mm)

Intramural edema

Stricture

   Without upstream bowel dilation

   With mild upstream bowel dilation (3–4 cm)

   With moderate to severe upstream bowel dilation (>4 cm)

Ulcerations

   Sacculations

   Diminished motility

Data from Bruining DH, Zimmermann EM, Loftus EV, et al. Consensus recommendations for evaluation, interpretation, and utilization of computed tomography and magnetic resonance enterography in patients with small bowel crohn's disease. Radiology 2018;286(3):778–9; and Bruining DH, Zimmermann EM, Loftus EV, et al. Consensus recommendations for evaluation, interpretation, and utilization of computed tomography and magnetic resonance enterography in patients with small bowel crohn's disease. Gastroenterology 2018;154(4):1173–5.

annular or nodular mass, or there is perforation.[32] Unfortunately, both the sensitivity and specificity of imaging in distinguishing an unusual stricture from a tumor are low.

Asymmetric wall changes of active inflammation (enhancement, wall thickening, edema, and ulceration) are considered pathognomonic of Crohn's disease. Asymmetry implies more than skip lesions or patchy involvement in the luminal direction. It means asymmetric mesenteric inflammation greater than the antimesenteric involvement, especially early in the disease. Thus, the emerging interdisciplinary consensus is that asymmetric bowel inflammation is diagnostic for small bowel Crohn's disease, even in the absence of clinical, endoscopic, or pathologic confirmation. Symmetric involvement is nonspecific, requiring imaging findings be correlated with clinical and endoscopic findings, because other possibilities exist, particularly in

patients without known Crohn's disease. In patients with known Crohn's disease, mural enhancement and wall thickening alone are sufficient to diagnose active inflammation, even when symmetric.

Ulcerations are focal extensions of gas or fluid into the thickened bowel wall, and are a marker of severe active inflammation. Sinus tracts generally extend outside the wall into the mesenteric fat, but can rarely run parallel to the bowel lumen.

Sacculations occur along the antimesenteric border and are secondary to preserved or relatively spared portions of small bowel, although the areas that are retracted toward the mesentery are involved with Crohn's inflammation, muscular hypertrophy, or fibrosis. The inflamed mesenteric border will be thickened and hyperenhancing, or may contain ulcers or intramural edema.

Intramural edema is present in moderate and severe active inflammation and is most accurately assessed with fat-saturated, T2-weighted MR imaging. On non–fat-saturated T2-weighted pulse sequences, it is difficult to distinguish intramural fat from edema. CT cannot reliably identify intramural edema, as because -attenuation wall changes can occur with variable amounts of fat deposition. In cases where intravenous contrast cannot be administered at MRE, intramural edema as demonstrated on T2-weighted images with fat saturation can be used as diagnostic of active inflammation. The additional presence of restricted diffusion adds confirmation of this conclusion.[33,34] Restricted diffusion itself is a nonspecific finding for enteric inflammation. However, when other pulse sequences demonstrate diagnostic findings of active inflammatory Crohn's disease, restricted diffusion correlates with the presence of endoscopic ulcerations.[33] When intramural edema and restricted diffusion are present, moderate or severe enteric inflammation is likely, and this should be explained in the body of the radiologic report.

Diminished motility can only be assessed with dynamic MR techniques that create multiple, rapidly acquired images that can be viewed as a cine-loop (ie, MR fluoroscopy). MR fluoroscopy is useful in evaluating bowel segments that are collapsed, and normal motility on fluoroscopic images should reassure the radiologist that inflammation is not present.[35–38]

When there is wall thickening, there is almost always some degree of luminal narrowing. As luminal narrowing progresses, upstream dilation will eventually develop, at which point a stricture can be diagnosed with a high degree of certainty. When a stricture is present, one should determine the degree of upstream dilation and the presence or absence of imaging signs of inflammation. Thus, strictures can be classified as a stricture with findings of active inflammation or a stricture without findings of active inflammation. When a stricture is present, stricture length and the degree of proximal small bowel dilation should be reported. Stricture formation is the subject of much ongoing investigation.[18,21,31,39-44] Ultimately, one of the major contributions that imaging may make is determining the potential reversibility of strictures using biologic agents.

There are several instances in which upstream dilation will not be associated with a stricture. First, if there is no upstream dilation, and luminal narrowing is present on multiple pulse sequences or serial imaging studies, it is appropriate to mention that a probable stricture is present: the degree of upstream dilation depends on many factors, including the degree of luminal narrowing, wall compliance, and preexisting and ingested fluid and food. Second, multiple upstream strictures limit the degree to which downstream strictures manifest proximal bowel dilation, because they limit the distal delivery of enteric contents. Third, when penetrating disease is present, especially with complex fistulae, upstream dilation to the stricture may be absent, because the proximal flow has been decompressed through the fistula.

EXTRAMURAL FINDINGS: PENETRATING DISEASE AND MESENTERIC INFLAMMATION

Penetrating disease is present when there is a sinus tract, a simple or complex fistula, abscess formation, or free, intraperitoneal perforation[45] (Box 2). A sinus tract is a wall defect that extends outside the entire small bowel wall and into the surrounding mesenteric fat or abscess, but not into other adjacent structures. Simple fistulae appear as a soft tissue linear tract extending from an inflamed bowel loop to another bowel loop or adjacent structures such as skin, psoas muscle, or urinary bladder. On MR imaging, the tract may or may not contain fluid on T2-weighted sequences. Complex fistulae are visualized as multiple linear tracts that extend to multiple adjacent structures, often with an asterisk, cloverleaf, or star shape. Involved bowel loops are angulated and seem to be fixed, tethered, or nonmobile (terms used in fluoroscopy can be applied to CTE/MRE). Small, interloop collections/abscesses are often seen with complex fistulas. Inflammatory masses are identified as poorly defined, mixed fat and soft tissue attenuation/signal, masslike structures in the mesenteric fat that arise from inflamed bowel segments.

It is important to realize that nearly all penetrating disease is associated with strictures with active inflammation.[18,21] In 1 large pathologic series,

Box 2

Terms for imaging findings of penetrating disease and mesenteric inflammation that should be used as descriptors in the body of the report

Fistulas

  Simple fistula

  Complex fistulas

  Sinus tract

  Perianal fistulas

Inflammatory mass

Abscess

Perienteric edema/inflammation

Engorged vasa recta

Fibrofatty proliferation

Mesenteric venous thrombosis and chronic mesenteric venous occlusion

Adenopathy

Data from Bruining DH, Zimmermann EM, Loftus EV, et al. Consensus recommendations for evaluation, interpretation, and utilization of computed tomography and magnetic resonance enterography in patients with small bowel crohn's disease. Radiology 2018;286(3):785–6; and Bruining DH, Zimmermann EM, Loftus EV, et al. Consensus recommendations for evaluation, interpretation, and utilization of computed tomography and magnetic resonance enterography in patients with small bowel crohn's disease. Gastroenterology 2018;154(4):1180–1.

93% of fistulas were associated with strictures, with 93% of the fistulae arising from the proximal or mid aspect of the stricture.[19] In another series, 96% of patients with fistulas had strictures, with 97% of fistulae also arising from a stricture.[20] Presence of a stricture should prompt a careful search for penetrating disease, and vice versa.

There are other findings in the mesenteric fat that should be noted. Perienteric edema is identified as increased attenuation/signal in the mesenteric fat adjacent to an affected loop of active inflammation, indicating more severe inflammation. The vessels adjacent to an inflamed loop are often engorged. We recommend that engorged vasa recta replace the use of the term comb sign. The fat adjacent to an affected loop may be increased, causing mass effect, displacing adjacent loops of small bowel. Generally, radiologists should use the term fibrofatty proliferation rather than creeping fat, which is identified by the surgeon or pathologist and much more subtle. Last, lymph nodes are commonly present in the mesentery (usually 1.0–1.5 cm in short axis, but sometimes larger with severe inflammation).

An important mesenteric finding is mesenteric venous thrombosis and occlusion. Mesenteric vein thrombosis is fortunately uncommon, even in the perioperative/postoperative state, when it is more often identified.[46] Thrombi can be peripheral or central, and can extend into the intrahepatic system. When central, they generally resolve. When peripheral, if they often do not recanalize; they appear as narrowed, truncated, or cutoff vessels with consequent serpiginous, tortuous mesenteric varices.[47] The term thrombosis should be used only in veins that are acutely occluded with thrombus. When chronic changes are present, it is best to use the term chronic mesenteric occlusion.

PERIANAL DISEASE

Perianal disease is a distinct entity from enteric penetrating Crohn's disease. Standard CTE and MRE images should include the perineum, and perianal fistulas and abscesses should be mentioned in the report. Adult MRE generally cannot include concomitant focused MR imaging perianal examination owing to machine time constraints,[48] but this factor is institution dependent.

EXTRAINTESTINAL FINDINGS RELEVANT TO CROHN'S DISEASE

Extraintestinal manifestations of Crohn's disease are visible on CTE and MRE and should be described (Box 3). These findings include sacroiliitis,

---

Box 3
Terms for extraintestinal findings relevant to Crohn's disease the presence or absence of which should be mentioned in the body of the report.

Imaging Findings

Sacroiliitis

Primary sclerosing cholangitis

Avascular necrosis

Pancreatitis

Nephrolithiasis and cholelithiasis

Cutaneous findings

Data from Bruining DH, Zimmermann EM, Loftus EV, et al. Consensus recommendations for evaluation, interpretation, and utilization of computed tomography and magnetic resonance enterography in patients with small bowel crohn's disease. Radiology 2018;286(3):790; and Bruining DH, Zimmermann EM, Loftus EV, et al. Consensus recommendations for evaluation, interpretation, and utilization of computed tomography and magnetic resonance enterography in patients with small bowel crohn's disease. Gastroenterology 2018;154(4):1185.

---

primary sclerosing cholangitis, avascular necrosis (most often of the femoral heads), pancreatitis, nephrolithiasis, and cholelithiasis.[49,50]

MORPHOLOGIC PHENOTYPES OF CROHN'S DISEASE ON ENTEROGRAPHY: RECOMMENDED IMPRESSIONS SUMMARIZING THE IMAGING FINDINGS

To synthesize these findings, the consensus panel developed the following terms that use the morphologic phenotypes of Crohn's disease originally described by Baker and colleagues.[11] These terms should be used in the impression section of the radiographic report (Box 4).

Box 4
Morphologic phenotypes as identified on computed tomography enterography/magnetic resonance enterography that should be used in the impression of the report

Inflammation

- Nonspecific small bowel inflammation
- Active inflammatory small bowel Crohn's disease
  - Without luminal narrowing
  - With luminal narrowing
- Crohn's disease with no imaging signs of active inflammation (known prior active inflammatory Crohn's disease with residual radiologic findings)
- No imaging signs of active inflammation

Stricture

- With imaging findings of active inflammation
- Without imaging findings of active inflammation
- Penetrating Crohn's disease (added in addition to determination of inflammatory Crohn's disease and stricture)
- Perianal Crohn's disease
- Other complications and important actionable information

Data from Bruining DH, Zimmermann EM, Loftus EV, et al. Consensus recommendations for evaluation, interpretation, and utilization of computed tomography and magnetic resonance enterography in patients with small bowel crohn's disease. Radiology 2018;286(3):793; and Bruining DH, Zimmermann EM, Loftus EV, et al. Consensus recommendations for evaluation, interpretation, and utilization of computed tomography and magnetic resonance enterography in patients with small bowel crohn's disease. Gastroenterology 2018;154(4):1187.

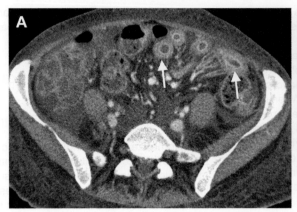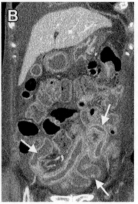

Fig. 1. Nonspecific small bowel inflammation. Axial (*A*) and coronal (*B*) images from a computed tomography enterography in a patient with gluten enteropathy and ulcerative jejunoileitis, demonstrating thick walled loops of small bowel with mural hyperenhancement (*arrows*) associated with extensive edema in the mesenteric fat and ascites. Imaging findings reflect nonspecific inflammation and not active inflammatory Crohn's disease owing to confluent and symmetric involvement of the bowel wall without luminal narrowing or mesenteric findings.

Inflammation: Nonspecific Small Bowel Inflammation

This term should be used when there is segmental, symmetric, mural thickening and hyperenhancement in a patient without known Crohn's disease (Fig. 1). The differential diagnosis of segmental mural thickening and hyperenhancement includes backwash ileitis, infectious enteritis, mucositis, graft versus host disease, radiation enteritis, nonsteroidal anti-inflammatory drug enteropathy, angioedema, vasculitis, and ischemia.

Active Inflammatory Small Bowel Crohn's Disease Without Luminal Narrowing

This term should be used when there are asymmetric wall changes, mural edema, ulcerations, perienteric stranding, engorged vasa recta, and the lumen is not narrowed (Fig. 2). It can also be used when there are

symmetric changes of active inflammation in a patient with known Crohn's disease (Fig. 3).

Active Inflammatory Small Bowel Crohn's Disease with Luminal Narrowing

This term should similarly be used when there are imaging findings of active inflammation in a patient with Crohn's disease, or when inflammation is asymmetric or concomitant penetrating or structuring complications are present, and there is concomitant upstream bowel dilation (Figs. 4 and 5).

Crohn's Disease with No Imaging Signs of Active Inflammation

This term should only be used in a patient with known Crohn's disease, with prior findings of active inflammation that are now absent on the current CTE/MRE (see Fig. 4, Fig. 6). Even with complete transmural healing, there may be patchy

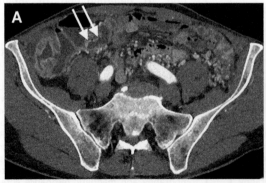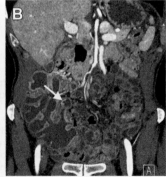

Fig. 2. Active inflammatory small bowel Crohn's disease without luminal narrowing. Axial (*A*) and coronal (*B*) computed tomography enterography images shows asymmetric, subtle stratified hyperenhancement in the terminal ileum (*arrows*) without luminal narrowing. There was endoscopic confirmation of active inflammation.

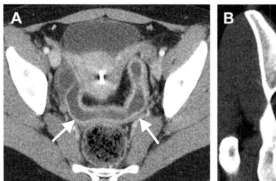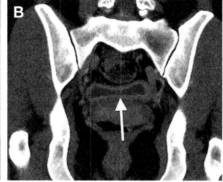

Fig. 3. Active inflammatory small bowel Crohn's disease without luminal narrowing. Axial (*A*) and coronal (*B*) computed tomography enterography images show symmetric, stratified hyperenhancement and wall thickening (*arrows*) in the distal ileum without luminal narrowing in a patient with known Crohn's disease.

residual intramural fat, residual sacculations/scarring, and mild wall thickening (3–4 mm). Using the suggested term assists the treating physician in continuing important and appropriate therapy.

Stricture with Imaging Findings of Active Inflammation

This term should be used when there is persistent luminal narrowing in a segment with findings of active inflammation, and there is upstream bowel dilation (**Figs. 7–9**). We strongly recommended

that if there is moderate to severe dilation (>4 cm) that "with small bowel obstruction" be added to this terminology. A careful search should be made for coexisting penetrating complications.

Stricture Without Imaging Findings of Active Inflammation

This term should be used when there is persistent luminal narrowing with proximal dilation, but no imaging findings of active inflammation, other than mild wall thickening (see **Fig. 7**, **Fig. 10**).

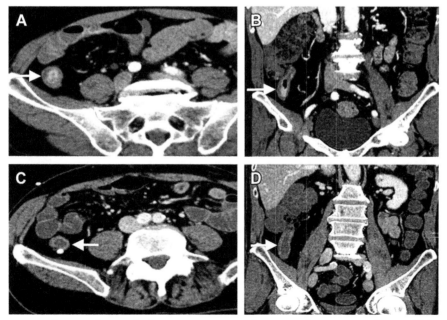

Fig. 4. Response to therapy after medical treatment computed tomography enterography. Axial (*A*) and coronal (*B*) computed tomography enterography images show active inflammatory Crohn's disease with mural hyperenhancement and wall thickening (*arrow*) in the distal ileum in a patient with newly diagnosed Crohn's disease. There was no upstream bowel dilation. After medical treatment, images from repeat computed tomography enterography (*C, D*) show normal luminal diameter and only mild wall thickening and only minimal stratified hyperenhancement. Endoscopy confirmed mucosal healing.

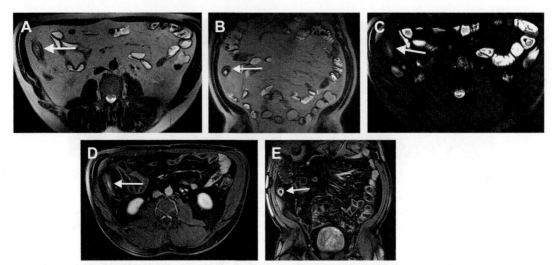

Fig. 5. Active inflammatory small bowel Crohn's disease with luminal narrowing magnetic resonance enterography. Axial (*A*) and coronal (*B*) half-Fourier acquisition single-shot turbo spin-echo (HASTE) images show wall thickening, luminal narrowing and increased mural T2 signal in distal ileum (*arrow*), demonstrated to be intramural edema on fat saturated axial HASTE image (*C, arrow*). Axial (*D*) and coronal (*E*) postcontrast images show wall thickening and stratified mural hyperenhancement (*arrow*).

Penetrating Crohn's Disease

Virtually all penetrating disease is associated with stricture formation with imaging findings of active inflammation (**Fig. 11**). It is very important to remember that, with complex fistulae, there may not be upstream bowel dilation (**Figs. 12** and **13**), and it is appropriate to indicate that a stricture with inflammation is likely present.

No Imaging Signs of Active Inflammation

This term should be used when the study is normal (**Fig. 14**). If prior CTE or MRE demonstrated active inflammatory Crohn's disease, then transmural healing has occurred without residual sequela.

Perianal Crohn's Disease

Radiologists should always image and comment on the appearance of the anus and any associated

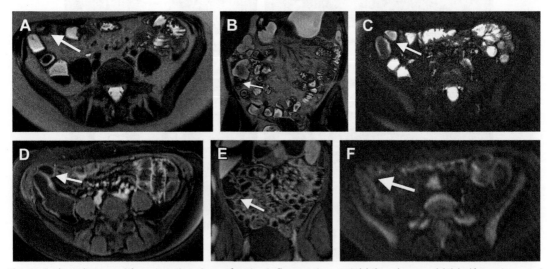

Fig. 6. Crohn's disease with no imaging signs of active inflammation. Axial (*A*) and coronal (*B*) half-Fourier acquisition single-shot turbo spin-echo (HASTE) image in a Crohn's patient show wall thickening (*arrow*) in the terminal ileum without increased intramural T2 signal (*arrow*), which is confirmed on the axial (*C*) fat-saturated HASTE image, indicating the absence of intramural edema. Axial (*D*) and coronal (*E*) postcontrast images show no mural hyperenhancement in the neoterminal ileum (*arrow*). (*F*) Diffusion-weighted image shows no restricted diffusion in the wall (*arrow*). Findings likely represent luminal collapse and do not represent inflammation.

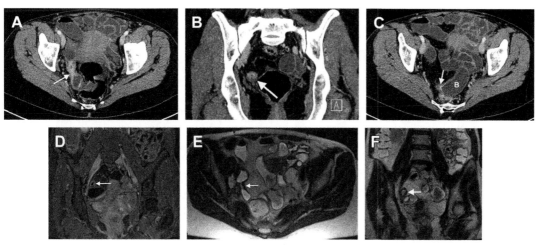

Fig. 7. Stricture with imaging findings of active inflammation evolving to stricture without imaging findings of active inflammation. Initial axial (*A*) and coronal (*B*) computed tomography enterography images show mural hyperenhancement and thickening, with luminal narrowing (*arrow*) and upstream small bowel dilation (*C*; *B* = upstream bowel dilation) (*A–C*). After medical therapy, only mild wall thickening and upstream dilation remains, with no mural hyperenhancement (*arrow*) (*D*) or intramural edema (*arrow*) (*E*, axial image; *F*, coronal image), indicating a stricture without imaging findings of active inflammation.

perianal disease in as much detail as possible (**Fig. 15**).

Other Complications

Box 3 lists extraenteric complications that should be noted in the impression (see **Figs. 11** and **12**,

Fig. 16). If a complicating small bowel tumor is suspected, this finding should be highlighted.

CROHN'S DISEASE REPORTING TEMPLATE

Most sites with an active inflammatory bowel disease group using CTE and/or MRE have found that

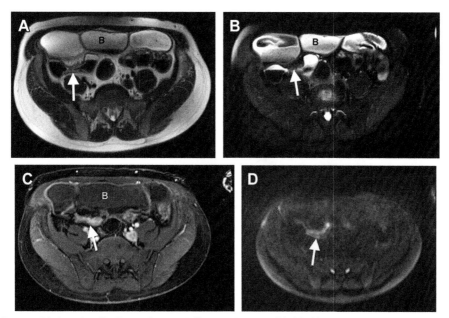

Fig. 8. Stricture with imaging findings of active inflammation. Axial (*A*) half-Fourier acquisition single-shot turbo spin-echo (HASTE) image shows increased mural T2 signal (*arrow*), confirmed on axial (*B*) fat-saturated HASTE image to represent intramural edema (*arrow*). There is luminal narrowing and a small bowel obstruction (*B*). (*C*) Axial postcontrast image shows wall thickening and mural stratified hyperenhancement (*arrow*). (*D*) Axial diffusion-weighted image shows restricted diffusion in the wall (*arrow*).

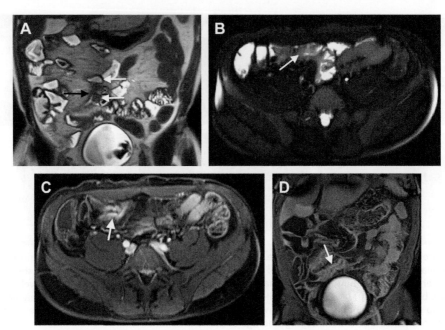

Fig. 9. Stricture with imaging findings of active inflammation. (*A*) Coronal T2-weighted image shows luminal narrowing and asymmetric ileal inflammation with effacement of mesenteric border folds (*black arrow*) and sacculations along the antimesenteric border (*white arrows*). (*B*) Axial fat-saturated half-Fourier acquisition single-shot turbo spin-echo image shows intramural edema (*arrow*). (*C*) Axial postcontrast image performed at 45 seconds after injection of contrast shows wall thickening and hyperenhancement (*white arrow*), reflecting active inflammation. (*D*) Coronal delayed postcontrast image 7 minutes later shows homogeneous enhancement (*white arrow*), probably reflecting coexisting fibrosis.

creating and using a standard reporting template assists gastroenterologists and colorectal surgeons in caring for their patients.[3,11,15,51] An example of a recommended reporting template is found in **Box 5**. The impression should include one of the recommended phrases relevant to the findings. Further,

any other actionable findings and/or impressions should be stated as with all reports.

A standard CT or MR imaging report template can be set to autolaunch in voice recognition systems when the examination is interpreted. These reports can be designed with drop-down menus

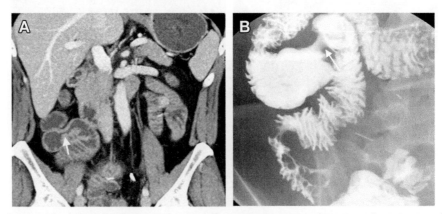

Fig. 10. Stricture with no imaging findings of active inflammation computed tomography enterography/barium. (*A*) Coronal computed tomography enterography image shows mild wall thickening, and a luminal narrowing with upstream dilation, without mural hyperenhancement (*arrow*). (*B*) An overhead image from a small bowel barium study performed 4 months earlier shows the stricture (*arrow*) and the upstream dilation with distal intramural sinus tracts and other strictures.

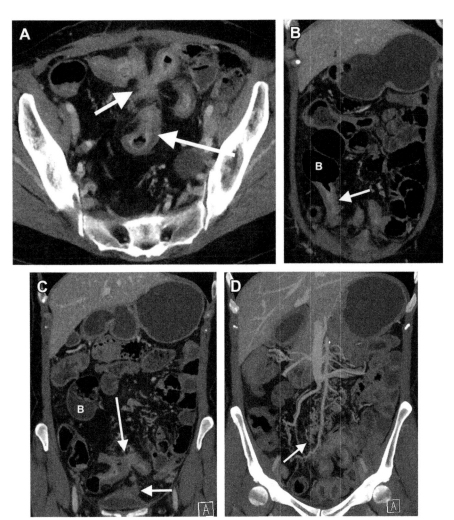

Fig. 11. Stricture with imaging findings of active inflammation and penetrating disease (complex fistula), small bowel obstruction, and chronic mesenteric occlusion. (A) Axial computed tomography enterography (CTE) image shows a complex enteroenteric fistula (*short white arrow*) arising from inflamed ileal loops (*long white arrow*). (B) Coronal CTE image shows the stricture upstream to the fistula with findings of active inflammation (*white arrow*). (C) Coronal CTE image shows the complex fistula (*long white arrow*) and an enterovesicular fistula (*short white arrow*) and associated urinary bladder wall thickening. (D) Coronal thick (1 cm) maximum intensity projection image demonstrates the tortuous, serpiginous, and dilated mesenteric veins (*white arrows*) from chronic mesenteric occlusion.

containing standardized phrases for sites of disease, and the extent and characterization of disease. In the impression portion of the report, drop-down menus containing the imaging-based morphologic phenotypes can also be inserted. In this way, terms can be standardized across multiple sites and radiologists.

DISEASE MONITORING PARADIGMS WITH CROSS-SECTIONAL ENTEROGRAPHY: IMPLICATIONS FOR PATIENT CARE

The routine description of active inflammation, its length, location, severity, presence of a stricture, and penetrating complications on cross-sectional enterography guide individualized treatment and follow-up decisions.[9] Objective markers of bowel wall healing may also predict future outcomes. The SONIC (Study of Biological and Immunomodulator Naive Patients in Crohn's Disease) trial investigators found that mucosal healing and endoscopic response at week 26 predicted corticosteroid remission at week 50.[52] MRE estimates of disease severity, response, and healing are highly correlated with endoscopic healing.[53] Inflammation on CTE is associated with ulcers at endoscopy, and an absence of inflammation is associated with mucosal healing.[54]

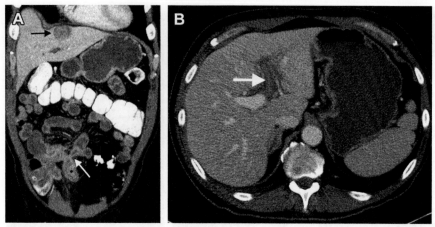

Fig. 12. Penetrating disease (complex fistula) arising from stricture with inflammation, left portal vein thrombosis and liver abscess. (*A*) Coronal computed tomography enterography (CTE) image shows a complex fistula (*white arrow*) associated with a stricture with imaging findings of active inflammation, and a complicating liver abscess (*black arrow*). The vasa recta are also dilated. (*B*) Axial CTE image in the mid liver shows a thrombus in the left portal vein (*white arrow*).

Cross-sectional enterography itself, which displays the full thickness of the bowel wall and proximal inflammation often unseen at endoscopic assessment,[4] can be used to measure objective endpoints. Sauer and colleagues[55] defined transmural healing as resolution of bowel wall thickening and intramural T2 signal at MRE, and found that transmural healing predicted clinical

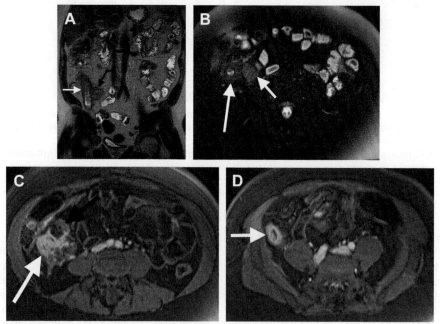

Fig. 13. Penetrating disease (abscess). Stricture with imaging findings of active inflammation likely despite absence of upstream dilation-coronal (*A*) half-Fourier acquisition single-shot turbo spin-echo (HASTE) image shows wall thickening with increased T2 signal (*white arrow*) upstream to a distal ileal stricture with and adjacent abscess (*black arrow*). (*B*) Axial fat-saturated HASTE upstream to the stricture shows increased mural T2 signal (*long white arrow*) and abscess (*short white arrow*). At the level of the stricture, axial (*C*) postcontrast image shows wall thickening, homogeneous mural hyperenhancement (*long white arrow*), and the abscess (*black arrow*). Just upstream to the stricture, axial (*D*) postcontrast volumetric interpolated breath-hold examination image shows stratified mural hyperenhancement (*arrow*).

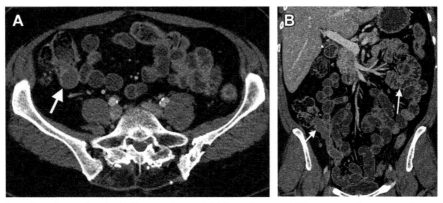

Fig. 14. No imaging signs of active inflammation-axial (*A*) and coronal (*B*) computed tomography enterography images show a normal terminal ileum (*white arrow*) and normal jejunal folds (*long white arrow*).

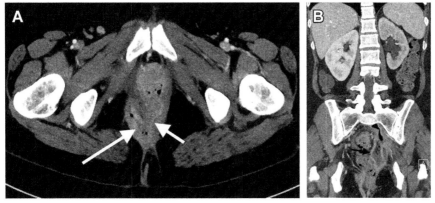

Fig. 15. Perianal fistula and abscess. Axial (*A*) and coronal (*B*) computed tomography enterography images show a perianal fistula (*short white arrow, A*) extending into a ramification (*long white arrow* in *A*) connecting to an ischiorectal fossa abscess (*black arrow* in *B*). A right nonobstructing caliceal tip stone is also shown (*B*).

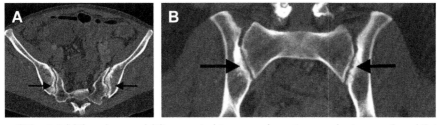

Fig. 16. Sacroiliitis. Axial (*A*) and coronal (*B*) computed tomography enterography images show bilateral sacroiliitis (*arrows*). Contrary to historical teaching, sacroiliitis is often asymmetric (here, *left* worse than *right*).

remission at a median clinical follow-up of 2 years. Response assessment by enterography can predict other outcomes as well. In 1 study, complete responders were defined as patients with a decrease in length or severity of inflammation of all inflamed bowel segments, and partial responders as those with an improvement in some but not all inflamed bowel segments.[56] These investigators found that complete and partial responses were associated with a 50% reduction in risk for corticosteroid use, and that complete response was associated with a decreased risk of hospitalizations and surgery.

Cross-sectional enterography findings can also be used to describe transitions between and coexistence of morphologic phenotypes, for example,

Box 5
Suggested format for CTE/MRE dictation report

Title: CTE with intravenous contrast or MRE without and with intravenous contrast

History: Appropriate entry

CT/MR technique: Appropriate entry

Oral contrast media: Type and volume

IV contrast media: Type and volume

Other medications: Glucagon, Buscopan dose, and method of delivery

Radiation exposure: DLP and/or CTDI$_{vol}$ for CTE

Comparison:

Findings:

- Bowel disease anatomic location
- Number of disease segments
  - Disease type(s) per disease segments (particularly important if disease segments have different findings)
  - Inflammation findings (see **Box 1**)
  - Location, length, and severity and any change from prior
  - Mesenteric findings (see **Box 2**)
- Stricture (see **Box 2**)
  - Without or with findings of inflammation
  - Length, location, and severity
  - Presence/absence of upstream bowel dilation
- Penetrating disease (see **Box 2**)
  - Site
  - Complexity or extent
  - Relationship to bowel and whether arises from inflamed and/or stricture
- Perianal disease
  - Site
  - Complexity/classification (best performed with a focused MR and generally not possible with standard, adult CTE or MRE)
  - Presence/absence of abscess
- Response to therapy
- Extraintestinal findings (see **Box 3**)

Impressions (see **Box 4**):

- Inflammation statement: Location, length, severity, or change
  - Nonspecific small bowel inflammation
  - Active inflammatory small bowel Crohn's disease without or with luminal narrowing
  - Crohn's disease with no imaging signs of active inflammation
  - No imaging signs of small bowel inflammation
- Stricture statement:
  - Stricture with signs of active inflammation—length of stricture and degree of proximal obstruction
  - Stricture without signs of active inflammation—length of stricture and degree of proximal obstruction

- Penetrating statement
  - Sinus tract, fistula (simple or complex), abscess and association with inflamed bowel segment and/or stricture
  - Perianal disease (if present)
- Other complications or important findings
  - Extraintestinal findings
  - Acute mesenteric vein thrombosis
  - Hepatic abscess
  - Potential for complicating small bowel carcinoma
  - Other actionable, incidental findings not related to Crohn's disease

Abbreviations: CTDI$_{vol}$, computed tomography dose index volume; CTE, computed tomography enterography; DLP, dose length product; IV, intravenous; MRE, magnetic resonance enterography.
Data from Refs.[1,11,15,51,58]

active small bowel inflammation may progress to stricture with findings of active inflammation or regress to transmural healing. For example, in 1 case-control study, patients with a stricture were more than 3 times more likely to develop a complication such as perforation or abscess than those without a stricture, but those with coexisting stricture and active inflammation were 15 times more likely to do so.[18] Cross-sectional enterography can demonstrate not only response and healing of active enteric inflammation,[57] but also healing of internal fistulas and regression and progression of inflammatory strictures.

SUMMARY

Crohn's disease is often a progressive and debilitating disease, generally affecting younger patients and leading to a lifetime of suffering. The addition of CT and MR imaging of this disease has opened new directions in guiding clinical treatment decisions and research. Some of the important questions to be answered are: (1) How can transmural healing be used to guide therapeutic decisions? (2) How will imaging help in the evaluation of antifibrotic therapy? and (3) How is it best to treat a patient with a stricture—medically or surgically? Some investigators believe that imaging rather than symptoms should be used as the endpoint of therapy, or be used as an important endpoint for clinical trials.[3,4,55] Because imaging identifies both the mural and the extramural manifestations of Crohn's disease, radiology may offer great insight into these important clinical questions. To do so, however, there must be both agreement and consistency in communicating/reporting the findings and impressions of imaging studies. We have provided the imaging community with the terms and tools to accomplish these essential tasks.

REFERENCES

1. Baker ME, Fletcher JG, Megibow AJ, et al. ACR-SAR-SPR practice parameter for the performance of CT enterography. 2015. Available at: https://www.acr.org/~/media/ACR/Documents/PGTS/guidelines/CT_Enterography.pdf?1a=en. Accessed May 29, 2018.
2. Deepak P, Fletcher JG, Fidler JL, et al. Computed tomography and magnetic resonance enterography in Crohn's disease: assessment of radiologic criteria and endpoints for clinical practice and trials. Inflamm Bowel Dis 2016;22(9):2280–8.
3. Deepak P, Park SH, Ehman EC, et al. Crohn's disease diagnosis, treatment approach, and management paradigm: what the radiologist needs to know. Abdom Radiol (NY) 2017;42(4):1068–86.
4. Faubion WA Jr, Fletcher JG, O'Byrne S, et al. EMerging BiomARKers in Inflammatory Bowel Disease (EMBARK) study identifies fecal calprotectin, serum MMP9, and serum IL-22 as a novel combination of biomarkers for Crohn's disease activity: role of cross-sectional imaging. Am J Gastroenterol 2013;108(12):1891–900.
5. Panes J, Bouhnik Y, Reinisch W, et al. Imaging techniques for assessment of inflammatory bowel disease: joint ECCO and ESGAR evidence-based consensus guidelines. J Crohns Colitis 2013;7(7):556–85.
6. Panes J, Bouzas R, Chaparro M, et al. Systematic review: the use of ultrasonography, computed tomography and magnetic resonance imaging for the diagnosis, assessment of activity and abdominal complications of Crohn's disease. Aliment Pharmacol Ther 2011;34(2):125–45.
7. Bruining DH, Siddiki HA, Fletcher JG, et al. Benefit of computed tomography enterography in Crohn's disease: effects on patient management and physician level of confidence. Inflamm Bowel Dis 2012;18(2):219–25.

8. Higgins PD, Caoili E, Zimmermann M, et al. Computed tomographic enterography adds information to clinical management in small bowel Crohn's disease. Inflamm Bowel Dis 2007;13(3): 262–8.

9. Rimola J, Rodriguez S, Garcia-Bosch O, et al. Magnetic resonance for assessment of disease activity and severity in ileocolonic Crohn's disease. Gut 2009;58(8):1113–20.

10. Samuel S, Bruining DH, Loftus EV Jr, et al. Endoscopic skipping of the distal terminal ileum in Crohn's disease can lead to negative results from ileocolonoscopy. Clin Gastroenterol Hepatol 2012; 10(11):1253–9.

11. Baker ME, Hara AK, Platt JF, et al. CT enterography for Crohn's disease: optimal technique and imaging issues. Abdom Imaging 2015;40(5): 938–52.

12. Grand DJ, Guglielmo FF, Al-Hawary MM. MR enterography in Crohn's disease: current consensus on optimal imaging technique and future advances from the SAR Crohn's disease-focused panel. Abdom Imaging 2015;40(5):953–64.

13. Levine A, Griffiths A, Markowitz J, et al. Pediatric modification of the Montreal classification for inflammatory bowel disease: the Paris classification. Inflamm Bowel Dis 2011;17(6):1314–21.

14. Silverberg MS, Satsangi J, Ahmad T, et al. Toward an integrated clinical, molecular and serological classification of inflammatory bowel disease: report of a Working Party of the 2005 Montreal World Congress of Gastroenterology. Can J Gastroenterol 2005;19(Suppl A):5A–36A.

15. Bruining DH, Zimmermann EM, Loftus EV, et al. Consensus recommendations for evaluation, interpretation, and utilization of computed tomography and magnetic resonance enterography in patients with small bowel crohn's disease. Gastroenterology 2018;154(4):1172–94.

16. Adler J, Punglia DR, Dillman JR, et al. Computed tomography enterography findings correlate with tissue inflammation, not fibrosis in resected small bowel Crohn's disease. Inflamm Bowel Dis 2012; 18(5):849–56.

17. Zappa M, Stefanescu C, Cazals-Hatem D, et al. Which magnetic resonance imaging findings accurately evaluate inflammation in small bowel Crohn's disease? A retrospective comparison with surgical pathologic analysis. Inflamm Bowel Dis 2011;17(4): 984–93.

18. Chaudhry NA, Riverso M, Grajo JR, et al. A fixed stricture on routine cross-sectional imaging predicts disease-related complications and adverse outcomes in patients with Crohn's disease. Inflamm Bowel Dis 2017;23(4):641–9.

19. Kelly JK, Preshaw RM. Origin of fistulas in Crohn's disease. J Clin Gastroenterol 1989;11(2):193–6.

20. Oberhuber G, Stangl PC, Vogelsang H, et al. Significant association of strictures and internal fistula formation in Crohn's disease. Virchows Arch 2000; 437(3):293–7.

21. Orscheln ES, Dillman JR, Towbin AJ, et al. Penetrating Crohn disease: does it occur in the absence of stricturing disease? Abdom Radiol (NY) 2017. [Epub ahead of print].

22. Baker ME, Walter J, Obuchowski NA, et al. Mural attenuation in normal small bowel and active inflammatory Crohn's disease on CT enterography: location, absolute attenuation, relative attenuation, and the effect of wall thickness. AJR Am J Roentgenol 2009;192(2):417–23.

23. Bodily KD, Fletcher JG, Solem CA, et al. Crohn disease: mural attenuation and thickness at contrast-enhanced CT enterography–correlation with endoscopic and histologic findings of inflammation. Radiology 2006;238(2):505–16.

24. Park SH. DWI at MR enterography for evaluating bowel inflammation in Crohn disease. AJR Am J Roentgenol 2016;207(1):40–8.

25. Rimola J, Ordas I, Rodriguez S, et al. Magnetic resonance imaging for evaluation of Crohn's disease: validation of parameters of severity and quantitative index of activity. Inflamm Bowel Dis 2011;17(8): 1759–68.

26. Steward MJ, Punwani S, Proctor I, et al. Non-perforating small bowel Crohn's disease assessed by MRI enterography: derivation and histopathological validation of an MR-based activity index. Eur J Radiol 2012;81(9):2080–8.

27. Tielbeek JA, Makanyanga JC, Bipat S, et al. Grading Crohn disease activity with MRI: interobserver variability of MRI features, MRI scoring of severity, and correlation with Crohn disease endoscopic index of severity. AJR Am J Roentgenol 2013;201(6):1220–8.

28. Tielbeek JA, Ziech ML, Li Z, et al. Evaluation of conventional, dynamic contrast enhanced and diffusion weighted MRI for quantitative Crohn's disease assessment with histopathology of surgical specimens. Eur Radiol 2014;24(3):619–29.

29. Church PC, Turner D, Feldman BM, et al. Systematic review with meta-analysis: magnetic resonance enterography signs for the detection of inflammation and intestinal damage in Crohn's disease. Aliment Pharmacol Ther 2015;41(2):153–66.

30. Makanyanga J, Punwani S, Taylor SA. Assessment of wall inflammation and fibrosis in Crohn's disease: value of T1-weighted gadolinium-enhanced MR imaging. Abdom Imaging 2012;37(6):933–43.

31. Rimola J, Planell N, Rodriguez S, et al. Characterization of inflammation and fibrosis in Crohn's disease lesions by magnetic resonance imaging. Am J Gastroenterol 2015;110(3):432–40.

32. Weber NK, Fletcher JG, Fidler JL, et al. Clinical characteristics and imaging features of small bowel

adenocarcinomas in Crohn's disease. Abdom Imaging 2015;40(5):1060–7.

33. Kim KJ, Lee Y, Park SH, et al. Diffusion-weighted MR enterography for evaluating Crohn's disease: how does it add diagnostically to conventional MR enterography? Inflamm Bowel Dis 2015;21(1): 101–9.

34. Seo N, Park SH, Kim KJ, et al. MR Enterography for the evaluation of small-bowel inflammation in Crohn disease by using diffusion-weighted imaging without intravenous contrast material: a prospective noninferiority study. Radiology 2016;278(3):762–72.

35. Froehlich JM, Waldherr C, Stoupis C, et al. MR motility imaging in Crohn's disease improves lesion detection compared with standard MR imaging. Eur Radiol 2010;20(8):1945–51.

36. Menys A, Atkinson D, Odille F, et al. Quantified terminal ileal motility during MR enterography as a potential biomarker of Crohn's disease activity: a preliminary study. Eur Radiol 2012;22(11):2494–501.

37. Menys A, Helbren E, Makanyanga J, et al. Small bowel strictures in Crohn's disease: a quantitative investigation of intestinal motility using MR enterography. Neurogastroenterol Motil 2013;25(12):967-e775.

38. Wnorowski AM, Guglielmo FF, Mitchell DG. How to perform and interpret cine MR enterography. J Magn Reson Imaging 2015;5(42):1180–9.

39. Bouhnik Y, Carbonnel F, Laharie D, et al. Efficacy of adalimumab in patients with Crohn's disease and symptomatic small bowel stricture: a multicentre, prospective, observational cohort (CREOLE) study. Gut 2018;67(1):53–60.

40. Higgins PD, Fletcher JG. Characterization of inflammation and fibrosis in Crohn's disease lesions by magnetic resonance imaging. Am J Gastroenterol 2015;110(3):441–3.

41. Rieder F, Fiocchi C, Rogler G. Mechanisms, management, and treatment of fibrosis in patients with inflammatory bowel diseases. Gastroenterology 2017;152(2):340–50.e6.

42. Rieder F, Latella G, Magro F, et al. European Crohn's and colitis organisation topical review on prediction, diagnosis and management of fibrostenosing Crohn's disease. J Crohns Colitis 2016;10(8):873–85.

43. Rieder F, Zimmermann EM, Remzi FH, et al. Crohn's disease complicated by strictures: a systematic review. Gut 2013;62(7):1072–84.

44. Stidham RW, Higgins PD. Imaging of intestinal fibrosis: current challenges and future methods. United European Gastroenterol J 2016;4(4):515–22.

45. Booya F, Akram S, Fletcher JG, et al. CT enterography and fistulizing Crohn's disease: clinical benefit and radiographic findings. Abdom Imaging 2009; 34(4):467–75.

46. Baker ME, Remzi F, Einstein D, et al. CT depiction of portal vein thrombi after creation of ileal pouch-anal anastomosis. Radiology 2003;227(1):73–9.

47. Violi NV, Schoepfer AM, Fournier N, et al. Prevalence and clinical importance of mesenteric venous thrombosis in the Swiss Inflammatory Bowel Disease Cohort. AJR Am J Roentgenol 2014;203(1):62–9.

48. Gecse KB, Bemelman W, Kamm MA, et al. A global consensus on the classification, diagnosis and multidisciplinary treatment of perianal fistulising Crohn's disease. Gut 2014;63(9):1381–92.

49. Bruining DH, Siddiki HA, Fletcher JG, et al. Prevalence of penetrating disease and extraintestinal manifestations of Crohn's disease detected with CT enterography. Inflamm Bowel Dis 2008;14(12): 1701–6.

50. Paparo F, Bacigalupo L, Garello I, et al. Crohn's disease: prevalence of intestinal and extraintestinal manifestations detected by computed tomography enterography with water enema. Abdom Imaging 2012;37(3):326–37.

51. Al-Hawary MM, Kaza RK, Platt JF. CT enterography: concepts and advances in Crohn's disease imaging. Radiol Clin North Am 2013;51(1):1–16.

52. Ferrante M, Colombel JF, Sandborn WJ, et al. Validation of endoscopic activity scores in patients with Crohn's disease based on a post hoc analysis of data from SONIC. Gastroenterology 2013;145(5): 978–86.e5.

53. Ordas I, Rimola J, Rodriguez S, et al. Accuracy of magnetic resonance enterography in assessing response to therapy and mucosal healing in patients with Crohn's disease. Gastroenterology 2014;146(2): 374–82.e1.

54. Hashimoto S, Shimizu K, Shibata H, et al. Utility of computed tomographic enteroclysis/enterography for the assessment of mucosal healing in Crohn's disease. Gastroenterol Res Pract 2013;2013: 984916.

55. Sauer CG, Middleton JP, McCracken C, et al. Magnetic resonance enterography healing and magnetic resonance enterography remission predicts improved outcome in pediatric Crohn disease. J Pediatr Gastroenterol Nutr 2016;62(3):378–83.

56. Deepak P, Fletcher JG, Fidler JL, et al. Radiological response is associated with better long-term outcomes and is a potential treatment target in patients with small bowel CROHN's disease. Am J Gastroenterol 2016;111(7):997–1006.

57. Bruining DH, Loftus EV Jr, Ehman EC, et al. Computed tomography enterography detects intestinal wall changes and effects of treatment in patients with Crohn's disease. Clin Gastroenterol Hepatol 2011;9(8):679–83.e1.

58. Bruining DH, Zimmermann EM, Loftus EV, et al. Consensus recommendations for evaluation, interpretation, and utilization of computed tomography and magnetic resonance enterography in patients with small bowel crohn's disease. Radiology 2018; 286(3):776–99.

Low-Dose Computed Tomography Colonography Technique

Kevin J. Chang, MD[a],*, Judy Yee, MD[b]

KEYWORDS

- Computed tomography colonography • Virtual colonoscopy • Radiation dose reduction
- Automatic dose modulation • Iterative reconstruction • kVp

KEY POINTS

- The role of radiation is of debatable importance for computed tomography (CT) colonography in the screening age population (generally over the age of 50) but consistent with the As Low As Reasonably Achievable (ALARA) principle only a very low radiation dose is necessary for colonic polyp detection.
- A wide variety of CT scan parameters can be adjusted or utilized to significantly reduce radiation dose such as reducing tube current (mAs), reducing tube voltage in smaller patients (kVp), using automatic dose modulation, and incorporating iterative reconstruction.
- Other practical approaches can also be used to help reduce radiation dose such as proper patient isocentering, optimizing colonic distension to minimize scan phases, limiting the scan volume to the colon, and varying view settings to reduce the impact of image noise.

INTRODUCTION

For much of the past 2 decades, computed tomography (CT) colonography (CTC) has fought an uphill battle to become an accepted option for colorectal screening. One of the major impediments to the eventual acceptance of CT colonography as a screening test has been the perceived risk of radiation associated with CT. In fact, theoretic radiation risks were specifically used by the US Preventative Services Task Force to delay the eventual "A" recommendation of CTC for colorectal screening[1] and are still used as an argument by the Centers for Medicare and Medicaid Services (CMS) against a national coverage determination (NCD) to include CTC as a Medicare/Medicaid-reimbursed

colorectal screening option.[2] Patients, the lay press, referring physicians, and even some radiologists have also expressed concern about CT radiation.[3–5]

PUTTING RADIATION RISKS IN PERSPECTIVE

The theoretic risks of a small dose of radiation associated with a low-dose examination such as CTC need to be weighed realistically against the benefits of colorectal screening. The theoretic risks associated with medical sources of radiation are based on a linear extrapolation of the cancer-induction risks associated with ultrahigh doses of radiation from atomic bomb exposures in Japan. This linear no-threshold model (BEIR VII)[6] remains

Disclosure Statement: K.J. Chang has no disclosure of any relationship with a commercial company that has a direct financial interest in subject matter or materials discussed in article or with a company making a competing product. J. Yee has research grants from Echopixel and Philips.

[a] Department of Radiology, Newton-Wellesley Hospital, Brown University Alpert Medical School, 2014 Washington Street, Newton, MA 02462, USA; [b] Department of Radiology, Montefiore Medical Center, Albert Einstein College of Medicine, 111 East 210th Street, Bronx, NY 10467, USA
* Corresponding author.
E-mail address: Kevin.J.Chang@gmail.com

Radiol Clin N Am 56 (2018) 709–717
https://doi.org/10.1016/j.rcl.2018.04.008

radiologic.theclinics.com

highly controversial and unproven at low doses associated with medical imaging.[7] The Health Physics Society in 2016 stated that below an exposure of 100 mSv, the observed radiation effects in people are not statistically different from zero."[8] If one assumes a CTC dose of 5 mSv, the theoretic risk of cancer induction at the initial screening age of 50 is 0.04%, dropping to 0.02% by age 70,[9] numbers difficult to compare much less prove when the comparable lifetime risk of developing cancer is 39%.[10] Compared with a 5% lifetime risk of developing colon cancer in particular, the benefits of preventing colon cancer vastly outweigh the theoretic risks of cancer induction, even when accounting for surveillance imaging at 5-year intervals. When compared with the real risks of colonic perforation at optical colonoscopy of 0.1% to 0.2%,[11] these theoretic risks of radiation are put into even greater perspective. These unproven risks are likely to be even lower, with average CTC doses at many institutions now lower than 3 mSv, a dose comparable to annual environmental background radiation exposure in the Unites States and a fraction of the dose associated with a routine abdomen/pelvis CT. With further vendor advances in CT radiation dose-reduction techniques, there is room for even further reductions, as one only needs enough photons to resolve a soft-tissue/gas interface for detection of polyps measuring larger than 5 mm in size.

Regardless of exactly what risks, if any, may be associated with such low doses of radiation, out of concern for patients and the public, it behooves the medical community to keep CT radiation dose As Low As Reasonably Achievable (the ALARA principle),[12] especially when it comes to a screening examination repeated at regular intervals that potentially every person of average risk qualifies for.

RADIATION DOSE METRICS AND TARGETS

All CT manufacturers are required to provide dose metrics, including a CT dose index ($CTDI_{vol}$) measured in mGy and a dose length product (DLP) in mGy-cm (the $CTDI_{vol}$ integrated over the scan length) for each scan series (see an example in **Fig. 1**). For a CTC, this includes summing doses for each scan position such as supine and prone, and occasionally a third position when troubleshooting an underdistended colonic segment. The $CTDI_{vol}$ is a measure of the average radiation output intensity of the CT scanner for a particular scan, whereas the DLP is a quantitative measure of the total radiation output when accounting for the scan length. To convert these measures of CT scan output to estimated patient-absorbed radiation doses, a conversion factor (k) based on the use of standardized body phantoms is multiplied by the total summed DLP to generate the estimated effective dose in mSv. Currently, the k value used to estimate effective dose in abdomen/pelvis CT examinations is 0.0171.[13,14] However, this k value can also be size-corrected for each particular patient to more closely estimate the dose absorbed, as this estimate is highly dependent on each patient's body habitus.[15,16] Nevertheless, multiplying the total summed DLP by approximately 1.5% serves as an easy estimate for the dose of each examination. An initial goal would be to reduce the dose to less than that of a double-contrast barium

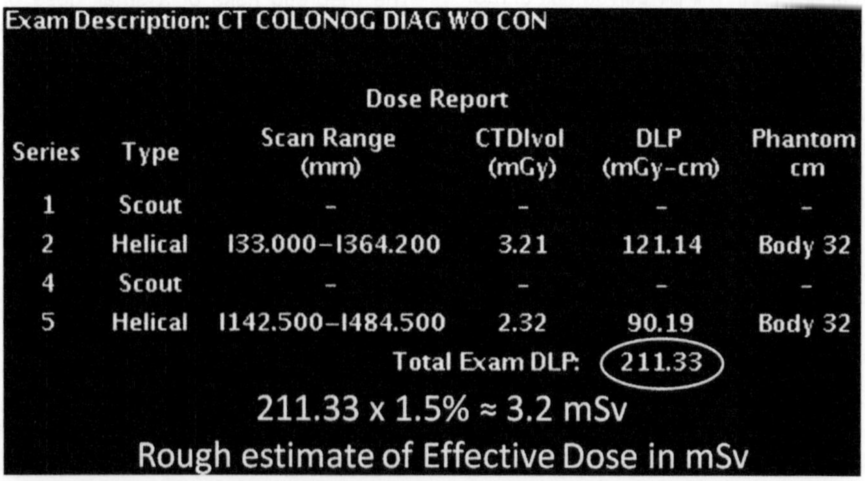

Exam Description: CT COLONOG DIAG WO CON

Dose Report

Series	Type	Scan Range (mm)	CTDIvol (mGy)	DLP (mGy–cm)	Phantom cm
1	Scout	–	–	–	–
2	Helical	133.000–1364.200	3.21	121.14	Body 32
4	Scout	–	–	–	–
5	Helical	1142.500–1484.500	2.32	90.19	Body 32
			Total Exam DLP:	211.33	

211.33 x 1.5% ≈ 3.2 mSv
Rough estimate of Effective Dose in mSv

Fig. 1. Using the CT dose page to estimate radiation dose. Adding the dose-length product (DLP) of the 2 CTC scan positions (series 2 and 5 above) and multiplying this by a k factor of approximately 1.5% yields a rough estimate of the estimated effective dose in mSv.

enema. However, optimized low-dose protocols should be able to bring doses even lower to between 2 and 5 mSv, with the use of iterative reconstruction algorithms on newer scanners capable of bringing these doses down to even 1 mSv or less.[17–20] A comparison of doses to other radiologic examinations is provided in **Table 1**.

COMPUTED TOMOGRAPHY PARAMETER CHANGES TO REDUCE RADIATION DOSE
Reduce Tube Current (mAs)

The easiest and most straightforward way to reduce radiation dose is by reducing the tube current (mAs), as the dose decreases linearly with a reduction in mAs (**Box 1**). However, the limitation of tube current reduction is the concomitant increase in image noise that results with noise, varying by a function of $1/\sqrt{mAs}$. There is significant opportunity for dose reduction in CTC analogous to the low doses employed in CT protocols used for renal stone detection and lung cancer screening, as relatively low amounts of radiation are needed to visualize the colonic air-mucosal interface on 2-dimensional images and in 3-dimensional endoluminal volume renders. The amount of image noise tolerated is largely a function of the particular 3-dimensional rendering software used as well as individual reader preference. It is important to note that noisy images will decrease the ability to identify incidental extracolonic findings, arguably a limitation that may be seen to be of greater benefit than harm in the context of a colorectal screening examination. Multiple studies have shown aggressive reductions in mAs, to as low as 10 mAs, are possible without an effect on the accuracy of polyp detection.[21–24]

Automatic Dose Modulation

A more judicious use of radiation can be incorporated into CTC by using automatic dose modulation

> **Box 1**
> **Strategies to reduce computed tomography colonography radiation dose**
>
> CT scan parameter adjustments
> - Reduce tube current (mAs)
> - Use automatic dose modulation (automatic exposure control)
> - Reduce tube voltage (kVp)
> - Use iterative reconstruction to reduce noise in low dose images
>
> Other practical methods to reduce radiation dose
> - Only perform CTC when bowel preparation is adequate, and indication is appropriate
> - Properly isocenter the patient in the CT gantry
> - Minimize additional scan phases by optimizing colonic distension
> - Limit scan volume to the colon
>
> Ways to reduce the visual impact of increased image noise
> - Increase slice thickness when reading extracolonic structures
> - Widen window settings to decrease the conspicuity of image noise

(also known as automatic exposure control), which varies radiation output on the basis of the size, shape, and composition of the patient. More specifically, this technique varies the radiation output by the position of the CT tube in relation to the patient, with the largest reductions in same output made in the lateral versus AP projections and in the bony pelvis versus gas-filled lung base, variations usually based on attenuations inferred from the initial AP and lateral scout topograms. CT projections through the densest tissues contribute the most to overall image noise; therefore, tube current can be reduced in less-attenuated projections without as significant an effect on noise.[25,26] This feature is known by many vendor-specific trade names including Smart mA, Auto mA, CARE Dose, D-DOM, Z-DOM, and SureExposure, and can be utilized in the X-Y/angular axis (reducing radiograph output in the AP dimension rather than the lateral projection) and/or along the Z-axis (reducing radiograph output in radiolucent portions of the body such as lung bases). A variation of automatic dose modulation is organ-based tube current modulation, where radiographs incident upon more radiosensitive portions of the body (such as in the anterior projection for breast tissue or testes) are

Table 1
Radiation dose comparison table

Examination	Dose (mSv)
KUB	0.6
Intravenous pyelogram (IVP)	3
Barium enema	8
CT abdomen/pelvis	10
CT abdomen/pelvis multiphase	20
CT colonography	1–6
US annual background radiation	3 (≤12)

Data from www.RadiologyInfo.org. Accessed October 31, 2017.

reduced and compensated by increases in the opposite projection (ie, posterior). A nonhardware variant of this technique is the controversial use of bismuth shields over the breasts or testes, although their use has been associated with additional imaging artifacts and noise. Breast surface doses have been shown to be reduced by as much as 40% without a qualitative impact on image quality.[27]

Particular to CTC, it is important to note that the use of hyperdense fecal/fluid tagging agents such as iodinated contrast and barium do not significantly alter radiation dose when using dose modulation[28] but may result in more beam-hardening artifact and inaccurate measurement of submerged polyp attenuation at low doses. In addition, when varying other CT parameters (such as kVp) while using automatic dose modulation, automatic adjustments in mAs may partially counteract attempts at dose reduction to maintain a constant prescribed level of image noise. Finally, at extremes in body habitus, automatic dose modulation may occasionally lead to over-radiating larger patients (a larger volume of intra-abdominal fat decreases reliance on reducing image noise to maintain soft tissue contrast) and under-radiating smaller patients (resulting in too much image noise). Setting minimum and maximum mA ranges will help constrain photon flux in these scenarios (eg, a minimum of 50 mA and a maximum of 450 mA).

Reduce Tube Voltage (kVp)

Although radiation dose decreases linearly with tube current, it decreases to a near exponential extent (by a power of 2.6) with reductions in peak tube voltage (kVp).[29,30] In addition to dose reduction, reducing tube voltage also increases the measured attenuation of fecal/fluid tagging agents as the kVp more closely approaches the K-edge of iodine and barium (33.2 and 37.4 keV, respectively). This increases the contrast between and conspicuity of submerged polyps and tagged fluid. However, decreasing kVp also leads to a proportionately greater increase in image noise compared with reducing mAs. However, contrast to noise ratio (CNR) between tagged fluid and polyps is largely maintained.[31] This technique becomes more limited in larger patients, as increases in image noise become more pronounced with a larger body habitus.[32] In fact, when combined with automatic dose modulation, occasionally radiation dose may counterintuitively increase with a decrease in kVp in very large patients as automatic increases in mAs attempt to compensate for increases in image noise. Because of this, some CT manufacturers vary the selected kVp by

the size of the patient and specific examination type in order to achieve a specified CNR. Alternatively, kVp may be selected based on body size (body mass index, body width on scout topogram, or patient weight); for example, 100 kVp can be used for patients weighing less than 150 lbs, 120 kVp for patients between 150 to 300 lbs, and even 140 kVp for patients over 300 lbs.[33] An even more simplified and binary protocol would be to reduce kVp to 100 when AP diameter on the lateral scout topogram measures 25 cm or less (Kevin Chang, MD, unpublished data, 2013). Varying tube voltage is a technique that is widely applicable on all CT scanners, even older scanners lacking automatic dose modulation features.

Iterative Reconstruction

Iterative reconstruction techniques have now become available on most current generation CT scanners and results in significantly lower image noise in CT image reconstruction over traditional filtered back-projection techniques, a technique previously not feasible due to limitations in computational power (Fig. 2).[34] This technique goes by various trade names including ASiR, ASiR-V, Veo, iDose4, IMR, IRIS, SAFIRE, ADMIRE, AIDR, and FIRST. Using iterative reconstruction allows for significantly greater opportunities for radiation dose reduction through reducing tube current and/or tube voltage than previously possible. As the image is iteratively reconstructed using sophisticated statistical and algebraic reconstruction algorithms, significant computational power and time are required depending on the algorithm employed, usually ranging between 5 and 45 minutes for an abdomen/pelvis CT. When used for CTC, a 50% to 75% reduction in radiation dose is possible without an effect on image quality.[19,35,36] For example, when reducing kVp from 120 to 100 for CTC on a GE scanner, an adaptive statistical iterative reconstruction (ASiR) setting of approximately 50% can mitigate the resultant increase in image noise to a level comparable to filtered back-projection.[37] Reductions in beam hardening and streak artifacts related to tagged fluid and bone are also possible, as is a future potential to increase spatial resolution.

OTHER PRACTICAL APPROACHES TO REDUCE RADIATION DOSE

Other practical strategies that do not necessarily involve changes to scan hardware or scanner protocols can also be applied to reduce radiation dose. Basic strategies such as only performing CTCs in indicated patients and only performing CTC when the colonic preparation is sufficient

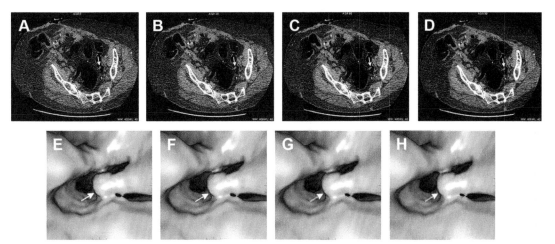

Fig. 2. Adaptive statistical Iterative reconstruction in CT colonography. Axial 2-dimensional (*A–D*) and 3-dimensional endoluminal renders (*E–H*) of a pedunculated polyp in the sigmoid colon (*arrow*) with no iterative reconstruction (*A, E*), with 30% ASiR (*B, F*), 60% ASiR (*C, G*), and 90% ASiR (*D, H*).

can limit radiation to appropriate individuals. Other approaches include proper isocentering of the patient in the CT gantry, minimizing additional scan phases through optimization of colonic distension, limiting additional scans to the segment of interest, limiting overall scan lengths to just the colon, and varying reading methods to minimize the perception of image noise.

Patient Isocentering

Proper centering of the patient in the CT gantry permits accurate estimation of body size on the scout topograms and automated selection of proper automatic dose modulation technique for the correct radiation dose. Positioning the patient too high or too low in the CT gantry can lead to magnification or minification of the patient on the scout topogram, leading to an overestimate or underestimate of the radiation dose necessary to generate images of desired image quality (**Fig. 3**). Use of the scanner laser alignment guides to center the patient is critical, as off-center positioning can result in surface radiation doses up to 30% higher than optimal.[38]

Minimize Additional Phases by Optimizing Colonic Distension

CTC typically involves imaging the entire colon in at least 2 positions, most commonly supine and prone (although many institutions now substitute a right lateral decubitus position for the prone position for more reliable distension of the sigmoid

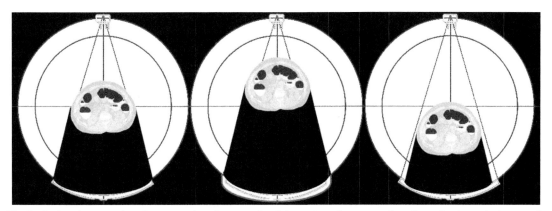

Fig. 3. Patient isocentering. Proper patient isocentering is important for proper function of automatic dose modulation (*left*). Positioning the patient too far from the detector array (*center*) will lead to an overestimate of patient size and greater than necessary radiation dose. Conversely, positioning the patient too close to the detector array (*right*) will lead to an underestimate of size and less than optimal radiation dose. In these images, the topogram is being acquired in an AP projection.

and transverse colon[39]) to allow for redistribution of residual fluid and to optimize visualization of the entire colonic wall circumference. The better and more consistently the colon is distended, the less often a third scan position will be necessary to troubleshoot underdistended segments. Strategies to optimize colonic distension include having the patient evacuate his or her colon prior to getting on the CT table (to reduce residual rectal fluid and minimize the incidence of a fluid block inhibiting colonic insufflation), using automated carbon dioxide insufflation, and possibly incorporating the right lateral decubitus position instead of the prone position. The use of spasmolytics such as glucagon has not been shown to reliably improve colonic distension.[40–43]

Z-Axis Collimation, Limit Scan Volume to Colon

Scan volumes should be limited to just the colon (1 cm above the highest colonic flexure to 1 cm below the anus), as structures such as the liver dome do not need to be fully evaluated in a colorectal screening examination (although it may be included when a CTC is being performed with intravenous contrast as part of a staging examination for a known obstructing colonic malignancy). When a third position needs to be acquired, limiting the scan to just the underdistended segment of interest will also limit additional radiation. A few scanners also have the capability of Z-axis collimation, which limits overscanning at the superior and inferior extent of the scan volume to further limit absorbed dose.[44]

Varying Slice Thickness and Widening Window Settings When Reading Extracolonic Findings

To reduce image noise when evaluating unenhanced extracolonic structures with lower inherent soft tissue contrast, slice thickness can be increased from the routine 0.625 to 1.25 mm slices typically reviewed in CTC to 3 to 5 mm, similar to that of routine diagnostic abdomen/pelvis CTs (**Fig. 4**). This can be performed at the CT scanner with a separate series sent to PACS for workstation review, or reformatted as a thicker multiplanar reformat on the 3-dimensional workstation for separate review before or after colonic evaluation. Similarly, a wider window setting can

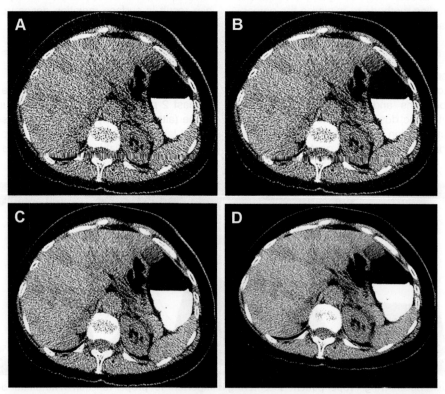

Fig. 4. Reading extracolonic findings at a higher slice thickness decreases image noise and improves soft tissue contrast. Axial 2-dimensional images from a CT colonography illustrating colon cancer metastases to the liver at (*A*) 0.6 mm, (*B*) 1.8 mm, (*C*) 3.0 mm, and (*D*) 6.6 mm slice thicknesses. Liver metastases are easier to resolve at thicker slice thickness.

also decrease the conspicuity of image noise.[45] Third-party vendors also offer noise filters that can be applied to reconstructed images. Some 3-dimensional software vendors also offer a noise filter function specifically for use with 3-dimensional endoluminal renders using lower dose images.

BENCHMARKING AGAINST PEERS

While radiation dose optimization should be specifically tailored to a particular practice using a specific combination of scan hardware and interpretation software, an important metric to judge the success of radiation dose reduction efforts is not only a before-and-after comparison for a specific scanner but a comparison against other institutions that also perform CTC. This is most easily achieved through site registration with the American College of Radiology's National Radiology and Data Registry (NRDR.ACR.org), specifically the CT Colonography Registry and the Dose Index Registry (DIR, applicable to all types of CT scans). Both registries monitor $CTDI_{vol}$, while the DIR also monitors DLP. Biannual feedback reports compare doses on a per-scanner or per-institution basis against regional and national standards.

SUMMARY

Incorporating and finding the most appropriate combination of the various strategies discussed previously is essential when performing screening CTC. It is helpful to take an incremental approach in implementing each method, as overuse of any of these strategies can result in overly noisy and potentially nondiagnostic images. As CTC involves 2 scans on the same patient, it naturally lends itself as a prime test bed for evaluating the effect of varying any single CT parameter on image quality. By varying 1 parameter at a time on only 1 of 2 CTC scan positions, each change can be compared with baseline image quality and radiation dose in the other scan position. With this method, changes can be evaluated on an intrapatient basis without a significant threat to the diagnostic adequacy of the overall examination. Image quality should be assessed on both the 2-dimensional images and the 3-dimensional endoluminal images as well, since each 3-dimensional workstation vendor may handle image noise in different ways, with image noise often manifesting as an increase in the mucosal graininess or nodularity of the rendered colonic wall, with a potential impact in not only polyp detection but also computer-aided detection (CAD) algorithms.

In summary, there are a wide variety and combination of strategies that can be employed in reducing radiation dose while maintaining diagnostic image quality and accuracy of polyp detection in CT colonography. In addition to variations in CT scan parameters and significant advances in scan and reconstruction technique, practical considerations specific to CTC include optimizing colonic distension, choosing the appropriate scan volume, and reducing the need for additional scan positions. Similar to other low-dose CT examinations (such as in lung cancer screening and renal stone detection), there is much room for more aggressive attempts at dose reduction in CTC without a significant sacrifice in the ability to detect and characterize clinically relevant colonic polyps and masses.

REFERENCES

1. Bibbins-Domingo K, Grossman DC, Curry SJ, et al. Screening for colorectal cancer: US preventive services task force recommendation statement. JAMA 2016;315(23):2564–75.
2. Jensen T, Salive M, Larsen W, et al. Centers for Medicare and Medicaid services: decision memo for screening computed tomography colonography (CTC) for colorectal cancer (CAG-00396N). 2009. Available at: https://www.cms.gov/medicare-coverage-database/details/nca-decision-memo.aspxAId=220&TAId=58&NcaName=Screening+Computed+Tomography+Colonography+(CTC)+for+Colorectal+Cancer. Accessed October 31, 2017.
3. Brenner DJ, Hall EJ. Computed tomography–an increasing source of radiation exposure. N Engl J Med 2007;357(22):2277–84.
4. Redberg RF, Smith-Bindman R. We are giving ourselves cancer. New York Times 2014. Opinion: A27.
5. Berrington de Gonzalez A, Mahesh M, Kim KP, et al. Projected cancer risks from computed tomographic scans performed in the United States in 2007. Arch Intern Med 2009;169(22):2071–7.
6. National Research Council. Health risks from exposure to low levels of ionizing radiation: BEIR VII Phase 2. Washington, DC: The National Academies Press; 2006.
7. Tubiana M, Aurengo A, Averbeck D, et al. The debate on the use of linear no threshold for assessing the effects of low doses. J Radiol Prot 2006; 26(3):317–24.
8. Burk RJ. Radiation risk in perspective: position statement of the Health Physics Society. 2016. Available at: http://hps.org/documents/risk_ps010-3.pdf. Accessed October 31, 2017.
9. Berrington de Gonzalez A, Kim KP, Knudsen AB, et al. Radiation-related cancer risks from CT colonography screening: a risk-benefit analysis. AJR Am J Roentgenol 2011;196(4):816–23.

10. SEER cancer statistics review 1975-2014. Available at: http://seer.cancer.gov/csr/1975_2014. Accessed October 31, 2017.

11. Gatto NM, Frucht H, Sundararajan V, et al. Risk of perforation after colonoscopy and sigmoidoscopy: a population-based study. J Natl Cancer Inst 2003; 95(3):230–6.

12. Standards for protection against radiation. U.S. code of federal regulations. Title 10, Section 20.1003; 2014.

13. Huda W, Randazzo W, Tipnis S, et al. Embryo dose estimates in body CT. AJR Am J Roentgenol 2010; 194(4):874–80.

14. Israel GM, Cicchiello L, Brink J, et al. Patient size and radiation exposure in thoracic, pelvic, and abdominal CT examinations performed with automatic exposure control. AJR Am J Roentgenol 2010;195(6):1342–6.

15. Huda W, He W. Estimating cancer risks to adults undergoing body CT examinations. Radiat Prot Dosimetry 2012;150(2):168–79.

16. Ogden K, Huda W, Scalzetti EM, et al. Patient size and x-ray transmission in body CT. Health Phys 2004;86(4):397–405.

17. Lee ES, Kim SH, Im JP, et al. Effect of different reconstruction algorithms on computer-aided diagnosis (CAD) performance in ultra-low dose CT colonography. Eur J Radiol 2015;84(4):547–54.

18. Lubner MG, Pooler BD, Kitchin DR, et al. Sub-milli-Sievert (sub-mSv) CT colonography: a prospective comparison of image quality and polyp conspicuity at reduced-dose versus standard-dose imaging. Eur Radiol 2015;25(7):2089–102.

19. Nagata K, Fujiwara M, Kanazawa H, et al. Evaluation of dose reduction and image quality in CT colonography: comparison of low-dose CT with iterative reconstruction and routine-dose CT with filtered back projection. Eur Radiol 2015;25(1):221–9.

20. Shin CI, Kim SH, Im JP, et al. One-mSv CT colonography: effect of different iterative reconstruction algorithms on radiologists' performance. Eur J Radiol 2016;85(3):641–8.

21. Cohnen M, Vogt C, Beck A, et al. Feasibility of MDCT colonography in ultra-low-dose technique in the detection of colorectal lesions: comparison with high-resolution video colonoscopy. AJR Am J Roentgenol 2004;183(5):1355–9.

22. Iannaccone R, Catalano C, Mangiapane F, et al. Colorectal polyps: detection with low-dose multi-detector row helical CT colonography versus two sequential colonoscopies. Radiology 2005;237(3):927–37.

23. Iannaccone R, Laghi A, Catalano C, et al. Detection of colorectal lesions: lower-dose multi-detector row helical CT colonography compared with conventional colonoscopy. Radiology 2003;229(3):775–81.

24. van Gelder RE, Venema HW, Serlie IW, et al. CT colonography at different radiation dose levels: feasibility of dose reduction. Radiology 2002; 224(1):25–33.

25. Haaga JR, Miraldi F, MacIntyre W, et al. The effect of mAs variation upon computed tomography image quality as evaluated by in vivo and in vitro studies. Radiology 1981;138(2):449–54.

26. Kalender WA, Wolf H, Suess C. Dose reduction in CT by anatomically adapted tube current modulation. II. Phantom measurements. Med Phys 1999;26(11):2248–53.

27. Yilmaz MH, Albayram S, Yasar D, et al. Female breast radiation exposure during thorax multidetector computed tomography and the effectiveness of bismuth breast shield to reduce breast radiation dose. J Comput Assist Tomogr 2007;31(1):138–42.

28. Lim HK, Lee KH, Kim SY, et al. Does the amount of tagged stool and fluid significantly affect the radiation exposure in low-dose CT colonography performed with an automatic exposure control? Eur Radiol 2011;21(2):345–52.

29. GE Healthcare. Lightspeed VCT technical reference manual. Revised 9th edition. Waukesha (WI): General Electric Company; 2007. p. 25 [Chapter 12].

30. Elojeimy S, Tipnis S, Huda W. Relationship between radiographic techniques (kilovolt and milliampere-second) and CTDI(VOL). Radiat Prot Dosimetry 2010;141(1):43–9.

31. Chang KJ, Caovan DB, Grand DJ, et al. Reducing radiation dose at CT colonography: decreasing kVp to 100 kilovolts. Radiology 2013;266:801–11.

32. Guimaraes LS, Fletcher JG, Harmsen WS, et al. Appropriate patient selection at abdominal dual-energy CT using 80 kV: relationship between patient size, image noise, and image quality. Radiology 2010;257(3):732–42.

33. McCollough CH. Automatic kVp selection. Paper presented at: MGH Radiation Safety in CT Symposium. Boston, MA, January 31, 2012.

34. Thibault JB, Sauer KD, Bouman CA, et al. A three-dimensional statistical approach to improved image quality for multislice helical CT. Med Phys 2007; 34(11):4526–44.

35. Flicek KT, Hara AK, Silva AC, et al. Reducing the radiation dose for CT colonography using adaptive statistical iterative reconstruction: a pilot study. AJR Am J Roentgenol 2010;195(1):126–31.

36. Millerd PJ, Paden RG, Lund JT, et al. Reducing the radiation dose for computed tomography colonography using model-based iterative reconstruction. Abdom Imaging 2014;40(5):1183–9.

37. Chang KJ, Heisler MA, Mahesh M, et al. CT colonography at low tube potential: using iterative reconstruction to decrease noise. Clin Radiol 2015;70(9):981–8.

38. Li J, Udayasankar UK, Toth TL, et al. Automatic patient centering for MDCT: effect on radiation dose. AJR Am J Roentgenol 2007;188(2):547–52.

39. Pickhardt PJ, Bakke J, Kuo J, et al. Volumetric analysis of colonic distention according to patient position at CT colonography: diagnostic value of the right lateral decubitus series. AJR Am J Roentgenol 2014;203(6):W623–8.

40. de Haan MC, Boellaard TN, Bossuyt PM, et al. Colon distension, perceived burden and side-effects of CT-colonography for screening using hyoscine butylbromide or glucagon hydrochloride as bowel relaxant. Eur J Radiol 2012;81(8): e910–6.

41. Morrin MM, Farrell RJ, Keogan MT, et al. CT colonography: colonic distention improved by dual positioning but not intravenous glucagon. Eur Radiol 2002;12(3):525–30.

42. Rogalla P, Lembcke A, Ruckert JC, et al. Spasmolysis at CT colonography: butyl scopolamine versus glucagon. Radiology 2005;236(1):184–8.

43. Yee J, Hung RK, Akerkar GA, et al. The usefulness of glucagon hydrochloride for colonic distention in CT colonography. AJR Am J Roentgenol 1999;173(1): 169–72.

44. Christner JA, Zavaletta VA, Eusemann CD, et al. Dose reduction in helical CT: dynamically adjustable z-axis X-ray beam collimation. AJR Am J Roentgenol 2010;194(1):W49–55.

45. Nakayama Y, Awai K, Funama Y, et al. Abdominal CT with low tube voltage: preliminary observations about radiation dose, contrast enhancement, image quality, and noise. Radiology 2005;237(3):945–51.

Computed Tomography Colonography
Pearls and Pitfalls

David H. Kim, MD[a],*, Courtney C. Moreno, MD[b],
Perry J. Pickhardt, MD[a]

KEYWORDS

- Screening • Colorectal cancer • CT colonography • CT

KEY POINTS

- Computed tomography colonography (CTC) is an optimal test among the accepted screening options. It is highly effective like colonoscopy yet safe similar to stool tests.
- CTC is a multicomponent examination where high-quality technique in bowel preparation, colonic distention, image acquisition, and interpretation lead to accurate polyp detection.
- Contrast coating of the mucosal surface of polyps is a key phenomenon that aids in polyp detection, particularly for those of a flat morphology.
- Active infusion of carbon dioxide during image acquisition is needed to maintain good distention.
- A learning curve exists for accurate polyp detection but is easily achievable with a solid cross-sectional imaging background.

Computed tomography colonography (CTC) is a low radiation dose CT examination with a specialized protocol to optimize detection of intraluminal polyps and masses. Patients typically ingest cathartic and tagging agents in preparation for the examination. The colon is distended with continuous carbon dioxide (CO_2) infusion and the patient is scanned in multiple positions with low radiation dose technique. Images are reviewed in both two-dimensional (2D) and 3D perspectives. The use of CTC in colorectal cancer (CRC) screening has proved to be effective both in detecting the important polyp targets that develop into cancer and for detecting early cancers. Observational studies have shown that the addition of CTC to the existing options can markedly improve CRC screening rates.[1,2] This article serves as a practical reference to optimize CTC performance in the detection of colorectal neoplasia. A specific protocol in use in 2 clinical programs as well as defined interpretation strategies will be described. Within this framework, various clinical pearls as well as pitfalls to avoid will be a major focus of this article.

CASE FOR THE OPTIMAL SCREENING TEST

Currently, there are several screening options for CRC screening (Table 1). In part, this has developed because no one test is perfect, each holding certain advantages and disadvantages. For example, proponents of colonoscopy have

---

Disclosure Statement: D.H. Kim: Cofounder of VirtuoCTC; shareholder for Elucent and Cellectar. C.C. Moreno: none. P.J. Pickhardt: Cofounder of VirtuoCTC; consultant for Bracco, Check-Cap; shareholder Elucent, Cellectar, Shine.
[a] Department of Radiology, University of Wisconsin School of Medicine and Public Health, E3/311 Clinical Science Center, 600 Highland Avenue, Madison, WI 53792-3252, USA; [b] Department of Radiology and Imaging Sciences, Emory University School of Medicine, 1365 Clifton Road, Northeast, Atlanta, GA 30322, USA
* Corresponding author.
E-mail address: dkim@uwhealth.org

Radiol Clin N Am 56 (2018) 719–735
https://doi.org/10.1016/j.rcl.2018.05.004

Table 1
Options for colorectal cancer screening

Screening Method	Frequency	Comments
Fecal occult blood test	Every y	Primarily detects early cancers not precancerous lesions; lowest risk profile
Fecal immunochemical test	Every y	Primarily detects early cancers not precancerous lesions; lowest risk profile
Stool DNA	Every 3 y	Primarily detects early cancers not precancerous lesions; lowest risk profile
Colonoscopy	Every 10 y	Detects precancerous lesions and cancers; risk present albeit low for perforations and sedation-related complications
Flexible sigmoidoscopy	Every 5 y	Detects precancerous lesions and cancers; only left colon examined
CTC	Every 5 y	Detects precancerous lesions and cancers; risk profile minimal

advocated for this test due to its better performance compared with stool studies. On the other hand, stool studies have been touted as the better option due to its noninvasive nature without the perforation and sedation complications that are possible at colonoscopy.

The recent inclusion of CTC to the United States Preventive Services Task Force (USPSTF) list of approved tests may change this situation over time.[3] The case can be made that CTC represents the optimal test for CRC screening where the balance between test effectiveness versus test safety is best achieved by CTC. Regarding effectiveness, CTC is similar to colonoscopy where it can detect both benign polyp precursors that may develop into cancer in the future as well as early CRC. The sensitivity and specificity for large polyps ($\geq$10 mm) ranges between 90% to 94% and 86% to 96%, respectively.[4,5] For cancer detection, CTC has a sensitivity of 96.1%.[6] In contrast, although stool studies can detect early cancers, the sensitivity for large polyps/advanced adenomas by fecal occult blood test (FOBT)/fecal immunochemical test (FIT) is poor at 22% to 40%.[7] This is not surprising because polyps do not typically bleed. Likewise, stool DNA tests have similar poor sensitivity at 42%.[8] There is little doubt that the ability to detect these precursor lesions markedly leverages CTC effectiveness over those tests that can only detect early cancers (ie, FOBT/FIT).

CTC has an excellent safety profile, closer to stool tests than that of colonoscopy. The low-pressure insufflation used for CTC carries a very low risk for perforation. Whereas rates for perforation at colonoscopy are at about 1 per thousand procedures, the rate at CTC is near nonexistent at 0.04% for screening patients.[9] Furthermore, CTC does not require sedation like colonoscopy, obviating the potential complications related to anesthetic medications. There have been initial theoretic concerns regarding future cancer induction from radiation, but similar dose exposures in other populations strongly suggest that clinically significant risk likely does not exist.[10–12] The Health Physics society argues against estimating health risks for exposure similar or below background levels (which would include levels for CTC screening) because the statistical uncertainties at these low levels are great.[13] For these reasons, a case can be made that CTC represents the optimal test within the menu of options for CRC screening.

THE TECHNICAL ASPECTS OF THE COMPUTED TOMOGRAPHY COLONOGRAPHY EXAMINATION

CTC is a multicomponent examination that includes specific patient activities before actual scanning is undertaken. The examination can be divided into bowel preparation, colonic distention, and image acquisition. There are numerous protocols in current use in undertaking CTC, each with advantages and various trade-offs. The specific protocol described in the following paragraphs has been validated in 2 large-scale clinical programs (n >16,000 patients). The protocol is optimized for average risk CRC screening in the healthy asymptomatic individual. With this framework in place, clinical observations and specific pitfalls to avoid gained from daily clinical use will be discussed to help shorten the CTC learning curve for optimal polyp detection.

Bowel Preparation

The bowel preparation begins 1 day before the scheduled examination (Table 2). The purpose is two-fold: (1) to clear the colon of any bulk material

Table 2	
Bowel preparation schedule	
Time (Beginning 1 d Prior to Scheduled Examination)	**Preparation**
12:00 AM	Liquid diet only
11:00 AM	2 bisacodyl tablets (stool softener)
3:00–5:00 PM	1 bottle (296 mL) magnesium citrate
6:00–8:00 PM (3 h after prior step)	1 bottle (296 mL) magnesium citrate 1 bottle (225 mL) 2% w/v barium sulfate
9:00–11:00 PM (3 h after prior step)	1 bottle (60 mL) iohexol

that may mimic or obscure a polyp or mass and (2) to tag any residual material or fluid in the colon. The patient is on a liquid-only diet beginning at midnight the day before the scheduled CTC examination. At 11:00 AM, 2 tablets of bisacodyl, a stool softener, are given. The patient is encouraged to maintain hydration throughout the day. At 3 to 5 PM, the patient begins the cathartic portion of the preparation with ingestion of one bottle of 10 ounces (296 mL) magnesium citrate. Three hours later, the second bottle of 10 ounces of magnesium citrate is ingested. In addition, the first contrast tagging agent of 2% w/v barium (225 mL) is taken at this time. Three hours later, the second tagging iodine-based agent is taken, and the bowel preparation is complete.

There are a few important points to highlight with the bowel preparation. First, because the cathartic portion does not begin until the afternoon (eg, this could be as late as 5 PM), the patient does not need to take a day off before the CTC examination for the bowel preparation. For working patients, it is a large benefit not to have to take multiple days off for the screening examination. Second, magnesium citrate is a cathartic agent that works by drawing fluid into the colonic lumen due to its osmotic nature. Thus, it is important that the patient is well hydrated for the agent to work optimally. Otherwise, the catharsis will be poor leading to adherent residual stool (see Pearls and Pitfalls section).

Colonic Distention

The second major technical component of CTC is colonic distention. Filling the colon with a gas separates opposing mucosal surfaces to allow detection of soft tissue lesions. This is best accomplished with automated CO_2 insufflation via a dedicated CTC insufflator (see Clinical Pearls section). The patient is placed in a left lateral decubitus position on the CT scanner table. A soft rectal catheter is placed, and the balloon is carefully inflated. The patient remains in a left lateral decubitus position for infusion of a volume of about 1.5 to 2.0 L and then patient is rolled to a right lateral decubitus position for infusion of another 1.5 to 2.0 L. At this point when the volume infused is about 4 L, the patient is then rolled supine. During the insufflation, the pressures will measure 13 to 18 mm Hg during filling and may transiently increase to 30 to 40 mm Hg with colonic spasm. When the pressures settle in the mid-20's mm Hg range and the volumes are greater than 4 L, the patient is likely optimally filled (**Fig. 1**). These values represent the trigger to scout and to

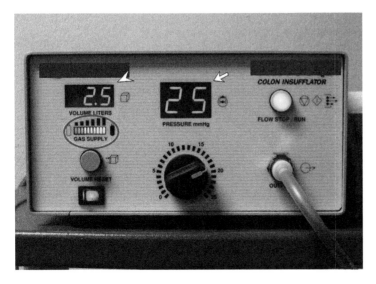

Fig. 1. Automated colonic insufflator. Image of the control panel shows the volume (*arrowhead*) and pressure (*arrow*) readings that give real-time feedback and allow easy determination when the colon is optimally distended. Note the "gas supply" meter (*open red circle*), which shows the status of the CO_2 tanks. When in the red range, the tank is nearly empty and often the insufflation is suboptimal (see Pearls and Pitfalls section).

perform the supine scan. The acquired images are assessed for adequacy of distention and coverage while the patient is rolled to a prone position. The rectal balloon should be deflated to allow one series where the distal rectum is not obscured. After a short delay, if the pressure values remain in the mid-20's mm Hg range, the prone scout and scan can be obtained with subsequent assessment for quality. Additional decubitus series can be undertaken if needed.[14]

Some points to note about insufflation. The ability to use pressure and volume measurements as surrogate measures to determine distention adequacy to begin scanning leads to reproducibly excellent distention. Relying on a set number of puffs and/or patient feedback to determine distention, as is done with manual room air administration, is not consistently reliable. In addition, the absolute volume displayed on the insufflator device control panel does not reflect how much is in the colon. The displayed volume simply reflects how much has passed through the machine (see Clinical Pearls section). The number typically ranges up to 6 to 8 L but 10 to 12 L can occur. And finally, the use of CO_2 minimizes postprocedure discomfort, because this gas is actively resorbed across the colonic mucosa. In the authors' experience, any discomfort that the patient is experiencing from distention almost immediately abates as soon as the machine is turned off. This is unlike room air administration where the patient can feel bloated and uncomfortable for several hours after distention.

Image Acquisition

The third technical component involves image acquisition and scanning parameters. Breath-held volumetric acquisition with thin collimation (1–1.25 mm with overlap) with isotropic or near isotropic voxels is key for a quality examination. No intravenous contrast is given for screening CTC, and scans are obtained in end expiration to minimize pressure effects on the transverse colon by the inflated lungs. The patient is typically scanned in 2 positions, once supine and the second prone.[15] Additional decubitus imaging is performed as needed.

There are a few points to highlight with image acquisition. The hardware and scanning requirements for CTC are forgiving, allowing even older scanners to be useful for this examination. The organ of interest (ie, the colon) is relatively static and does not require high temporal resolution such as in cardiac applications. In addition, there is high contrast between the soft tissue polyp target of 6 mm or greater in size and the air-filled lumen.

Thus, even older 16 slice scanners can perform high-quality CTC with thin imaging yet reasonable length breath-holds. And second, because of the low dose technique, beam hardening can create artifacts leading to characteristic imaging pitfalls (see Pitfalls section).

Interpretation at Computed Tomography Colonography

Interpretation strategies have evolved over time. There is now general consensus that the images should be viewed from both 2D and 3D perspectives to optimize the detection and characterization of colorectal polyps and masses. The reasons will be discussed further in the Clinical Pearls section. The primary 2D approach involves interactively scrolling through a stack of thin-slice CTC transverse images in polyp windows (Window 2000 HU, Level 0 HU), in a manner similar to reading standard CT. The colon is traced in a retrograde fashion from the rectum to the cecum for all obtained series. The reader searches for focal soft tissue projections into the lumen, which may represent polyps while excluding haustral folds, which protrude into the colonic lumen.

The primary 3D approach involves viewing postprocessed data that are presented from a 3D perspective. Some examples include the endoluminal fly-through, perspective filet, unfolded cube, and band view with the endoluminal fly-through as the most commonly used and validated view. The reader "flies" from the rectum to the cecum and then from the cecum to the rectum. This allows visualization of both sides of colonic folds. The process is repeated for all series. A 3D view radically changes the perspective of the dataset from the 2D approach where it is easier to recognize polypoid morphology as a mental 3D translation that is required for 2D viewing is not needed.

All potential polyps that are identified by 2D and 3D approaches are ultimately evaluated for 2 basic criteria: (1) a fixed position from the colonic mucosa and (2) a soft tissue core (Fig. 2). If a candidate does not meet these requirements, then a pseudopolyp due to stool is a possibility. Several pitfalls can affect this determination. Herein lies the learning curve and ultimately determinates the skill of the reader. For example, some colonic segments can shift in position between supine and prone positioning, such as the sigmoid colon that is tortuous and on a mesentery. Thus, it can be difficult to determine if the polyp candidate is moving in relation to gravity within the colon or if fixed in location arising from the same point in the sigmoid where underlying colon has moved.

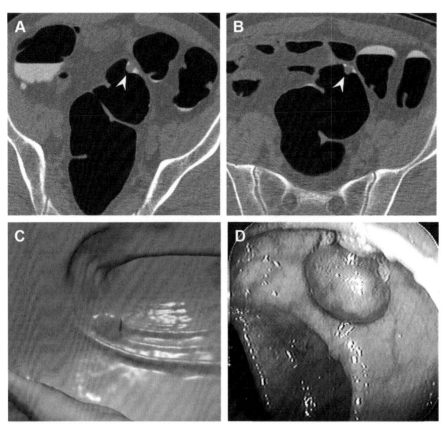

Fig. 2. A 55-year-old man with potential polyp detected in sigmoid colon at CTC. 2D transverse images (*A*, supine; *B*, prone) show that the polyp candidate (*arrowhead*) is fixed in location along the left anterior wall of the proximal sigmoid. If stool, this should fall to a dependent location. The 2D images both show a gray soft tissue core as would be expected with a true polyp. 3D CTC image (*C*) shows the sessile morphology. Colonoscopic image (*D*) mirrors the CTC finding, which was a tubular adenoma at histology.

It requires a strong cross-sectional skill set to make this determination accurately, using the few internal landmarks (ie, distance from similar bends, from a specific diverticulum, etc.) as reference points (Fig. 3).

PEARLS AND PITFALLS OF COMPUTED TOMOGRAPHY COLONOGRAPHY

More than a decade of clinical use has highlighted important observations and developed best practices regarding CTC. Along with knowledge of various pearls and pitfalls to avoid, these tips will help improve CTC interpretation. These pointers involve both technical and interpretative topics. Knowledge of these issues should help decrease the learning curve for expertise in CTC interpretation.

Mucosal Surface Oral Contrast Coating of Polyps

This serendipitous phenomenon is perhaps the most important gleaned clinical pearl that was

not expected early in the CTC experience. A not uncommon occurrence is adherence of the oral tagging agent on the mucosal surface of polyps. Initially, this was considered a potential pitfall where a polyp may be obscured by the contrast or mistaken as partially tagged stool. Over time, it has become apparent that contrast coating is an important aid for the detection of polyps, particularly of flat morphology. It allows easy detection of polyps as well as increases confidence that a true soft tissue lesion exists.

With experience, it becomes evident that polyps with a sessile or pedunculated morphology are easy to detect and do not pose interpretative difficulty without the need for contrast coating. Most polyps are of this protruding morphology as most cancers arise from an adenomatous lineage[16] (which tend to be of this morphology). Flat polyps, however, can be subtle as they are plaquelike lesions only minimally raised from the colonic surface (ie, 3 mm or less) (Fig. 4). Contrast coating is the main way that these lesions are detected. It is important to detect flat polyps because it is

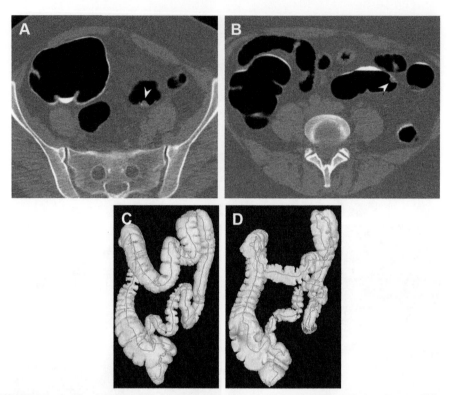

Fig. 3. Difficulties in confirming a true polyp. Supine 2D transverse CTC image (*A*) shows a possible soft tissue polyp in the sigmoid colon (*arrowhead*). Note how it is on the posterior wall, which could be in a dependent location in relation to gravity. Prone 2D transverse CTC image (*B*) shows the possible polyp (*arrowhead*) on the anterior wall, suggesting that it has moved to a dependent location from gravity. This candidate represents a true polyp that is fixed in position with the underlying colon moving on a mesentery. Note shift and rotation of the sigmoid colon between supine (*C*) and prone (*D*) 3D maps. The red dot marks the position of the polyp that remains at the same bend.

now known that around 25% of cancers arise from serrated lesions, which typically present as flat polyps.[17] The sessile serrated polyp (SSP) is a recently discovered cancer precursor separate from the main precursor lesion of the adenomatous polyp (ie, tubular adenoma, tubulovillous adenoma, and villous adenoma). Unfortunately, the terminology is confusing where SSPs are also called sessile serrated adenomas, which suggest an adenomatous histologic lineage, which they are not.[18] SSPs are in the serrated polyp family that includes the benign hyperplastic polyp. In fact, this lesion previously had been mistaken histologically for a hyperplastic polyp but is now recognized as a discrete entity. SSPs are typically flat, large (greater than 10 mm in size), and reside in the right colon.[19,20]

Mucin produced by polyps (particularly villous lesions or flat polyps of serrated histology) plays a major role in this coating phenomenon (see **Fig. 4**). Serrated polyps are known to elaborate various mucoproteins that adhere to the surface

of the polyp.[21] It is theorized that the tagging agents in the CTC bowel preparations interact with this mucin to then create an adherent contrast plaque overlying the polyp (**Fig. 5**). This coat can range from a thin film of contrast to several millimeters thick with an average thickness of 1.5 mm.[22] It is not certain which of the tagging agents contribute to the contrast coat—although it is surmised that barium is the major component. Furthermore, it is unknown whether a dry or wet cathartic agent affects the incidence of coating. What is known is that a specific protocol of a dry osmotic cathartic agent (ie, magnesium citrate) paired with dual tagging of 2% w/v barium sulfate and water-soluble iodine (ie, diatrizoate or iohexol) is the bowel regimen that has demonstrated that this phenomenon consistently occurs and can be used to optimize interpretation.[22] Studies from the barium enema era have suggested an interaction between the magnesium cation and barium sulfate that could promote coating.[23] Although other CTC bowel preparations may lead to this

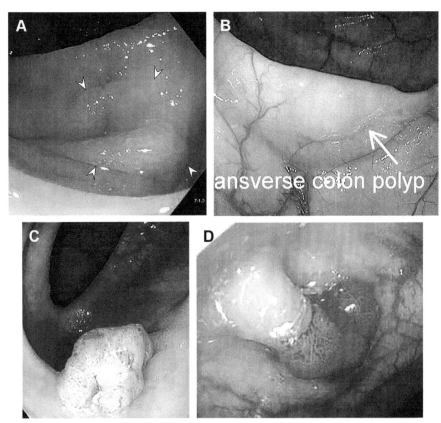

Fig. 4. CTC-detected polyps of various morphologies. Colonoscopic image (*A*) shows a polyp (*arrowheads*) with flat morphology initially detected at CTC. Note how this polyp is only mildly raised from the mucosal surface with minimal soft tissue bulk. If not for contrast coating (which has been washed off before the colonoscopic image), it would be difficult to detect this polyp. Colonoscopic image (*B*) shows overlying adherent yellowish mucin on the flat polyp, which plays a role in contrast coating. In contrast, polyps of sessile (*C*) or pedunculated (*D*) morphologies are easily detected without contrast coating given their soft tissue bulk.

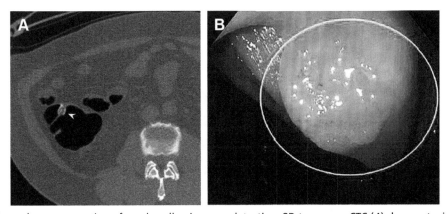

Fig. 5. Mucosal contrast coating of a polyp allowing easy detection. 2D transverse CTC (*A*) shows a typical case of a coated SSP (*arrowhead*) in the ascending colon. Note how this plaque draws attention to this area from the rest of the colon to allow later scrutiny and confirmation. Without this plaque, it would be difficult to detect subtle mucosal thickening of flat polyps. After confirmation, the patient was sent to colonoscopy (*B*) for removal of the flat SSP (*circle*) later that afternoon.

phenomenon, there have been no published series to date. The substitution for a wet-based preparation such as polyethylene glycol or use of a single iodinated tagging agent such as iohexol and the occurrence of contrast coating is unknown.

Without contrast coating, the detection of flat polyps is difficult, tedious, and less accurate, requiring careful scrutiny for minimal focal thickening of the colonic surface. These lesions are similarly subtle at 3D. However, the presence of contrast coating transforms the interpretative process into an easy stepwise process where these lesions are easily detected and confirmed. At 2D, the colon can be quickly scanned for flat plaques of contrast in a soft tissue window setting. The white contrast plaques are obvious against the gray soft tissue wall. These are easily seen without tedious concentration unlike if the colon was scanned for minimal mucosal irregularities of similar attenuation. At 3D, these lesions seem sessile in appearance with the combination of the overlying adherent contrast. Once a contrast plaque is seen, it can be put into a queue for further evaluation.

To confirm the presence of a coated flat polyp and distinguish from tagged stool, the candidate must fulfill a few criteria where again the phenomenon of contrast coating is helpful. First, like any possible polyp, the candidate must be fixed in location on the supine and prone series. Tagged stool typically slides to a dependent location although can be adherent to the wall at times. If fixed in position, the contrast plaque needs to be carefully scrutinized for minimal soft tissue thickening undermining the contrast on both views. When present, this then represents a true coated flat polyp (**Fig. 6**). In short, although there is a learning curve, the interpretative process is straightforward and accurate.

Pitfalls that can affect interpretation related to contrast coating are technical in nature. The use of lesional contrast coating is hampered in situations where the normal colonic mucosa is lined by residual contrast tagged stool (**Fig. 7**). Thus, the search for contrast plaques is difficult if not impossible. For an osmotic "dry" cathartic, this can occur if the patient is relatively dehydrated, affecting the cleansing ability of the cathartic. The effluent that cleanses the colon in part is made up of these fluids. It is important that the patient be well hydrated before starting the bowel preparation and remains hydrated during the preparation. The patients are urged to ingest 4 to 6 glasses of water before starting the bowel preparation and to continue to ingest a similar amount over the course of the preparation. Contrast lining

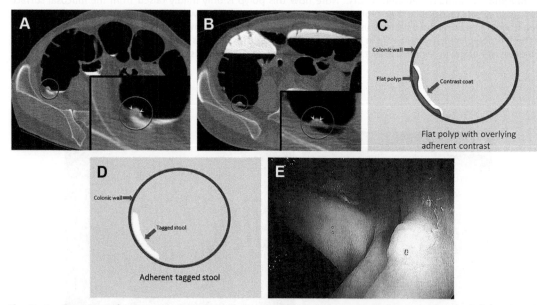

Fig. 6. Confirmation of suspected coated polyp. Transverse 2D CTC images (*A*, supine; *B*, prone) show that the contrast plaque (*red circles*) are in the same location despite changes in patient positions. Note the minimal soft tissue undermining the coat (*arrowheads in inset*). The presence of this border (*red line* in diagram, *C*) confirms a coated polyp and excludes the main differential entity of tagged stool where it is not present where the border parallels the concave surface of the colonic lumen (*yellow line*, *D*). An SSP was resected at colonoscopy (*E*). (*From* Kim DH, Lubner MG, Cahoon AR, et al. Flat serrated polyps at CT colonography: relevance, appearance, and optimizing interpretation. Radiographics 2018;38:70; with permission.)

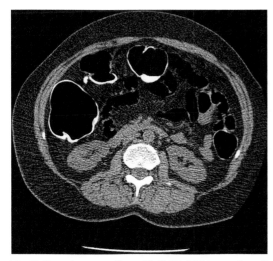

Fig. 7. Bowel preparation pitfall. 2D CTC image in soft tissue windows shows tagging contrast agents lining the colonic mucosa in the right colon. This occurs when there is poor cleansing with adherent tagged stool in the right colon or when the tagging agents are reversed in order. Note how it becomes impossible to use the presence of contrast plaques to help identify flat polyps in this situation.

normal mucosa can also happen in a situation where the patient reverses the order of the tagging agents (iodine-based agent before the barium). The reasoning behind this phenomenon is not known but often leads to a characteristic smooth coating of the right colon (see **Fig. 7**).

Distention and Tips on Carbon Dioxide Use

Colonic distention is key for quality CTC interpretation. Underdistention can obscure polyps as well as create pseudolesions. The use of automated low-pressure CO_2 insufflation has resulted in a marked improvement from prior manual administration of room air.[24,25] Room air often led to poorly distended colons because it was difficult to determine when the patient was optimally filled, given individual variability in colonic volume. Because direct monitoring was not available at CT as with fluoroscopy during a barium enema, distention adequacy was assessed in part by patient tolerance that may not correlate with maximal colonic distention. Automated CO_2 instillation allows for more consistency in distention where volume measurements and pressure measurements serve as useful surrogate markers for colonic distention.[25] When certain levels are reached (ie, volume measurements of 4 L and pressure equilibrium of mid-20's), the scan can be initiated with confidence that the colon will be optimally distended (see **Fig. 1**). In general, for optimal colonic

distention, it is helpful to wait until at least 4 L have passed through the machine. Often, pressure measurements suggesting equilibrium are seen at 2 L but often the colon is not maximally distended and needs to be distended to a greater degree, leading to easier interpretation of the examination (**Fig. 8**).

There are a few important observations to highlight regarding CO_2 use to maximize distention. Perhaps most important is that CO_2 should be actively infusing while the CTC images are acquired. Unlike room air, which is composed mainly of nitrogen that is unable to be effectively absorbed by the colonic mucosa, CO_2 is resorbed across the colonic mucosa and into the bloodstream, ultimately eliminated via exhalation.[26] Thus, active infusion is needed to balance CO_2 loss even if there is no reflux into the small bowel or loss around the rectal catheter. An equilibrium is ultimately achieved between infusion and loss. Consequently, if CO_2 is not continually infusing during image acquisition and is instead stopped for several seconds/minutes before imaging, the colon will be underdistended at imaging. On the other hand, adequate distention can be achieved even in the face of an ileocecal anastomosis with ongoing reflux into the small bowel. As long as the CO_2 is continuously infusing, an equilibrium can be reached for good colonic distention (**Fig. 9**).

Secondly, it is important not to equate the volume recorded by the machine with the amount in the colon. Some have erroneously conflated the two and thought that certain volume levels would increase the risk for perforation. The number is simply the volume that passed through the machine but not the amount in the colon because there is a continuing ongoing loss of CO_2 as discussed earlier. Instead, the pressure measurements are important to monitor (along with patient discomfort). During the filling phase, the pressures typically measure 13 to 19 mm Hg. There may be transient spasm with pressures ranging from 30 to 40 mm Hg, but this typically decreases after several seconds. At equilibrium the pressures are in the mid-20's mm Hg. If there are continued constant pressure increases in the 30 to 50's, then decreasing CO_2 instillation or stopping the infusion is suggested. As a side note, there are safety mechanisms built in where the insufflator should stop instilling after several seconds at 50 mm Hg with a mechanical pressure valve release at 75 mm Hg to prevent colonic perforation.

And finally, it is important to not mistake the phenomenon of asymptomatic colonic pneumatosis for perforation. This observed event has

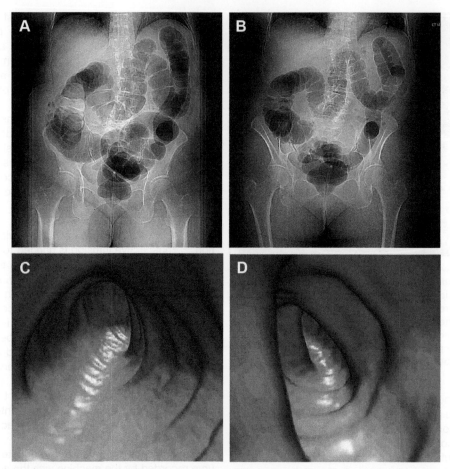

Fig. 8. Colonic distention. CTC scout (*A*) from a screening CTC demonstrates excellent distention where scanning was begun when pressures equilibrated at 22 to 25 mm Hg with volume at 4 L. Note the widely open lumen at 3D (*B*). The patient returned for routine screening 5 years later. CTC scout (*C*) shows a less distended colon where the pressure and volume measurements were 22 to 25 mmHG and 2 L, respectively. Because the scan was started earlier at the 2 L mark, the colon is less distended. Note that although diagnostic, the examination becomes more difficult to read because the haustral folds are not as effaced and crowded together (*D*).

been seen at a rate of 0.1% in screening patients with CO_2 distention.[27] These patients show curvilinear air in the bowel wall in the right colon of varying circumferential degree. Unlike true colonic perforation, the patients are asymptomatic and do not require any treatment. This finding is thought to be related to the increased diffusability of CO_2, possibly augmented by mucosal microtrauma from cathartic preparation (**Fig. 10**).

Pitfalls leading to decreased distention are often obvious but some situations are not initially apparent. The most common cause is obstruction of the CO_2 inflow from a fluid column in the tubing that manifests by a frozen number on the machine panel. Typically, there is variation in pressure measurements and slowly increasing volume numbers with insufflation. Problem solving requires an assessment of the tubing from the patient to the machine. If there is too much fluid in the tubing obstructing inflow, then milking the fluid back to the collection bag to clear the tubing will then allow CO_2 infusion. It may be helpful to stop the scan to allow the patient to use the restroom to attempt to expel any residual fluid in the rectum and distal colon (**Fig. 11**). Although the cause for decreased distention can often easily be determined with systematic problem solving, another situation that may not be readily obvious is a low-pressure tank (see **Fig. 1**). When nearly empty, the tanks do not generate enough pressure and can lead to underdistention. It can be a confusing situation where no obvious block or narrowing in the tubing is seen and there are no intrinsic patient factors that could leave to decreased colonic distensibility such as diverticular myochosis. If the control panel confirms that the tanks are low, it may be helpful to switch out to full tanks. In many cases, the

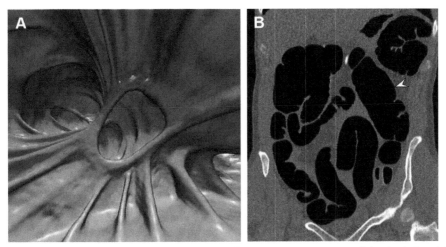

Fig. 9. Screening CTC in an individual with a prior ileocolonic anastomosis. 3D endoluminal view (A) shows a widely patent anastomosis. Coronal 2D CTC image (B) shows excellent distention of the colon (*arrowhead*, transverse colon) despite ongoing reflux into the small bowel.

distension will improve as more instillation pressure is generated.

Distension and Use of Decubitus Series

Decubitus series may be added to the standard supine and prone positions or can even primarily substitute for the standard series in specific situations.[14,28] Decubitus series allow evaluation of a segment of colon that is collapsed and unable to be evaluated on the standard views. The positioning on a person's side takes off the pressure effects on the colon from the body (particularly seen on the prone series), leading to improved distention. Initially, the authors attempted to select the decubitus view (right lateral or left lateral) that would be optimal to evaluate a collapsed segment. For example, if the descending colon was collapsed, a right lateral decubitus was selected to place the descending colon in the nondependent position, whereas a left lateral decubitus was used for the right colon. However, a right lateral decubitus (right side down) works well for any segment of the colon, including, paradoxically, the cecum. The cecal apex fills on this view despite being in a dependent location due to its small mesentery that allows mobility within the abdomen (Fig. 12). Thus, when there is a collapsed segment, there is no need to decide which decubitus view to select. Instead, once the decision is made for additional sequences, the authors start with a right lateral decubitus followed by a left lateral decubitus if needed.

Although decubitus views are typically used as additional problem solving series, they can be used primarily to replace one or both of the

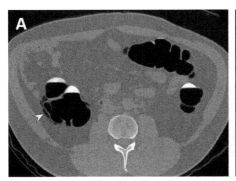
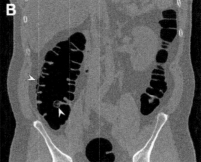

Fig. 10. Asymptomatic colonic pneumatosis. Transverse (A) and coronal (B) 2D CTC images show a typical right-sided distribution of pneumatosis (*arrowheads*) that can infrequently occur in otherwise asymptomatic persons. If not for this imaging finding, the patient would be completely unaware. No interventions or supportive measures are needed as was the case for this patient.

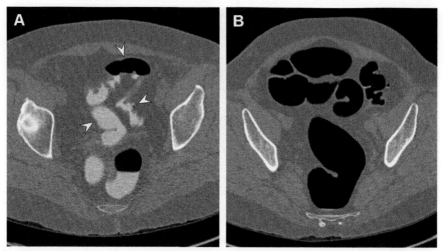

Fig. 11. Fluid block. Transverse 2D CTC image (*A*) shows large amounts of residual contrasted fluid in the colon. This typically occurs because the bowel preparation was started late. Note the poor sigmoid distention (*arrowheads*) due to the intracolonic fluid blocks. Fluid in the colon or tubing can cause obstruction to CO_2 inflow because the infusion is low pressure in nature. 2D CTC image (*B*) after allowing the patient after a delay of a few hours and use of the restroom shows clearance of the fluid and excellent distention.

standard supine/prone series. Common situations include patients who cannot tolerate prone positioning either due to a stoma or due to obesity. For obesity, often the prone series is limited by underdistension by the pressure exerted by the patient's girth, particularly on the transverse colon. There is one major drawback for a primary supine/right lateral decubitus series. The lack of "opposite positioning" as present in a supine/prone combination minimizes intraluminal movement where it can be difficult to determine if the lack of movement of an object is due to a fixed location of a polyp or of adherent stool. Thus, if a right lateral

decubitus is substituted, it can be helpful to have the patient rotate in the opposite direction 270° as opposed to simply turning 90°. And finally, when patients are morbidly obese, it may be worthwhile to substitute bilateral decubiti series for the standard series primarily.

Use of Both 2D and 3D Imaging for Interpretation

The optimal strategy involves evaluating the CTC supine and prone datasets (and decubitus when obtained) from both a 2D and a 3D perspective.

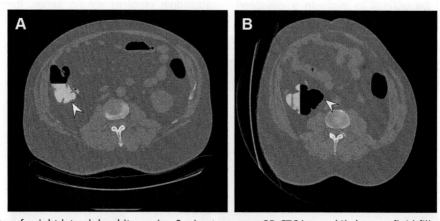

Fig. 12. Use of a right lateral decubitus series. Supine transverse 2D CTC image (*A*) shows a fluid-filled underdistended cecum (*arrowhead*), which was collapsed on the prone series (not shown). Although counter-intuitive, a right lateral decubitus (*B*) is the best option to evaluate the cecum and cecal apex (*B, arrowhead*). The right colon and particularly the cecum optimally fills due to the mobility of the cecal mesentery that allows CO_2 to collect as it rises to a nondependent area.

It is clearly evident that the 2 perspectives are complementary where some polyps are more easily seen at one perspective than the other where the polyp can be almost invisible. Specifically, polyps can project off a haustral fold in a manner that makes it easy to misperceive as an extension of the fold at 2D. Or, the polyp comes off at angle from the colonic mucosa relative to the 2D axial review that makes it look like a fold. In both cases, these polyps are easily recognized at 3D. Similarly, submerged polyps not visible at 3D (without electronic cleansing, which the authors avoid) are easily seen within the tagged fluid pool at 2D (Fig. 13). By combining both approaches, it is difficult to miss clinically significant polyps.

Workstations used to interpret CTC should be seamless to work in each environment, performing basic functions such as measuring, bookmarking locations of interest, changing window/level (2D), field of view (3D), percent mucosa seen (3D), etc. But perhaps the most important

functionality that may not be initially obvious relates to the need at CTC to work interactively between both environments. It is imperative that a workstation allows the ability to localize one point on the 2D image with the specific same point on the 3D image and the reverse. Currently, many CTC workstations can efficiently undertake the first situation but few can do the latter well. In other words, when a potential polyp is seen at 2D, most workstations can easily show what the area looks like at 3D. However, when an abnormality is seen at 3D, many workstations can show the axial slice that correlates with the identified area of interest at 3D but not the specific point on the 2D image that the 3D imaging is showing. It can be cumbersome to ultimately determine the specific correlative point at 2D. Without this easy functionality, it is difficult to incorporate the primary 3D perspective into the interpretation process (Fig. 14).

Of the interpretative pitfalls, there are 2 in particular to highlight because they are a not uncommon

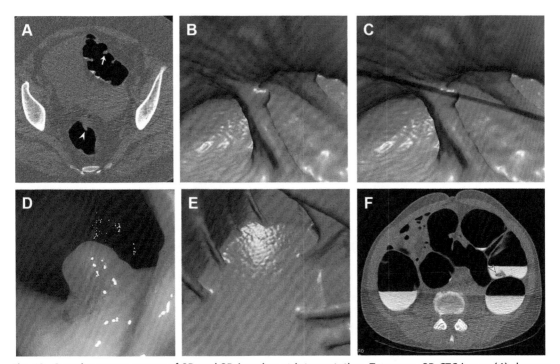

Fig. 13. Complementary nature of 2D and 3D imaging at interpretation. Transverse 2D CTC image (*A*) shows a structure projecting into the lumen (*arrowhead*), which could be easily mistaken as a rectal fold during 2D review. Note how it mirrors other folds such as in the sigmoid (*arrow*). However, this polyp is easily recognized at 3D (*B*). 3D endoluminal CTC image with 2D correlating line (*C*) reveals the reason for the difficulty at 2D, related to the orientation of the 2D images to the polyp. Interactive scrolling in this plane leads to the appearance that the polyp is a part of the fold. Colonoscopic image (*D*) shows the true polypoid nature of the polyp detected at CTC. 3D endoluminal CTC image (*E*) in a different patient misses a polyp submerged in a pool of residual contrasted fluid. Here, the 2D image compensates for the 3D "miss" where a 2D review would easily detect this soft tissue polyp (*arrowhead*) within the contrast fluid pool (*F*).

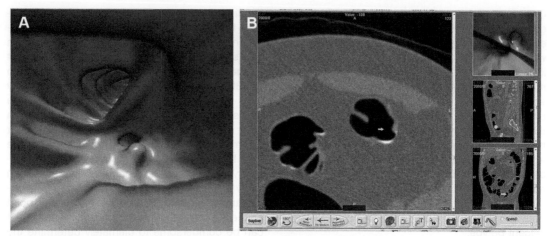

Fig. 14. 3D/2D correlation. 3D CTC endoluminal view (*A*) shows a possible polyp adjacent to a diverticulum. It is important that the specific point on 2D is easily determined. Image of a workstation (*B*) shows that the 2D correlate to the 3D finding is easily determined. The red line on the 3D image in the upper right corner determines that the axial slice is through the structure of concern and the blue arrow on the 2D image shows the specific point the 3D image is depicting.

occurrence. If unaware of these issues, erroneous conclusions can be easily drawn and negatively affect interpretations. Both are related to characterization or confirmation of suspected polyps.

The first is related to movement of the underlying colon. When a segment is on a mesentery such as the sigmoid, it is easy to see that the underlying colon may shift between patient positions.

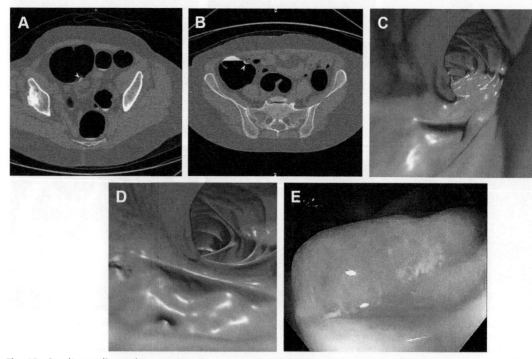

Fig. 15. Cecal/ascending colon rotation. Transverse 2D CTC images (*A*, supine; *B*, prone) show a coated polyp in the ascending colon (*arrowhead*). Note how the coated polyp is in a dependent location on both views, which could lead to the incorrect assessment that the abnormality is tagged stool moving in response to gravity. 3D endoluminal CTC image (*C*) from the supine series shows the relationship between the polyp and ileocecal valve, which remains constant on the prone 3D image (*D*). Thus, cecal/ascending counterclockwise rotation accounts for the 2D images. Colonoscopic image (*E*) shows the SSP resected later that afternoon.

However, the cecum and ascending colon can also move, which may not be initially obvious without careful scrutiny. *There is a characteristic rotation of the right colon in a counter-clockwise direction when the patient moves from a supine position to prone position*[29,30] (**Fig. 15**). It often makes a polyp appear to move to a dependent location from gravity. If unaware that this actually represents rotation of the underlying colon, then the conclusion that the polyp represents mobile stool could be made. It is important to recognize this as colonic movement to come to the correct determination that the polyp candidate represents a true polyp. Given the right-sided propensity of serrated neoplasms, this is an important observation because removal of these lesions can prevent a future cancer.

The second pitfall is related to the low radiation dose nature of the CTC examination. It requires only a fraction of the dose of the typical CT examination, given the target size of 6 mm in a high contrast environment. The lowered dose, however, can affect on the appearance of the polyp where the typical homogenous soft tissue core is not seen. Instead, the polyp can be heterogenous or even fatty in appearance due to volume averaging or streak artifact. This is accentuated for flat polyps where there is minimal bulk to the polyp (**Fig. 16**). Once recognized, this pitfall is easily compensated by the phenomenon of lesional contrast coating where such lesions that exhibit an overlying coat represent a true polyp despite a heterogeneous, streaky appearance without an apparent soft tissue core.

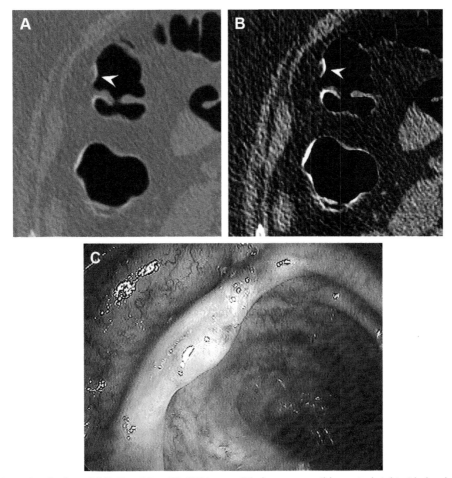

Fig. 16. Beam hardening pitfall. Decubitus 2D CTC image (*A*) shows a possible coated right-sided polyp (*arrowhead*). Note the marked low attenuation core (*arrowhead*) on soft tissue windows (*B*). A SSP seen at colonoscopy (*C*). Recognition of this artifact in combination with the presence of an overlying contrast coat should prevent an incorrect interpretation of lipoma or stool. (*From* Kim DH, Lubner MG, Cahoon AR, et al. Flat serrated polyps at CT colonography: relevance, appearance, and optimizing interpretation. Radiographics 2018;38:70; with permission.)

SUMMARY

CTC is a powerful tool in CRC screening. An argument can be made that it represents the best test out of the menu of options, given its ability to prevent cancer from polyp detection as well as to detect early cancers. CTC is as effective as colonoscopy yet holds a safety profile similar to noninvasive stool tests. The clinical experience over the past decade has helped to develop best practices and recognize clinical pearls to avoid pitfalls that negatively affect interpretation. The phenomenon of lesional contrast coating is key in improving detection and confirmation of polyps, particularly those with a flat morphology. A specific bowel preparation using a dry cathartic and dual tagging has been shown to promote this coating. Optimizing distention includes continuous infusion of CO_2 during image acquisition in order to maintain an equilibrium of inflow versus loss. Decubitus imaging can be helpful for problem solving. And finally, both 2D and 3D imaging is required for effective interpretation. Knowledge of these topics will shorten the CTC learning curve and help to optimize performance.

REFERENCES

1. Weiss JM, Kim DH, Smith MA, et al. Predictors of primary care provider adoption of CT colonography for colorectal cancer screening. Abdom Radiol (NY) 2017;42:1268–75.
2. Benson M, Pier J, Kraft S, et al. Optical colonoscopy and virtual colonoscopy numbers after initiation of a CT colonography program: long term data. J Gastrointestin Liver Dis 2012;21:391–5.
3. Bibbins-Domingo K, Grossman DC, Curry SJ, et al. Screening for colorectal cancer US preventive services task force recommendation statement. JAMA 2016;315:2564–75.
4. Johnson CD, Chen MH, Toledano AY, et al. Accuracy of CT colonography for detection of large adenomas and cancers. N Engl J Med 2008;359:1207–17.
5. Pickhardt PJ, Choi JR, Hwang I, et al. Computed tomographic virtual colonoscopy to screen for colorectal neoplasia in asymptomatic adults. N Engl J Med 2003;349:2191–200.
6. Pickhardt PJ, Hassan C, Halligan S, et al. Colorectal cancer: CT colonography and colonoscopy for detection-systematic review and meta-analysis. Radiology 2011;259:393–405.
7. Lin JS, Piper MA, Perdue LA, et al. Screening for colorectal cancer updated evidence report and systematic review for the US preventive services task force. JAMA 2016;315:2576–94.
8. Imperiale TF, Ransohoff DF, Itzkowitz SH, et al. Multitarget stool DNA testing for colorectal-cancer screening. N Engl J Med 2014;370:1287–97.
9. Bellini D, Rengo M, De Cecco CN, et al. Perforation rate in CT colonography: a systematic review of the literature and meta-analysis. Eur Radiol 2014;24:1487–96.
10. Hammar N, Linnersjo A, Alfredsson L, et al. Cancer incidence in airline and military pilots in Sweden - 1961-1996. Aviat Space Environ Med 2002;73:2–7.
11. Muirhead CR, O'Hagan JA, Haylock RGE, et al. Mortality and cancer incidence following occupational radiation exposure: third analysis of the National Registry for Radiation Workers. Br J Cancer 2009;100:206–12.
12. Pukkala E, Aspholm R, Auvinen A, et al. Incidence of cancer among Nordic airline pilots over five decades: occupational cohort study. Br Med J 2002;325:567–9.
13. Radiation risk in perspective. Position statement of the Health Physics Society 2016;PS010–3.
14. Buchach CM, Kim DH, Pickhardt PJ. Performing an additional decubitus series at CT colonography. Abdom Imaging 2011;36:538–44.
15. Fletcher JG, Johnson CD, Welch TJ, et al. Optimization of CT colonography technique: prospective trial in 180 patients. Radiology 2000;216:704–11.
16. Vogelstein B, Fearon ER, Hamilton SR, et al. Genetic alterations during colorectal-tumor development. N Engl J Med 1988;319:525–32.
17. Jass JR. Classification of colorectal cancer based on correlation of clinical, morphological and molecular features. Histopathology 2007;50:113–30.
18. East JE, Atkin WS, Bateman AC, et al. British Society of Gastroenterology position statement on serrated polyps in the colon and rectum. Gut 2017;66:1181–96.
19. Lash RH, Genta RM, Schuler CM. Sessile serrated adenomas: prevalence of dysplasia and carcinoma in 2139 patients. J Clin Pathol 2010;63:681–6.
20. Kim DH, Matkowskyj KA, Lubner MG, et al. Serrated polyps at CT colonography: prevalence and characteristics of the serrated polyp spectrum. Radiology 2016. https://doi.org/10.1148/radiol.2016151608.
21. Biemer-Huttmann AE, Walsh MD, McGuckin MA, et al. Immunohistochemical staining patterns of MUC1, MUC2, MUC4, and MUC5AC mucins in hyperplastic polyps, serrated adenomas, and traditional adenomas of the colorectum. J Histochem Cytochem 1999;47:1039–47.
22. Kim DH, Hinshaw JL, Lubner MG, et al. Contrast coating for the surface of flat polyps at CT colonography: a marker for detection. Eur Radiol 2014;24:940–6.
23. Conry BG, Jones S, Bartram CI. The effect of oral magnesium-containing bowel preparation agents on mucosal coating by barium-sulfate suspensions. Br J Radiol 1987;60:1215–9.
24. Shinners TJ, Pickhardt PJ, Taylor AJ, et al. Patient-controlled room air insufflation versus automated

carbon dioxide delivery for CT colonography. AJR Am J Roentgenol 2006;186:1491–6.

25. Burling D, Taylor SA, Halligan S, et al. Automated insufflation of carbon dioxide for MDCT colonography: distension and patient experience compared with manual insufflation. AJR Am J Roentgenol 2006;186:96–103.

26. Saltzman HA, Sieker HO. Intestinal response to changing gaseous environments- normobaric and hyperbaric observations. Ann N Y Acad Sci 1968; 150:31–9.

27. Pickhardt PJ, Kim DH, Taylor AJ. Asymptomatic pneumatosis at CT colonography: a benign self-limited imaging finding distinct from perforation. AJR Am J Roentgenol 2008;190:W112–7.

28. Siewert B, Morrin MM, Farrell R, et al. Impact of decubitus scanning on diagnostic quality of CT colonography (CTC). Am J Roentgenol 2005; 184:S21.

29. Chen JC, Dachman AH. Cecal mobility: a potential pitfall of CT colonography. Am J Roentgenol 2006; 186:1086–9.

30. Kim JY, Park SH, Lee SS, et al. Ascending colon rotation following patient positional change during CT colonography: a potential pitfall in interpretation. Eur Radiol 2011;21:353–9.

Current Status of Magnetic Resonance Colonography for Screening and Diagnosis of Colorectal Cancer

Marije P. van der Paardt, MD, PhD[a,b,*],
Jaap Stoker, MD, PhD[b]

KEYWORDS

- Magnetic resonance colonography • Colonography • MRI • Colorectal cancer screening
- Virtual colonoscopy • Magnetic resonance colonoscopy • Screening • Colorectal cancer

KEY POINTS

- MR colonography lacks the need for ionizing radiation and is therefore a potential screening tool for CRC.
- Few MR colonography studies evaluated its potential for colorectal cancer screening, because there is wide availability of and experience with other screening tools.
- Data on diagnostic performance and patient burden of MR colonography in colorectal cancer screening and future preference of MR colonography as a screening tool are promising, but still heterogeneous.
- MR colonography is a cost-effective screening tool compared with no screening, but to be cost-effective, MR colonography should have higher participation rates than CT colonography.
- MR colonography in its current state is not suitable for CRC screening.

INTRODUCTION

Magnetic resonance (MR) colonography was introduced in the 1990s, just after the widespread introduction of computed tomography (CT) colonography. Both techniques were explored for minimally invasive assessment (or virtual colonoscopy) of the complete colon and especially in the setting of screening for colorectal cancer (CRC) and its precursors.[1,2] Fecal occult blood tests (FOBT), barium contrast enema, sigmoidoscopy, and colonoscopy have been evaluated for CRC screening, with optical colonoscopy being the most accurate, with high sensitivity and specificity regarding the detection of CRC and its precursors. Major drawback of this technique is the cathartic bowel preparation; patient sedation for procedural discomfort; and, although small, risk of procedural complications.[3] Luboldt and colleagues[4] presented preliminary results on colonic polyp detection with MR colonography in a small group of 23 persons. Initial results were promising, but poor spatial resolution and the lack of adequate postprocessing were hurdles to overcome. Since then, the technique of MR colonography has improved.

Disclosure Statement: Dr M.P. van der Paardt has nothing to disclose. Dr J. Stoker is a research consultant for Robarts Clinical Trials concerning MRI in Crohn's disease.
[a] Department of Radiology, Albert Schweitzer Ziekenhuis, Postbus 444, Dordrecht 3300 AK, The Netherlands;
[b] Department of Radiology and Nuclear Medicine, Academic Medical Center, University of Amsterdam, Meibergdreef 9, Amsterdam 1105 AZ, The Netherlands
* Corresponding author. Postbus 444, Dordrecht 3300 AK, The Netherlands.
E-mail address: m.p.vanderpaardt@asz.nl

Radiol Clin N Am 56 (2018) 737–749
https://doi.org/10.1016/j.rcl.2018.04.007
0033-8389/18/© 2018 Elsevier Inc. All rights reserved.

In this paper, we provide an overview on the status and potential of MR colonography in the setting of detection and screening of CRC and its precursors. This article is an update of the paper: Magnetic Resonance Colonography for Screening and Diagnosis of Colorectal Cancer.[1]

COLORECTAL CANCER

Over the past decades CRC morbidity and mortality rates have declined in the United States because of screening and surveillance, improved treatment strategies, and lifestyle changes (reduction in smoking and consumption of meat). Yet, CRC is the third most common diagnosed malignancy in the United States. For 2017 it is estimated that more than 135,000 individuals will be diagnosed with CRC and more than 50,000 deaths from CRC.[5] Early detection of CRC is vital because survival rates rapidly decline after spread of the disease to regional surroundings or distant organs. The 5-year survival rate of localized tumor is 90% compared with 71% and 14% for regional and distant disease, respectively.[5] The development of CRC is believed to follow a certain pathway in which malignant degeneration of an adenomatous polyp advances in an invasive carcinoma: the adenoma-carcinoma sequence. Size is a major prognostic factor for malignant transformation of a polyp, with lesions greater than 10 mm harboring most malignant potential. Yet, size is not the only prognostic factor for malignant transformation of the polyp. Polyps that show high-grade dysplasia and/or a villous component after histologic evaluation, also display increased risk of malignant degeneration. Therefore, polyps larger than 10 mm or with high-grade dysplasia or a villous component have been defined as advanced.

Important evidence now shows that approximately 70% of CRC develop from advanced adenomas, the traditional adenoma-carcinoma pathway. The other 30% are believed to arise via the serrated neoplastic pathway.[6] The traditional serrated polyps used to be classified as harboring no malignant potential. Over time this view changed as molecular analysis of CRC showed that some tumors had similarities with the molecular basis of the sessile serrated adenomas, which were not shown in CRC that originated from advanced adenomas.[7] Clinical implications of this pathway are still being determined.[8] Treatment and surveillance strategies might differ from those of the traditional pathway. Also screening strategies might change because serrated polyps are less likely to bleed, so FOBT might be challenging.[7] Although most MR colonography studies have not yet included the serrated pathway in the evaluation of the technique, a recent study showed that inclusion of the serrated pathway hardly affected long-term predictions on mortality and incidence of the screening program, when serrated lesions were removed.[8]

From the 1970s to recent time periods, the 5-year relative survival rate for all CRC stages combined increased 10%, because of improvements in treatment and earlier detection.[5] Current guidelines for CRC screening include FOBT, colonoscopy, and radiologic imaging tests that enable evaluation of the entire colon. Most research has focused on CT colonography and therefore most data on diagnostic accuracy are available for CT colonography. CT colonography proved to be highly accurate in CRC detection and precursor lesions of 10 mm and larger and therefore CT colonography is implemented as a screening tool for CRC by the US Multi-Society Task Force on Colorectal Cancer.[9] MR colonography, however, is not part of the screening tool recommendation of this guideline, probably because heterogeneity in MR colonography data acquisition, patient preparation techniques, and accuracy data still exist. During the considerable progress over the years in optimizing the CT colonography technique, major steps were also made in CT colonography dose reduction, making it acceptable for screening purposes. Yet the advantage of MR colonography over CT colonography is the lack of ionizing radiation and the excellent soft tissue contrast.

MAGNETIC RESONANCE COLONOGRAPHY

The evaluation of the colon with colonography techniques is based on detection of intraluminal mucosal protrusions and, in the setting of CRC screening, protrusions caused by polyps or mass lesions (Figs. 1 and 2). As in colonoscopy, polys are morphologically subdivided into sessile lesions, pedunculated lesions, and flat lesions. Sessile polyps are defined as mucosal protrusions of more than 3 mm elevation, without a mucosal stalk. When a protuberance with a stalk is present, the polyp is defined as a pedunculated polyp. Different definitions are used for flat lesions. Flat lesions can either be slightly elevated, truly flat, or even depressed. The definition for a slightly elevated flat lesion is no more than 2 to 3 mm in intraluminal height or no more than half of its greatest diameter.[10]

Because the histologic component is not demonstrable with MR colonography, size is the major criterion. Generally, three polyp size categories are recognized: (1) diminutive (<6 mm), (2) small (6–9 mm), and (3) large (10 mm) polyps. Another criterion is the presence of fat that is readily demonstrated at either CT colonography or MR

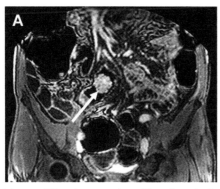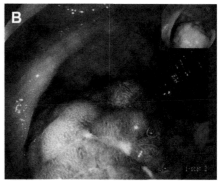

Fig. 1. Dark lumen MR colonography with automated carbon dioxide colon distention after iodinated oral fecal tagging. (*A*) Three-dimensional T1-weighted turbo field echo after intravenous paramagnetic contrast administration showed a contrast-enhanced intraluminal pedunculated lesion (*white arrow*) in the sigmoid colon. (*B*) Colonoscopy demonstrated a pedunculated polyp of 30 mm, which proved to be a tubulovillous adenoma at histopathology.

colonography. Although this is pathognomonic for a lipoma, this is a relative less common finding.

For adequate delineation of the colon wall, bowel preparation and colon distention are indispensable for MR colonography. We discuss both requirements next (**Box 1**).

Bowel Preparation

Dark and bright strategy

Delineation of the bowel wall is either achieved by high intraluminal signal intensity on T1-weighted images (bright lumen) or low intraluminal signal intensity (dark lumen) (**Boxes 2 and 3, Table 1**). In the latter strategy, a hypointense lumen on T1-weighted imaging is achieved either by rectal gas insufflation (room air or carbon dioxide)[11,12] or by rectal administration of water.[13] In one study the "dark" lumen strategy was evaluated after only oral ingestion alone of a polyethylene glycol–electrolyte solution.[14] One other study rectally administered a fat contrast medium for bowel distention.[15] Because the bowel lumen is "dark," the bowel wall is visualized after administration of a gadolinium-based intravenous contrast agent.

Therefore, polyps and mass lesions appear as bright protrusions in a dark lumen, whereas in the bright lumen strategy, the bowel wall and its lesions are hypointense against the "bright"-appearing lumen. A bright lumen is achieved by intraluminal water mixed with gadolinium administered either rectally, orally, or both.[16–18] A disadvantage of the bright lumen strategy is the large amount of contrast agent required for the water/gadolinium mixture in comparison with the dark lumen strategy. Also, residual air and stool can negatively influence diagnostic accuracy.

Bowel cleansing and fecal tagging

Normal bowel content is a complicating factor for detecting CRC and its precursors for colonoscopy and CT and MR colonography, because it can camouflage or mimic the target lesions. Therefore, as in colonoscopy, bowel preparation by means of colon cleansing or fecal tagging is required for MR colonography. Bowel cleansing for MR colonography generally consists of full cathartic preparation along with a clear liquid diet the day before, comparable with colonoscopy. In the earlier days of

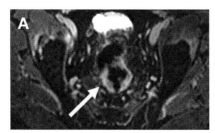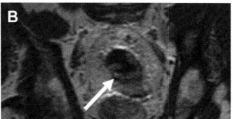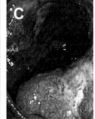

Fig. 2. Dark lumen MR colonography with automated carbon dioxide colon distention. Three-dimensional T1-weighted axial turbo field echo (*A*) and two-dimensional T2-weighted half-Fourier single-shot turbo spin-echo (*B*) demonstrated an almost circumferential colon wall lesion (*white arrow, A, B*) in the rectosigmoid. (*C*) Colonoscopy and histopathology demonstrated a circumferential carcinoma of the rectosigmoid.

Box 1
MR colonography requirements

- Bowel preparation either with cathartic cleansing or fecal tagging to reduce the negative influence of residual stool on diagnostic performance (see **Box 2**)
- Adequate colon distention for adequate delineation of the colon wall
- Dual positioning for adequate distention and to avoid false positive caused by residual stool or air
- Spasmolytics to reduce bowel cramping and motion artifacts
- Data acquisition during breath-hold (15–20 seconds) to reduce breathing artifacts

---

Box 3
Bowel preparation

Dark lumen
- Fecal tagging
  ○ Barium-based
  ○ Iodine-based
- Cathartic cleansing

Bright lumen
- Fecal tagging
  ○ Paramagnetic-based
- Cathartic cleansing

MR colonography performance trials, bowel cleansing was the strategy generally used most of the time because comparison with colonoscopy for lesion detection was performed at the same day.[19,20] Although bowel cleansing is generally accepted in clinical practice, cleansing is considered troublesome by patients and as one of the most unpleasant elements of colonoscopy.[21]

Fecal tagging strategies were developed alongside bowel cleansing strategies. In fecal tagging the signal intensity of the fecal material is altered by oral ingestion of a tagging agent. In contrast to colonoscopy, a cleansed colon is not a prerequisite for lesion detection, as long as adequate delineation of the bowel wall is accomplished

---

Box 2
MR colonography imaging strategies

Dark lumen strategy
- Low intraluminal signal intensity on T1-weighted imaging
  ○ Water
  ○ Air
  ○ Carbon dioxide
  ○ Fat mixture
- High signal of the colon wall after administration of an intravenous paramagnetic contrast agent

Bright lumen strategy
- High intraluminal signal intensity on T1-weighted imaging
  ○ Water/paramagnetic contrast agent mixture
- Low signal of the colon wall

---

and residual stool is easily distinguished from intraluminal bowel wall pathology. Hence, fecal tagging was introduced to reduce patient discomfort and increase patient acceptance of MR colonography. It is important for fecal tagging agents to blend easily with the fecal material and to be consumed without effort. The main goal is to render homogeneous signal distribution of the fecal material. However, as in CT colonography, fecal tagging does not necessarily have to encompass a similar signal intensity to that of the surrounding enema, as long as the delineation of the colon wall is differentiated from residual stool (**Fig. 3**). Hence, low to intermediate signal intensity of residual fecal material next to low signal intensity of the enema proved to be feasible and resulted in good to excellent image quality as long as the signal of the residual stool was homogeneous and liquid.[12]

Most fecal tagging strategies are in combination with dietary restrictions. Usually this includes a diet low in fiber, so as to allow homogenous tagging.[22] Dark lumen studies were initially performed with barium-based fecal tagging to achieve "dark" fecal material alongside a T1 hypointense water enema.[23] Fecal tagging with a paramagnetic contrast agent combined with a water/paramagnetic contrast enema is used for a homogeneous "bright" lumen.[16]

Initial studies showed good tolerance of barium-based tagging for dark lumen MR colonography,[23] yet Goehde and colleagues[24] demonstrated problems of constipation with barium-based fecal tagging even being rated worse than the cleansing strategy for colonoscopy. Moreover, poor image quality caused by high signal of the stool was found in 18% of the images.

Florie and colleagues[25] studied three strategies in 45 patients: (1) barium-based tagging with air enema (dark lumen), (2) barium-based tagging

Table 1
Overview of MR colonography studies in 50 or more human subjects on diagnostic accuracy of CRC detection

Authors, Ref., Year	No. of Patients	Patient Population	Bowel Preparation	Cleansing or Fecal Tagging	Colon Distention Method
Bright lumen MR colonography					
Luboldt et al,[19] 2000	132	Colonoscopy referral for excluding CRC	Preparation colonoscopy	Cleansing	Water/gadolinium mixture
Pappalardo et al,[54] 2000	70	Symptomatic, FOBT+	PEG solution	Cleansing	Water/gadolinium mixture
Florie et al,[17] 2007	200	Personal or family history of polyps and CRC	Lactulose, gadolinium	Tagging	Water/gadolinium mixture
Saar et al,[18] 2007	120	Symptomatic, FOBT+, history of polypectomy	PEG solution	Cleansing	Water/gadolinium mixture
Dark lumen MR colonography studies					
Ajaj,[55] 2003	122	Variety of reasons for colonoscopy	PEG solution	Cleansing	Water
Ajaj et al,[11] 2004	55[a]	Variety of reasons for colonoscopy and 5 volunteers	PEG solution	Cleansing	Room air or water
Leung et al,[43] 2004	156[b]	High-risk and average-risk	Sodium phosphate or PEG solution	Cleansing	Room air
Hartmann et al,[56] 2006	92	Symptomatic	PEG solution	Cleansing	Water
Kuehle et al,[13] 2007	315	Screening	Gastrografin, barium sulfate, locust bean gum	Tagging	Water
Rodriguez Gomez et al,[32] 2008	83	Clinical suspicion/high risk	Barium sulfate	Tagging	Water and room air[c]
Achiam et al,[57] 2009	56	First-time referral colonoscopy	Barium sulfate/ferumoxsil mixture	Tagging	Water
Bakir et al,[14] 2009	55	Symptomatic, FOBT+	Sodium phosphate solution	Cleansing	PEG solution[d]
Graser et al,[35] 2013	286	Asymptomatic[e]	Bisacodyl, sodium phosphate, PEG solution	Cleansing	Water
Van der Paardt et al,[29] 2014	98	Symptomatic	Meglumine- ioxithalamate	Tagging	Carbon dioxide

Abbreviations: FOBT+, positive fecal occult blood test; MRC, MR colonography; PEG, polyethylene glycol.
[a] Fifty patients and five volunteers.
[b] Seventy-six average risk and 80 high risk.
[c] Twenty-nine patients room air distention and 54 patients water distention.
[d] Oral administration only.
[e] Fifty years or older with average risk and 40 years or older with a family history of CRC.

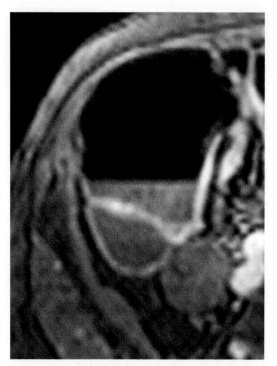

Fig. 3. T1-weighted axial turbo field echo of dark lumen MR colonography with the use of automated carbon dioxide insufflation for colon distention and iodinated oral contrast for fecal tagging. Iodine fecal tagging rendered a homogeneous signal distribution of the fecal material and after intravenous paramagnetic contrast administration adequate bowel wall differentiation of the fecal material is demonstrated.

with water enema (dark lumen), and (3) lactulose/gadolinium-based tagging with gadolinium/water mixture enema (bright lumen). Florie and colleagues[17] demonstrated better tolerance for gadolinium-based tagging than barium-based tagging although there was no significant difference comparing patient experiences of pain and embarrassment. Also, better signal homogeneity after gadolinium-based tagging was shown, but comparable overall image quality with the bright lumen strategy versus dark lumen strategy using air for rectal filling. The subsequent diagnostic accuracy study was performed according to the bright lumen technique as evaluated in this study.

Achiam and colleagues[26] compared barium sulfate/ferumoxsil and barium sulfate as fecal tagging agent. Barium sulfate/ferumoxsil showed significantly better tagging efficiency and less patient nausea. Moreover, in their patient acceptance study comparing colonoscopy and MR colonography, patients preferred fecal tagging over bowel purgation.[27]

Kinner and colleagues[28] introduced a fecal tagging agent containing Gastrografin, barium

sulfate, and locust bean gum without any dietary restrictions in a screening population. There was a significant difference between patient acceptance of the bowel preparations for colonoscopy and MR colonography in favor of MR colonography. Yet, overall there was no significant difference in patient acceptance of colonoscopy and MR colonography. In this strategy 4.4% of the colon segments had untagged stool, which impeded diagnostic evaluation.[13]

Our research group evaluated MR colonography with carbon dioxide insufflation for bowel distention after four different bowel preparation schemes: (1) gadolinium-based tagging, (2) bowel purgation, (3) barium-based tagging, and (4) iodine-based tagging.[12] The iodine tagging group showed the least residual stool, most homogenous liquid stool, and lowest signal intensity on T1-weighted images. Moreover, participants experienced the least burden of the preparation in the iodine tagging group. Hence, a subsequent diagnostic accuracy study of MR colonography versus colonoscopy was performed with iodine tagging bowel preparation.[21,29]

For now, no consensus is reached regarding the optimal bowel preparation scheme for MR colonography results on image quality and patient acceptance of the bowel preparation are varying.

Colon Distention

Bowel distention is the second requirement for MR colonography because it optimizes delineation of the bowel wall. Dual positioning (prone and supine) is helpful in facilitating the distention of all bowel segments (as is standard procedure in CT colonography) and, especially in bright lumen imaging, for distinguishing polyps from residual stool and air because those are gravity dependent (**Fig. 4**).

Depending on the chosen strategy (bright or dark lumen MR colonography), room air, water, carbon dioxide, and even a fat enema are used for colon distention, rendering the lumen dark, versus water spiked with gadolinium, which is used for bright lumen colon distention.

In general water-based colon distention is achieved after rectal administration of 2 to 2.5 L via a rectal cannula under hydrostatic pressure. Gaseous distending agents, room air or carbon dioxide, may be administrated with a rectal cannula either by manual insufflation or automated insufflation. The latter is used for CT colonography and provides superior distention.[30]

Morrin and colleagues demonstrated better acceptance of air distention than water distention

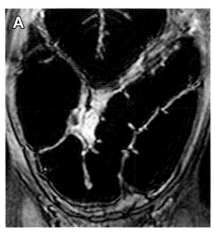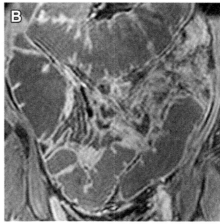

Fig. 4. T1-weighted coronal turbo field echo of lower abdomen in supine (A) and prone (B) position. Differences in colon distention are visible. Supine position (A) demonstrates superior distention of the sigmoid and descending colon than prone position (B). The gravity-dependent tagged fecal material has repositioned after change in abdominal position. The fecal material is homogeneously tagged and hypointense compared with the colon wall, which renders an adequate delineation of the colon wall.

in two patients who had undergone both distention techniques where early evacuation of the water enema was considered embarrassing.[31]

Florie and colleagues,[25] who compared three bowel distention strategies (water, room air, and water/gadolinium mixture) demonstrated sufficient to good distention in all three strategies. There was no significant difference between experienced pain and embarrassment. The subsequent bright lumen diagnostic accuracy study with water/gadolinium distention in 227 patients at increased risk for CRC demonstrated 40 colon segments insufficiently distended, which is less than 1% of the total of colon segments.[17]

Ajaj and colleagues[11] compared air distention with water distention in 55 patients and concluded that there were no significant differences between image quality and discomfort and that there were no artifacts caused by susceptibility in the air distended group; however, the distention with air was rated superior than water distention. A different study comparing air with water in 83 subjects at increased risk of CRC showed opposite results, where water distention was superior to room air distention and the latter showing significantly worse image quality.[32]

Zhang and colleagues[15] evaluated the use of a fat enema instilled under hydrostatic pressure with only 0.8% of poor distention. The authors stated that it provided less susceptibility artifacts than air. Tolerance of the fat enema was not evaluated in this study and diagnostic accuracy was modest (see later).

One prospective dark lumen study in 55 patients used an oral bowel preparation (polyethylene glycol solution) to cleanse and distend the bowel before MR colonography imaging without rectal administration of a distending agent. The aim was to evaluate bowel distention with the intention to improve patient acceptance.[14] Adequate distention was achieved in 91% to 96% of the patients. However, the diagnostic accuracy could only be evaluated in 50 of the 55 patients because of impaired image quality in five patients and showed moderate accuracy results (per-patient sensitivity 65%; specificity, 91%). MR colonography was experienced by patients to be comfortable (13%), moderately comfortable (71%), and uncomfortable (16%), but comparison with colonoscopy was not mentioned.

Carbon dioxide for bowel distention was evaluated in MR colonography by Lomas and colleagues[33] for better patient acceptance. Laparoscopic experience had shown that carbon dioxide is more comfortable for patients than room air because it is rapidly reabsorbed into the blood. Earlier attempts with gaseous distention methods were hampered by susceptibility artifacts and motion artifacts, but Lomas and colleagues had overcome these hurdles with faster data acquisition techniques and a high soft tissue contrast sequence. The feasibility study on automated carbon dioxide distention for MR colonography by our research group demonstrated adequate to optimal bowel distention in 93% of the colon segments. All the artifacts were attributed to motion artifacts and no susceptibility effects were encountered.[12] The subsequent diagnostic accuracy study showed similar results with 94% adequate to optimal distended colon segments.[29]

DATA ACQUISITION

For MR colonography the conventional contraindications for MR imaging also apply: claustrophobia, cardiac pacemakers, metallic implants, or foreign bodies. Depending on the strategy used (dark or bright lumen), allergy to gadolinium-based contrast agents and impaired renal function are relative contraindications.

Breathing artifacts can hamper image quality; therefore, data should be acquired during breath-hold and short repetition and echo times are required for acceptable breath-hold duration (15–20 seconds). Bowel motion and cramping during bowel distention are reduced after administration of a spasmolytic agent, which improves image quality and patient acceptance. As in colonoscopy, intravenous glucagon and butylscopolamine are the most frequently used spasmolytics. However, careful timing of data acquisition is important because with intravenous administration of the spasmolytics, half-life time is short. Butylscopolamine has been shown to result in better distention for CT colonography with carbon dioxide insufflation and lower patient burden but is not approved by the US Food and Drug Administration for this indication.[34]

MR colonography data acquisition is preferably performed with an MRI scanner of 1.5 T or higher. Although most MR colonography studies are performed with 1.5 T, tendency in the latest studies is the use of a 3-T MRI.[29,35,36] Signal-to-noise ratio is higher with 3 T, but specific absorption rate of energy, chemical shift artifacts, and prolonged relaxation times are drawbacks that temper the performance of 3-T MRI.

Phased array coils are used for simultaneous data acquisitioning of multiple points in the abdomen, allowing higher spatial resolution and faster imaging times. This can therefore decrease the breath-hold duration or improve image quality. However, the field of view of the scanner can be somewhat limited (40 × 40 cm), which sometimes limits the coverage of all distended colonic segments, and imaging of the upper abdomen and lower abdomen separately may be necessary. Fusion of the stacks is performed with postprocessing software.[12] Lesion detection is performed with a three-dimensional T1-weighted gradient echo and, with isotropic voxel size, is used for multiplanar reconstruction. Usually a two-dimensional T2-weighted half-Fourier acquisition single-shot turbo spin echo or two-dimensional T2-weighted true fast imaging with steady-state precession is used for problem solving when T1-weighted images are impaired by artifacts.

DIAGNOSTIC ACCURACY

In 2009 a systematic review on MR colonography in detection of colorectal lesions was performed to compare the diagnostic accuracy of MR colonography with colonoscopy as a reference standard.[37] A total of 13 studies was included with a total of 1285 patients. The patients were (nine studies) symptomatic and/or asymptomatic patients at increased risk of CRC, and in three studies referral was unexplained. Four MR colonography studies used the bright lumen technique. The sensitivity for CRC was 100% comprising 32 carcinomas in five studies. The per-patient sensitivity for lesions larger than 10 mm was 88% (95% confidence interval, 63%–97%) and specificity 99% (95% confidence interval, 95%–100%). The summary sensitivity estimate in detecting polyps 10 mm or larger was 84% (95% confidence interval, 66%–94%). However, heterogeneity of the studies was large, which impeded meta-analysis of overall per-patient diagnostic accuracy and per-polyp accuracy in the detection of polyps smaller than 6 mm and polyps 6 to 9 mm.

The largest study in this systematic review comprised 315 asymptomatic patients with a normal risk profile for CRC.[13] This encompassed a dark lumen MR colonography study after barium-based tagging and a water-based enema for distention. Kuehle and colleagues[13] demonstrated a per-patient sensitivity of 98.1% for lesions 10 mm and larger and 92% for lesions larger than 5 mm with six false-positive findings. A little more than 4% of the fecal material proved untagged and therefore they concluded that a good accuracy of MR colonography in a screening population for lesion detection was shown but optimization of image quality and fecal tagging are needed.

The only study to our knowledge including use of a fat enema for bowel distention showed a 95.5% sensitivity for neoplasm larger than 10 mm and 55.6% for 5 to 10 mm, with none of the lesions less than 5 mm detected in this study.[15] Haykir and colleagues[38] evaluated the accuracy of CT colonography and MR colonography in 42 patients symptomatic for CRC who underwent both CT colonography and MR colonography on the same day and compared it with colonoscopy as the reference standard. The sensitivity and specificity of MR colonography for colon pathologies were 96.4% and 100%, respectively, and were 92.8% and 100%, respectively, for CT colonography. To our knowledge, this is the only study evaluating both MR colonography and CT colonography in the same patient cohort.

One of the largest studies published after the systematic review on MR colonography diagnostic accuracy was the study of Graser and colleagues.[35] In 286 asymptomatic patients in a screening population dark lumen MR colonography after bowel cleansing was performed at 3-T MRI. Additionally, FOBT sampling was performed before MR colonography and colonoscopy. MR colonography showed a sensitivity for advanced neoplasia per patient of 83.8% and a specificity of 95.3%. The per-lesion sensitivity for advanced neoplasia was 76.2%. Accuracies for adenomas greater than 6 mm and advanced neoplasia were 96.9% and 51.7% for colonoscopy, 94.4% and 81.1% for MR colonography, and 82.8% and 87.5% for FOBT. They concluded that MR colonography diagnostic accuracy is high for colorectal adenomas greater than 6 mm and advanced neoplasia, and, moreover, MR colonography could outperform FOBT, because the latter is known to show good detection results for CRC but not for adenomas.

Since 2014, few MR colonography studies have been performed for CRC detection. Acay and colleagues[39] demonstrated reasonable accuracy results for dark lumen MR colonography after cleansing and water for distention in 38 patients symptomatic for CRC; 50% of the 6- to 9-m lesions were seen on MR colonography and 11 out of 13 lesions 10 mm and larger (84.6% per lesion sensitivity) were identified.

Our research group demonstrated in the aforementioned dark lumen MR colonography study with the use of oral iodine tagging and automated carbon dioxide distention, a per-patient sensitivity for lesions greater than or equal to 10 mm of 91.7% and specificity of 96.5% for an experienced reader in a symptomatic patient cohort (98 patients).[29] Sensitivity dropped to 75% when MR colonography was evaluated by less experienced readers (resident radiology and radiology research physician). The sensitivity for advanced neoplasia of greater than or equal to 10 mm and greater than or equal to 6 mm was both 88.9% and specificity for both of 98.9%.

A study published in 2016 evaluated diagnostic accuracy of MR colonography in detection of adenomas compared with colonoscopy in 25 patients at intermediate risk of CRC. Detection results of MR colonography were disappointing with five adenomas larger than 6 mm (four adenomas even larger than 10 mm) found with colonoscopy but missed on MR colonography. The authors concluded that MR colonography does not detect adenomas sufficiently.[36]

PATIENT ACCEPTANCE COMPARED WITH COLONOSCOPY

In the experience of the authors colonoscopy proved more burdensome than MR colonography for the dark lumen and bright lumen technique[21,40] and patients preferred MR colonography over colonoscopy for future examination. However, data on patient preference vary. Few studies demonstrated a tendency of lower patient burden for MR colonography,[21,27,40,41] whereas other studies demonstrated no difference in patient burden compared with colonoscopy.[20,32,42] Kinner and colleagues[28] showed better patient acceptance of MR colonography (using barium-based fecal tagging and water for colon distention) versus colonoscopy when evaluating bowel preparations only. However, they also demonstrated no difference in overall patient acceptance between MR colonography and colonoscopy and future preference for either colonoscopy or MR colonography was equal. Moreover, although no significant difference in burden was found, patients preferred colonoscopy over MR colonography in the study by Leung and colleagues.[43] Perhaps the use of analgesics and sedation during colonoscopy balances patient acceptance of MR colonography and colonoscopy. This is supported by a randomized controlled trial in CT colonography that demonstrated a clinically relevant reduction of pain when analgesics were used during the procedure.[44]

EXTRACOLONIC FINDINGS

In contrast to colonoscopy MR colonography, with its high soft tissue contrast, is able to detect extracolonic pathology. In CT colonography the consensus proposal for reporting of extracolonic findings recognizes four classifications of findings (E-rads)[45]: limited examination (E0), normal examination/anatomic variant (E1), clinically unimportant finding (E2), likely unimportant (E3), and potential important (E4). For E3 and E4 further diagnostic work-up is indicated or is necessary. This could have clinical implications in terms of increased costs and patient burden. Not all MR colonography studies evaluated extracolonic findings. In the authors experience the number of potential important extracolonic findings (E4) is limited; 4.8% in the bright lumen study[46] and 4.0% in the dark lumen study.[29] Ajaj and colleagues[47] reported 510 extracolonic findings in 69% of the subjects (total 375). However, 12% had therapeutically relevant findings.

In the study of Haykir and colleagues,[38] 42 patients underwent MR colonography followed by

CT and colonoscopy. MR colonography and CT identified 19 extracolonic lesions in 12 patients, benign and clinically relevant lesions were not differentiated, nor was it explained whether these lesions were identified by both MR colonography and CT or in combination of these examinations. Both MR colonography and CT examinations identified bladder cancer and MR colonography additionally recognized a recto vesical fistula.

COST-EFFECTIVENESS OF MAGNETIC RESONANCE COLONOGRAPHY AS A SCREENING TOOL

The study by Greuter and colleagues[8] evaluated the cost-effectiveness of colonoscopy, CT colonography, MR colonography, and fecal immunochemical test (FIT) as screening tools for CRC. This study is, to our knowledge, the first study to also include MR colonography as a CRC screening tool. Based on clinical trial population, this study analyzed, among others, the cost-effectiveness of CRC screening with CT colonography and MR colonography and compared it with no screening, colonoscopy screening, and FIT screening. It showed comparable results for colonoscopy, CT colonography, and MR colonography in reducing CRC deaths. CT colonography and MR colonography were cost-effective compared with no screening and three rounds of 10-year colonoscopy screening. FIT screening, however, proved to be the most effective and most cost-saving and compared with FIT, CT and MR colonography were no longer cost-effective. With an equal number of screening rounds, MR colonography led to similar health gains as CT colonography, yet the cost-savings were lower, which was mainly because of higher costs. It should be considered, however, that these results are based on clinical trial populations that may not reflect the screening population. Participation for MR colonography was based on CT colonography data, which may not reflect the actual participation rate because to date no randomized controlled trial has evaluated patient acceptance and yield of MR colonography and CT colonography. To be cost-effective, MR colonography should have higher participation rates than CT colonography.

Furthermore, costs of extracolonic findings were not evaluated in this study. This could lead to higher costs of CT colonography and MR colonography than considered in this analysis, although in the author's own experience, limited clinically relevant extracolonic findings were detected.[29,46]

SUMMARY UPDATE AND FUTURE PERSPECTIVE

In recent years not many additional studies have evaluated the use of MR colonography as a screening tool for CRC and its precursors (Box 4). This is probably because of the wide availability and experience with FOBT, sigmoidoscopy, colonoscopy, and CT colonography, with the latter largely having dealt with the drawback of ionizing radiation by means of dose reduction.

For practical and ethical reasons all MR colonography studies, to our knowledge, have used a tandem design in which MR colonography is performed before colonoscopy. However, a randomized controlled trial in 2012 showed a discrepancy in expected and perceived burden of CT colonography and colonoscopy, which was in favor of colonoscopy.[48] For that reason, future research should preferably be done in a randomized controlled design to evaluate patient acceptance and yield of MR colonography compared with colonoscopy, and even CT colonography. Especially because initial data on the cost-effectiveness of MR colonography are promising only when participation for MR colonography is higher than for CT colonography.

A different role for MR colonography might be in the setting of incomplete colonoscopy or in a perioperative setting of diagnostic work-up for CRC.[49–51] Furthermore, preoperative neoadjuvant therapy in colon cancer is increasingly studied and as a consequence, MRI might become important for preoperative local staging and has proven superior detection of liver metastasis over CT;

Box 4
Update summary

- Few studies have reported on MR colonography as a screening tool for CRC and its precursors, because of wide availability and experience with other screening tools (eg, colonoscopy).
- MR colonography still shows heterogeneous results for diagnostic performance and patient burden.
- MR colonography is a cost-effective screening tool compared with no screening or three rounds of 10-yearly colonoscopy.
- The cost-savings of MR colonography were lower compared with CT colonography.
- To be cost-effective, MR colonography should have higher participation rates than CT colonography.

however, the role of MR colonography has not been evaluated to date.[52,53]

Data on the diagnostic accuracy and patient acceptance of MR colonography are heterogeneous. No conclusions can be drawn on the differences in accuracy of the bright lumen versus the dark lumen technique, nor can any technical recommendations be given for MR colonography as a screening tool for CRC and its precursors. We therefore believe that MR colonography in its current state is not yet suitable for widespread CRC screening.

REFERENCES

1. Van Der Paardt MP, Stoker J. Magnetic resonance colonography for screening and diagnosis of colorectal cancer. Magn Reson Imaging Clin N Am 2014;22(1):67–83.
2. Levine MS, Yee J. History, evolution, and current status of radiologic imaging tests for colorectal cancer screening. Radiology 2014;273(2S): S160–80.
3. Levin B, Lieberman DA, McFarland B, et al. Screening and surveillance for the early detection of colorectal cancer and adenomatous polyps, 2008: a joint guideline from the American Cancer Society, the US Multi-Society Task Force on Colorectal Cancer, and the American College of Radiology. Gastroenterology 2008;134(5):1570–95.
4. Luboldt W, Steiner P, Bauerfeind P, et al. Detection of mass lesions with MR colonography: preliminary report. Radiology 1998;207:59–65.
5. Siegel RL, Miller KD, Fedewa SA, et al. Colorectal cancer statistics, 2017. CA Cancer J Clin 2017; 67(3):177–93.
6. Senore C, Bellisario C, Segnan N. Distribution of colorectal polyps: implications for screening. Best Pract Res Clin Gastroenterol 2017;31(4): 481–8.
7. Leggett B, Whitehall V. Role of the serrated pathway in colorectal cancer pathogenesis. Gastroenterology 2010;138(6):2088–100.
8. Greuter MJE, Berkhof J, Fijneman RJA, et al. The potential of imaging techniques as a screening tool for colorectal cancer: a cost-effectiveness analysis. Br J Radiol 2016;89(1063):20150910.
9. Rex DK, Boland CR, Dominitz JA, et al. Colorectal cancer screening: recommendations for physicians and patients from the U.S. Multi-Society Task Force on Colorectal Cancer. Gastroenterology 2017; 153(1):307–23.
10. Iafrate F, Hassan C, Pickhardt PJ, et al. Portrait of a polyp: the CTC dilemma. Abdom Imaging 2010; 35(1):49–54.
11. Ajaj W, Lauenstein TC, Pelster G, et al. MR colonography: how does air compare to water for colonic distention? J Magn Reson Imaging 2004;19(2): 216–21.
12. Zijta FM, Nederveen AJ, Jensch S, et al. Feasibility of using automated insufflated carbon dioxide (CO(2)) for luminal distension in 3.0T MR colonography. Eur J Radiol 2012;81(6):1128–33.
13. Kuehle CA, Langhorst J, Ladd SC, et al. Magnetic resonance colonography without bowel cleansing: a prospective cross sectional study in a screening population. Gut 2007;56(8):1079–85.
14. Bakir B, Acunas B, Bugra D, et al. MR colonography after oral administration of polyethylene glycol-electrolyte solution. Radiology 2009; 251(3):901–9.
15. Zhang S, Peng J-W, Shi Q-Y, et al. Colorectal neoplasm: magnetic resonance colonography with fat enema: initial clinical experience. World J Gastroenterol 2007;13(40):5371–5.
16. Weishaupt D, Patak MA, Froehlich JM, et al. Faecal tagging to avoid colonic cleansing before MRI colonography. Lancet 1999;354(9181):835–6.
17. Florie J, Jensch S, Nievelstein R, et al. MR colonography with limited bowel preparation compared with optical colonoscopy in patients at increased risk for colorectal cancer. Radiology 2007;243(1): 122–31.
18. Saar B, Meining A, Beer A, et al. Prospective study on bright lumen magnetic resonance colonography in comparison with conventional colonoscopy. Br J Radiol 2007;80(952):235–41.
19. Luboldt W, Bauerfeind P, Wildermuth S, et al. Colonic masses: detection with MR colonography. Radiology 2000;216(2):383–8.
20. Lam WWM, Leung WK, Wu JKL, et al. Screening of colonic tumors by air-inflated magnetic resonance (MR) colonography. J Magn Reson Imaging 2004; 19(4):447–52.
21. van der Paardt MP, Zijta FM, Boellaard TN, et al. Magnetic resonance colonography with automated carbon dioxide insufflation: patient burden and preferences. Eur J Radiol 2015;84(1):19–25.
22. Liedenbaum MH, Denters MJ, de Vries AH, et al. Low-fiber diet in limited bowel preparation for CT colonography: influence on image quality and patient acceptance. AJR Am J Roentgenol 2010;195(1): W31–7.
23. Lauenstein TC, Goehde SC, Ruehm SG, et al. MR colonography with barium-based fecal tagging: initial clinical experience. Radiology 2002;223(1): 248–54.
24. Goehde SC, Descher E, Boekstegers a, et al. Dark lumen MR colonography based on fecal tagging for detection of colorectal masses: accuracy and patient acceptance. Abdom Imaging 2005;30(5): 576–83.
25. Florie J, van Gelder RE, Haberkorn B, et al. Magnetic resonance colonography with limited bowel

preparation: a comparison of three strategies. J Magn Reson Imaging 2007;25(4):766–74.

26. Achiam MP, Chabanova E, Løgager VB, et al. MR colonography with fecal tagging: barium vs. barium ferumoxsil. Acad Radiol 2008;15(5):576–83.

27. Achiam MP, Løgager V, Chabanova E, et al. Patient acceptance of MR colonography with improved fecal tagging versus conventional colonoscopy. Eur J Radiol 2010;73(1):143–7.

28. Kinner S, Kuehle CA, Langhorst J, et al. MR colonography vs. optical colonoscopy: comparison of patients' acceptance in a screening population. Eur Radiol 2007;17(9):2286–93.

29. van der Paardt MP, Zijta FM, Boellaard TN, et al. Magnetic resonance colonography with automated carbon dioxide insufflation: diagnostic accuracy and distension. Eur J Radiol 2014;83(5):743–50.

30. Neri E, Halligan S, Hellström M, et al. The second ESGAR consensus statement on CT colonography. Eur Radiol 2013;23(3):720–9.

31. Morrin MM, Hochman MG, Farrell RJ, et al. MR colonography using colonic distention with air as the contrast material: work in progress. AJR Am J Roentgenol 2001;176(1):144–6.

32. Rodriguez Gomez S, Pagés Llinas M, Castells Garangou A, et al. Dark-lumen MR colonography with fecal tagging: a comparison of water enema and air methods of colonic distension for detecting colonic neoplasms. Eur Radiol 2008;18(7):1396–405.

33. Lomas DJ, Sood RR, Graves MJ, et al. Colon carcinoma: MR imaging with CO2 enema–pilot study. Radiology 2001;219(2):558–62.

34. de Haan MC, Boellaard TN, Bossuyt PM, et al. Colon distension, perceived burden and side-effects of CT-colonography for screening using hyoscine butylbromide or glucagon hydrochloride as bowel relaxant. Eur J Radiol 2012;81(8):e910–6.

35. Graser A, Melzer A, Lindner E, et al. Magnetic resonance colonography for the detection of colorectal neoplasia in asymptomatic adults. Gastroenterology 2013;144(4):743–50.e2.

36. Huneburg R, Kukuk G, Nattermann J, et al. Colonoscopy detects significantly more flat adenomas than 3-tesla magnetic resonance colonography: a pilot trial. Endosc Int Open 2016;4(2):E164–9.

37. Zijta FM, Bipat S, Stoker J. Magnetic resonance (MR) colonography in the detection of colorectal lesions: a systematic review of prospective studies. Eur Radiol 2010;20(5):1031–46.

38. Haykir R, Karakose S, Karabacakoglu A, et al. Three-dimensional MR and axial CT colonography versus conventional colonoscopy for detection of colon pathologies. World J Gastroenterol 2006;12(15):2345–50.

39. Acay MB, Bayramotlu S, Acay A. The sensitivity of MR colonography using dark lumen technique for detection of colonic lesions. Turk J Gastroenterol 2014;25(3):271–8.

40. Florie J, Birnie E, van Gelder RE, et al. MR Colonography with limited bowel preparation: patient acceptance compared with that of full-preparation colonoscopy. Radiology 2007;245(1):150–9.

41. Lim EJ, Leung C, Pitman A, et al. Magnetic resonance colonography for colorectal cancer screening in patients with Lynch syndrome gene mutation. Fam Cancer 2010;9(4):555–61.

42. Keeling AN, Morrin MM, McKenzie C, et al. Intravenous, contrast-enhanced MR colonography using air as endoluminal contrast agent: impact on colorectal polyp detection. Eur J Radiol 2010;81:31–8.

43. Leung WK, Lam WWM, Wu JCY, et al. Magnetic resonance colonography in the detection of colonic neoplasm in high-risk and average-risk individuals. Am J Gastroenterol 2004;99(1):102–8.

44. Boellaard TN, van der Paardt MP, Hollmann MW, et al. A multi-centre randomised double-blind placebo-controlled trial to evaluate the value of a single bolus intravenous alfentanil in CT colonography. BMC Gastroenterol 2013;13(1):94.

45. Zalis ME, Barish MA, Choi JR, et al. CT colonography reporting and data system: a consensus proposal 1. Radiology 2005;236:3–9.

46. Yusuf E, Florie J, Nio CY, et al. Incidental extracolonic findings on bright lumen MR colonography in a population at increased risk for colorectal carcinoma. Eur J Radiol 2011;78(1):135–41.

47. Ajaj W, Ruehm SG, Ladd SC, et al. Utility of dark-lumen MR colonography for the assessment of extra-colonic organs. Eur Radiol 2007;17(6):1574–83.

48. de Wijkerslooth TR, de Haan MC, Stoop EM, et al. Burden of colonoscopy compared to non-cathartic CT-colonography in a colorectal cancer screening programme: randomised controlled trial. Gut 2012;61(11):1552–9.

49. Hartmann D, Bassler B, Schilling D, et al. Incomplete conventional colonoscopy: magnetic resonance colonography in the evaluation of the proximal colon. Endoscopy 2005;37(9):816–20.

50. Ajaj W, Lauenstein TC, Pelster G, et al. MR colonography in patients with incomplete conventional colonoscopy. Radiology 2005;234(2):452–9.

51. Achiam MP, Løgager V, Lund Rasmussen V, et al. Perioperative colonic evaluation in patients with rectal cancer; MR colonography versus standard care. Acad Radiol 2015;22(12):1522–8.

52. FOxTROT Collaborative Group. Feasibility of preoperative chemotherapy for locally advanced operable

colon cancer: the pilot phase of a randomised controlled trial. Lancet Oncol 2012;13(11):1152–60.

53. Nerad E, Lambregts DMJ, Kersten ELJ, et al. MRI for local staging of colon cancer: can MRI become the optimal staging modality for patients with colon cancer? Dis Colon Rectum 2017;4(60): 385–92.

54. Pappalardo G, Polettini E, Frattaroli FM, et al. Magnetic resonance colonography versus conventional colonoscopy for the detection of colonic endoluminal lesions. Gastroenterology 2000;119(2):300–4.

55. Ajaj W. Dark lumen magnetic resonance colonography: comparison with conventional colonoscopy for the detection of colorectal pathology. Gut 2003; 52(12):1738–43.

56. Hartmann D, Bassler B, Schilling D, et al. Colorectal polyps: detection with dark lumen MRC versus conventional colonoscopy. Radiology 2006;238(1): 143–9.

57. Achiam MP, Løgager VB, Chabanova E, et al. Diagnostic accuracy of MR colonography with fecal tagging. Abdom Imaging 2009;34(4):483–90.

MR Imaging of Rectal Cancer

Natally Horvat, MD[a,b], Iva Petkovska, MD[a], Marc J. Gollub, MD[a],*

KEYWORDS

• Rectum • Rectal neoplasms • MR imaging • Anatomy • Neoplasm staging • Neoplasm recurrence

KEY POINTS

• Rectal MR imaging plays a pivotal role in the pretreatment and posttreatment assessment of rectal cancer, assisting the multidisciplinary team in tailoring treatment.
• The success of rectal MR imaging strictly depends on obtaining good image quality to evaluate the main anatomic structures and their relationships to the tumor.
• In primary staging, it is important to describe tumor location, T and N category, extramural venous invasion, tumor relationship to the sphincter complex, and circumferential resection margins.
• Neoadjuvant therapy is considered the standard of care for patients with locally advanced tumors, resulting in tumor downstaging and improved local control.
• At restaging, besides the T and N categories, it is important to assess treatment response, particularly with the emergence of nonoperative approaches.

INTRODUCTION

Colorectal cancer (CRC) is the third most common cancer in men and the second most common in women worldwide.[1] It is also the second leading cause of cancer death.[2] In 2017, an estimated 95,620 new cases of CRC will be diagnosed in the United States alone. Of all these cases, 39,910 will occur in the rectum. Overall, cancer prevention, screening programs, and improvements in early diagnosis and treatment have improved CRC survival rates in the last few years.[2] In addition, the emergence of a multidisciplinary team effort (with close cooperation among surgeons, oncologists, endoscopists, radiologists, and radiotherapists) as well as technological advances in surgical techniques, (CRT), and imaging techniques, especially in the field of MR imaging, have played a pivotal role for improving patients' outcomes.[3,4] However, despite improvements in

patient survival and the overall incidence rate, the incidence of CRC and rectal cancer (RC) in particular has increased among patients younger than 50 years old.[5]

RC is known to have a propensity to recur locally and to metastasize systemically. Up until the 1990s, surgery was considered the only type of treatment, and more than 50% of the patients had local recurrence (LR).[3] The prognosis of RC has been directly related to the infiltration into the mesorectum and the ability to surgically attain negative circumferential resection margins (CRM).[6] The introduction of the total mesorectal excision (TME) technique and CRT led to improvements in local disease control.[7–11] Moreover, pathologic complete response (pCR), observed in 15% to 27% of cases after CRT, has created the concept of minimally invasive surgeries and nonoperative management (ie, a watch-and-wait

Disclosure Statement: All authors declare no conflict of interest. All authors were partially supported through the NIH/NCI Cancer Center Support Grant P30 CA008748.
[a] Department of Radiology, Memorial Sloan Kettering Cancer Center, 1275 York Avenue, New York, NY 10065, USA; [b] Department of Radiology, Hospital Sírio-Libanês, Adma Jafet 91, São Paulo, São Paulo 01308-050, Brazil
* Corresponding author. Department of Radiology, Memorial Sloan Kettering Cancer Center, 1275 York Avenue, New York, NY 10065.
E-mail address: gollubm@mskcc.org

Radiol Clin N Am 56 (2018) 751–774
https://doi.org/10.1016/j.rcl.2018.04.004

approach), showing improvement in patient quality of life and outcome.[3,12–14]

To optimize patient outcomes in the current clinical scenario where different treatment approaches can be considered, rectal MR imaging plays a key role assisting the multidisciplinary team in treatment planning. This article aims to review current concepts in the management of patients with RC, focusing primarily on MR imaging for primary staging, restaging, and assessing LR. The authors also emphasize the use of a structured radiologic reporting system with standardized terminology, which reduces misinterpretation and enhances the communication process between radiologists and other specialists.[15]

IMAGING MODALITIES FOR STAGING RECTAL CANCER

Staging is important for determining the optimal treatment approach for RC. Several diagnostic modalities are available: digital rectal examination (DRE) and sigmoidoscopy, endorectal ultrasound (ERUS), high-resolution pelvic MR imaging, computed tomography (CT), and PET/CT.

DRE and sigmoidoscopy followed by biopsy with pathologic examination are themselves often used to diagnose RC. Sigmoidoscopy is also considered the method of choice to determine the location of the tumor based on the distance between the tumor and the anal verge (AV).[16,17] However, for local staging, both have limited impact.[18]

ERUS provides a clear evaluation of the layers of the bowel wall and can provide preoperative assessment of the depth of tumor penetration. ERUS can also evaluate the presence of local lymph node (LN) metastases.[19] However, its inability to assess the tumor relationship with CRM, tumors beyond the reach of the probe, stenotic tumors, and extra-mesorectal LNs, as well as to distinguish fibrosis from tumor, makes it limited for staging advanced RC in both primary and post-CRT settings.[20,21] For the specific differentiation between T1 and T2 tumors, ERUS is recommended.[16]

Compared with all imaging modalities, high-resolution pelvic MR imaging is considered the standard imaging modality for local staging of RC for both primary (preoperative) staging and restaging. Briefly, primary staging MR imaging can assist in (a) selecting patients suitable for neoadjuvant therapy, (b) guiding surgical planning, and (c) identifying poor prognostic factors, such as presence of extramural vascular invasion (EMVI) or mucin, and CRM positivity.[20] The Magnetic Resonance Imaging and Rectal Cancer

European Equivalence (MERCURY) study showed that high-resolution MR imaging can accurately assess the CRM preoperatively, differentiating low-risk from high-risk patients.[4] On the other hand, restaging MR imaging is important for (a) the evaluation of tumor regression, (b) tailoring surgical planning, (c) diagnosing clinical complete response in association with clinical and endoscopic examinations, and (d) monitoring of patients in a watch-and-wait program. Last, MR imaging is also important during follow-up by allowing an early diagnosis of recurrence and outlining disease extension within the pelvic compartments in order to help determine resectability and to plan the best treatment approach.[22]

CT is unreliable for local T and N staging. In regards to systemic staging, contrast-enhanced CT of the chest, abdomen, and pelvis is the modality of choice according to the National Comprehensive Cancer Network (NCCN) guidelines.[18]

PET/CT scan is not routinely indicated for staging RC according to the NCCN.[18] It should only be used to evaluate an equivocal finding on contrast-enhanced CT or in patients with strong contraindications to intravenous contrast media injection.[18] There are a few studies that have evaluated the use of PET/CT for detecting response to treatment[23]; however, no formal consensus has been established.[18] PET/CT can also be considered for surveillance and evaluation of recurrent disease.[18]

Early experience in PET/MR imaging has demonstrated higher accuracy in T staging and at least comparable accuracy in N and M staging to PET/CT, because of high soft tissue contrast provided by MR imaging; however, larger studies are needed to evaluate the added value of this modality.[24]

CURRENT CONCEPTS AND MANAGEMENT OF RECTAL CANCER

TNM staging is summarized in **Table 1**.[18] TNM staging is the most commonly used cancer staging system, whereby T describes the tumor, N describes the LNs near the tumor, and M describes whether the tumor has metastasized. The prefixes "c," "p," and "y" denote clinical, pathologic, and postneoadjuvant therapy, respectively.

In the United States, treatment of RC is based on NCCN guidelines, which adhere to the TNM staging set by the American Joint Committee on Cancer. According to this, patients without distant metastasis and with clinical stage cT1-2 and cN0 based on ERUS or MR imaging should undergo surgery. On the other hand, patients with locally advanced RC (cT3-4, cN0, or any cT and cN1-2),

Table 1
TNM classification with MR imaging subclassification for T3 category[a]

TNM	Definitions/Extension to
Primary tumor (T)	
TX	Primary tumor cannot be assessed
T0	No evidence of primary tumor
Tis	Carcinoma in situ: intraepithelial or invasion of lamina propria
T1	Submucosa
T2	Muscularis propria
T3	Subserosa/perirectal tissue
a[a]	<1 mm
b[a]	1–5 mm
c[a]	5–15 mm
d[a]	>15 mm
T4	
a	Tumor penetrates to the surface of the visceral peritoneum
b	Tumor invades of is adherent to other organs of structures
Regional LNs (N)	
NX	Regional LNs cannot be assessed
N0	No regional LN metastasis
N1	Metastasis in 1–3 regional LNs
a	1 LN
b	2–3 LNs
c	Tumor deposit(s) in the subserosa, mesentery, or nonperitonealized perirectal tissues
N2	Metastasis in 4 or more LNs
a	4–6 LNs
b	7 or more regional LNs
Distant metastasis (M)	
M0	No distant metastasis
M1	Distant metastasis
a	Metastasis confined to one organ or site (eg, liver, lung, nonregional LN)
b	Metastasis in more than one organ/site or to the peritoneum

[a] The subclassification of the T3 category is based on an MR imaging evaluation and is used in the European guidelines for treatment recommendations.[17]

who have locally unresectable tumor, or who are medically inoperable are managed with neoadjuvant CRT followed by surgery.[18]

On the other hand, in Europe, patients without distant metastasis are stratified based on rectal MR imaging into risk groups as follows: (a) low risk, treated with surgery alone; (b) intermediate risk, treated with neoadjuvant short course radiation or CRT followed by surgery; and (c) high risk, treated with neoadjuvant long-course CRT followed by surgery.[3,17,25]

- The low-risk patients ("the good," <10% risk for LR) are those with cT1-T3b (<5-mm tumor penetration into the mesorectal fat) in the middle or upper rectum, without EMVI, and with negative mesorectal fascia (MRF) or CRM, defined as the distance between the tumor edge and the surgical margin greater than or equal to 1 mm.
- The intermediate-risk patients ("the bad," 10%–20% risk for LR) are defined as cT2-3 in low rectal tumors, cT3c-4a (only posterior vaginal wall), any cT with cN1-2, or presence of EMVI, and all of which must have a negative CRM.
- The high-risk patients ("the ugly," >20% risk for LR) are characterized by cT4 other than posterior vaginal wall involvement, positive CRM, or lateral LNs, including common, internal and external iliac nodes, and obturator LNs.[3,17,25]

SURGICAL TECHNIQUES

Thus far, surgical resection continues to be the mainstay of curative therapy for RC with a variety of surgical approaches, depending on the location and extent of the disease. These techniques include minimally invasive procedures, such as transanal endoscopic microsurgery (TEM), and/or invasive transabdominal resection procedures, such as low anterior resection (LAR), proctectomy and coloanal anastomosis, abdominoperineal resection (APR), and pelvic exenteration.

Minimally invasive surgeries, including TEM (Fig. 1A), are reserved for selected cT1, cN0 early-stage tumors, less than 3 cm, well to moderately differentiated, that are within 8 cm of the AV and limited to less than 30% of the rectal circumference.[18,26] However, if in the resection specimen the patient presents pT2 disease or high-risk features, a subsequent transabdominal resection is indicated.[18]

Several transabdominal resection procedures are available. TME is the standard of care in transabdominal surgeries and results in better outcomes and improvement in patient quality of life.[18] It is characterized by an en bloc resection of the mesorectum through a sharp dissection along the MRF. TME allows the surgeon to excise the entire rectum with surrounding vessels and LNs within an intact visceral fascial envelope while sparing the autonomic nerves.[27]

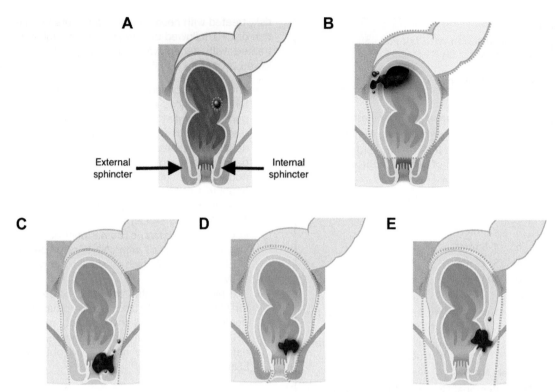

Fig. 1. Surgical techniques for RC. (A) TEM. (B) LAR. (C) Abdominoperineal resection. (D) Intersphincteric abdominoperineal excision. (E) Extralevator abdominoperineal excision.

The most commonly performed radical resection is the LAR, which is indicated for tumors in the mid to upper rectum. It is characterized by resection 4 to 5 cm below the distal edge of the tumor using TME, followed by the creation of a colorectal anastomosis, if feasible. In LAR, the following structures are excised: rectum, mesorectum, MRF, and sigmoid colon (or part of it) (Fig. 1B). Tumors in the mid to lower rectum are resected up to the level of the pelvic floor muscle, and if the anal function is intact and distal clearance is adequate, LAR/TME may be followed by coloanal anastomosis.

For distal tumors, a negative distal margin of 1 to 2 cm may be acceptable and must be confirmed by frozen section during the surgery. For those tumors, sphincter-sparing surgeries, such as ultra-LAR and intersphincteric resection, with coloanal anastomosis may be attempted, considering the substantial improvements in quality of life.[28]

Ultra-LAR is offered for patients with low RC above the anorectal junction (ARJ), and the anastomosis is done 1 cm distal to the tumor margin. The anal canal remains intact.

Standard APR with TME is performed (a) when the tumor infiltrates the anal canal or levator ani/ external sphincter muscle, (b) when the tumor is less than 1 cm from AV, or (c) in cases whereby the negative resection margins would result in incontinence. APR is characterized by en bloc resection of the rectosigmoid, the rectum, and the anus, as well as the surrounding mesentery and mesorectum followed by permanent colostomy (Fig. 1C). In APR, 2 incisions are made, one in the abdominal wall and the other in the perineum.

There are 2 variations to the standard APR: intersphincteric APR and the extralevator abdominoperineal excision (ELAPE). Intersphincteric APR can be considered when the intersphincteric plane is not infiltrated by the tumor and the external sphincter is spared (Fig. 1D). Thus, the external sphincter is preserved, avoiding the need for permanent colostomy. ELAPE, differently, extends the resection and includes the levator muscles with the other structures resected in APR (Fig. 1E). This technique avoids the "waist" seen in standard APR and creates a cylindrical specimen, with the purpose of reducing bowel/tumor perforation and positivity of CRM.[29] ELAPE is indicated in tumors that invade the intersphincteric plane, external sphincter/levator ani, but sparing adjacent structures.

For locally advanced tumors or extensive recurrent disease, pelvic exenteration can be performed and involves radical resection of the pelvic viscera and draining lymphatics.[30]

Finally, laparoscopic and robotic procedures have been maturing over recent years and can be considered by an experienced surgeon and for lower-risk tumors. These procedures have been shown to have less complications and better indicators of quality of life compared with open surgery.[31] However, there are some conflicting results regarding outcomes with some studies demonstrating higher rates of CRM positivity and incomplete TME.[32,33]

MR IMAGING TECHNIQUE

The success of high-resolution rectal MR imaging strictly depends on the ability of the radiological staff to obtain good imaging quality that allows the evaluation of the main anatomic structures and their relationships with the tumor.[16,34]

There is no recommendation for the systematic use of bowel preparation, filling the rectum with any contrast agent (eg, gel), air insufflation, or use of intravenous contrast agents.[16,34,35] The minimal recommended field of strength for adequate rectal MR imaging is 1.0 T, but ideally higher fields are preferred, either 1.5 T or 3.0 T with no current consensus for which is preferred. It is recommended to use a phased-array pelvic surface coil, and there is no indication for an endorectal coil.[16] MR imaging should be performed with the patients lying comfortably in the supine position, and patients must be informed about the scan duration, which may be up to 50 minutes. The standard MR protocol for (re)staging of RC includes 2-dimensional fast spin-echo (FSE) T2-weighted image (WI) sequences without fat suppression in the axial, sagittal, and coronal planes.

Axial T2WI with large field-of-view (FOV) of the entire pelvis, from the aortic bifurcation through the sphincter, allows the best view of inferior mesenteric, lateral, and inguinal LNs and enables comparison with other imaging modalities (Fig. 2A).

Sagittal T2WI from one side of the pelvic wall to the other. This sequence allows the localization of the primary tumor and enables the measurement

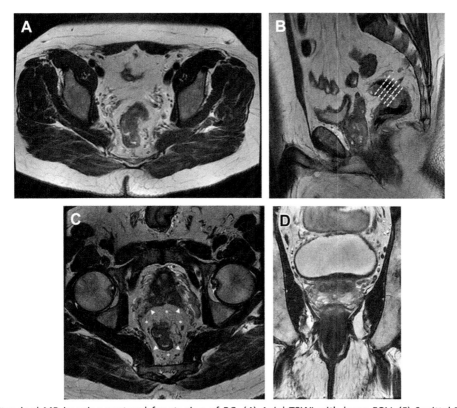

Fig. 2. Standard MR imaging protocol for staging of RC. (*A*) Axial T2WI with large FOV. (*B*) Sagittal T2WI. (*C*) High-resolution axial oblique T2WI perpendicular to the long axis of the rectum at the level of the tumor (*dashed lines* on *B*). MRF (*arrowheads*) is characterized as a thin line with low SI surrounding the mesorectal fat (*asterisks*). (*D*) Coronal oblique T2WI parallel to anal canal.

of its height and the relationship with the midline structures, such as the AV (Fig. 2B).

High-resolution, small FOV *axial oblique T2WI* is recommended to be perpendicular to the long axis of the rectum, at the level of the tumor and with a small FOV; the optimal slide thickness of this sequence varies between 1 and 3 mm (often 3-mm slices). This sequence is essential in the protocol, and the proper angulation is of vital importance, given that it provides the best imaging for evaluating the T category and the MRF involvement. However, it is also the most challenging sequence to acquire, because it requires training of the technicians and/or the presence of a radiologist at the time of imaging acquisition, but the training and engagement of the entire team lead to good results (Fig. 2C).

Coronal oblique T2WI is recommended to be acquired parallel to the tumor axis for lesions in the mid and upper rectum; although for low rectal tumors, the angulation varies depending on the extent of the tumor and may be performed perpendicular and parallel to either the tumor axis or the anal canal. The *coronal oblique parallel T2WI* to the anal canal is helpful to evaluate the relationship of the tumor with the anal canal structures (Fig. 2D).

Diffusion-weighted imaging (DWI) is optional at primary staging, but it is recommended for restaging. Dynamic contrast-enhanced MR imaging (DCE-MR imaging) and 3-dimensional T2WI sequences are not routinely recommended and are currently used mainly for research purposes.[16]

The main imaging parameters are summarized in **Table 2**.

COMMON DIFFICULTIES AND HOW TO OVERCOME

The proper angulation of the axial oblique plane is crucial for T staging; an incorrect plane may cause blurring of the muscularis propria that may lead to overstaging. Sometimes the tumor is not easily visible on sagittal plane, or the rectum is very redundant, or the tumor origin cannot be defined in large polypoid masses. In those cases, it is helpful to carefully review the clinical history and prior examinations of the patient. If the tumor remains unidentified, it may be necessary to cover the entire length of the rectum.[34,36]

Motion artifacts are also important limitations that cause misinterpretation in rectal MR imaging. The possible solutions are to ensure that the patient is comfortable, request that patient empty their bladder and rectum before getting in the scanner; swap the directions of phase- and frequency-encoding; reduce the duration of scanning; focus on oblique high-resolution T2WI, which is the most important sequence; and administer intravenous or intramuscular spasmolytic agents (eg, Glucagon or Buscopan).[37] There is no consensus regarding the routine use of spasmolytic agent,[16] but in the authors' institution, Glucagon 0.1 mg intravenously, intramuscularly, or subcutaneously is routinely used before the scan to reduce bowel motion.

Some artifacts in imaging quality can be caused by coil positioning. The coil should be positioned properly to guarantee coverage of the rectum, mesorectum, sphincter complex, and LN draining territory.[34]

ANATOMIC CONCEPTS FOR MR IMAGING

High-spatial-resolution MR imaging provides an accurate evaluation of the key anatomic landmarks important in the decision-making process in patients with RC, with good surgical correlation. Therefore, it is even more essential that radiologists be familiar with the anatomy of the pelvis in order to make proper tumor staging. The most important anatomic structures from caudal to cranial direction are the following:

- The *AV* is defined, surgically, as the lower edge of the anal canal (specifically the internal anal sphincter muscle). The inferior edge of the tumor is measured related to it.
  ○ Best sequence to be evaluated: sagittal T2WI.
- The *anal canal (anus)* is the caudal part of the gastrointestinal tract and measures approximately 4 cm in length (range, 3–5 cm). The dentate line divides the upper one-third (lined by glandular mucosa) and lower two-thirds of the anal canal (lined by squamous epithelium), but it is not visible on MR imaging. The anal canal extends from the histologic AV (junction of keratinizing and nonkeratinizing squamous epithelium; approximately the lower end of the external anal sphincter) to the ARJ.
  ○ Best sequence to be evaluated: coronal T2WI.
- The *sphincter complex* surrounds the anal canal and is divided into internal and external. The internal sphincter is a continuation of the inner circular muscular layer of the rectum (smooth muscle), whereas the external sphincter complex is composed of skeletal muscle, predominantly levator ani, puborectal sling, and external sphincter muscles (Fig. 3).
  ○ Best sequence to be evaluated: coronal oblique T2WI.

Table 2
MR imaging parameters among most common vendors

	GE		Siemens		Phillips	
	1.5 T	3.0 T	1.5 T	3.0 T	1.5 T	3.0 T
Axial T2						
Sequence name/ETL	FRFSE/19	FRFSE/19	FRFSE/24	TSE/29	TSE/32	TSE/29
FOV (mm)	200–240	200–240	380	200–240	200–240	200–240
Section thickness (mm)	5	5	5	5	5	5
Matrix	320 × 224	320 × 320	320 × 320	320 × 320	348 × 248	348 × 248
TR (ms)/TE (ms)	2500–3500/120	2500–3500/120	3500–5000/90–150	2500–3500/100	2500–3500/100	2500–3500/100
Bandwidth (kHz)/flip angle (°)	31/160	41/111	32/90	127/90	Min/90	Min
Sagittal T2						
Sequence name/ETL	FRFSE/19	FRFSE/19	FRFSE/24	TSE/29	TSE/32	TSE/29
FOV (mm)	200–240	200–240	380	200–240	250	200–240
Section thickness (mm)	4	4	4	4	4	4
Matrix	320 × 224	416 × 384	320 × 240	320 × 320	312 × 256	360 × 243
TR (ms)/TE (ms)	2500–3500/120	2500–3500/120	3500–5000/90–150	2500–3500/100	3000–5000/100	2500–3500/100
Bandwidth (kHz)/flip angle (°)	31/160	62/111	32/90	127/90	Min/90	Min
Frequency direction	AP	AP	AP	AP	AP	AP
Coronal T2						
Sequence name/ETL	FRFSE/19	FRFSE/19	FRFSE/24	TSE/29	TSE/32	TSE/29
FOV (mm)	180	180	180	200–240	250	200–240
Section thickness (mm)	3	3	3	3	3	3
Matrix	320 × 224	320 × 320	320 × 240	320 × 320	464 × 288	360 × 243
TR (ms)/TE (ms)	2500–3500/120	2500–3500/120	3500–5000/90–150	2500–3500/100	3000–5000/120	2500–3500/100
Bandwidth (kHz)/flip angle (°)	31/160	41/111	32/90	127/90	Min/90	Min

(continued on next page)

Table 2
(continued)

	GE		Siemens		Phillips	
	1.5 T	3.0 T	1.5 T	3.0 T	1.5 T	3.0 T
Oblique axial T2						
Sequence name/ETL	FRFSE/19	FRFSE/19	FRFSE	TSE/29	TSE/29	TSE/29
FOV (mm)	180	180	180	200–240	250	200–240
Section thickness (mm)	3	3	3	3	3	4
Matrix	320 × 224	320 × 320	256 × 256	320 × 320	416 × 266	360 × 243
TR (ms)/TE (ms)	4000–6000/120	4000–6000/120	3500–5000/90–150	2500–3500/100	3000–5000/120	2500–3500/100
Bandwidth (kHz)/flip angle (°)	31/160	41/111	32/18	127/90	Min/90	Minimum
Oblique coronal T2						
Sequence name/ETL	FRFSE/19	FRFSE/19	FRFSE	TSE/29	TSE/29	TSE/29
FOV (mm)	180	180	180	200–240	250	200–240
Section thickness (mm)	3	3	3	3	3	4
Matrix	320 × 224	320 × 320	256 × 256	320 × 320	416 × 266	360 × 243
TR (ms)/TE (ms)	2500–3500/120	2500–3500/120	3500–5000/90–150	2500–3500/100	3000–5000/120	2500–3500/100
Bandwidth (kHz)/Flip angle (°)	31/160	41/111	32/18	127/90	Min/90	Min
DWI						
Plane	Axial	Axial	Axial	Axial	Axial	Axial
Sequence name	DWI	DWI	DWI	DWI	DWI	DWI
FOV (mm)	240	240	240	240	180	180
Section thickness (mm)	5	5	5	5	5	5
Matrix	128 × 128	128 × 128	128 × 128	128 × 128	128 × 128	128 × 128
TR (ms)/TE (ms)	6000/Min	6000/Min	4000/Min	6000/Min	Min/Min	6000/Min
Bandwidth (kHz)/flip angle (°)	250/90	250/90	250/90	250/90	Min/90	Minimum

Abbreviations: ETL, echo train length; TE, echo time, TR, repetition time.

A

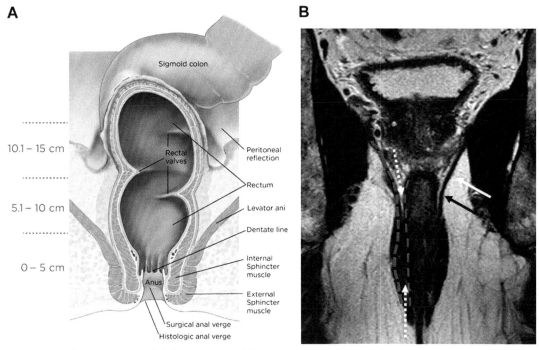

B

Fig. 3. Coronal view anatomy. (*A*) Illustration and (*B*) coronal T2WI showing the levator ani (LA) (*white arrow*), internal sphincter (*red line*), external sphincter/LA complex (*blue line*), intersphincteric plane (*dashed arrows*), and ARJ (*black arrow*).

- The *ARJ* (known surgically as the anorectal "ring") is situated in the plane of insertion of the levator ani into the fibers of the puborectalis, which continues with the external sphincter, and where the rectum is angled forward by the puborectalis sling[38] (see **Fig. 3**; **Fig. 4**).
  - Best sequences to be evaluated: coronal and sagittal T2WI.
- The *rectum* has a highly variable definition and is also dependent on the size and gender of the patient[39,40]; however, 15 cm from the AV

has been used as the standard on the rigid sigmoidoscope.[4] It is divided into 3 components: (a) lower (0–5 from the AV), (b) middle (5.1–10 cm from the AV), and (c) upper rectum (10.1–15 cm from the AV) (see **Figs. 3** and **4**).[38]
  - Best sequence to be evaluated: sagittal T2WI.
- The *rectal wall layer* or the rectum wall is composed of 5 layers and includes from the inside out: (a) mucosa, lined by columnar epithelium; (b) muscularis mucosa; (c)

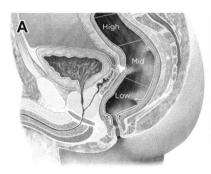
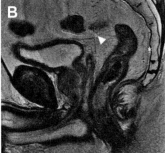
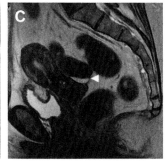

Fig. 4. Sagittal view anatomy. (*A*) Illustration, (*B*) sagittal T2WI in a man and (*C*) in a woman demonstrate the rectum, peritoneal reflection (*arrowheads*) above the top of the seminal vesicle and in the plane of cervical region. The retrorectal space, characterized as a virtual space between the MRF and presacral fascia, is also demonstrated (*asterisks*).

submucosa; (d) muscularis propria (consisting of inner circular and outer longitudinal layers); and (e) serosa. On MR imaging, usually 3 layers are visible on T2WI: mucosa (innermost thin hypointense layer), submucosa (middle hyperintense layer), and muscularis propria (outer hypointense layer) (**Fig. 5**).[41]

○ Best sequence to be evaluated: oblique axial high-resolution T2WI.

• The *perirectal fat and MRF.* The perirectal fat, also called mesorectum, tapers caudally (to become the intersphincteric spade), surrounds the rectum, and contains vessels and LNs. It is enclosed by the MRF, which appears as a thin line with low signal intensity (SI) on T2WI and corresponds to the surgical excision plane in TME.[41] The MRF completely surrounds the rectum only in the lower third; however, its recognition can be difficult in this segment due to the reduced quantity of mesorectum (see **Fig. 5**). The mid rectum is surrounded anteriorly by the peritoneum and laterally and posteriorly by the MRF. On the other hand, in the upper rectum, the peritoneum surrounds the anterior and lateral circumference, and the MRF surrounds the posterior aspect (**Fig. 6**).

○ Best sequence to be evaluated: oblique axial high-resolution T2WI.

• The *Denonvillier's fascia* is the anteroinferior component of the MRF characterized by a dense tissue band more pronounced in men, which separates the rectum from the prostate and bladder. The rectovaginal fascia is its homologue in women.[41]

○ Best sequence to be evaluated: sagittal T2WI and oblique axial high-resolution T2WI.

• The *anterior peritoneal reflection* consists of a thin line of peritoneum, hypointense on T2WI, attaching to the anterior wall of the rectum. It is usually found at the level above the top of the seminal vesicles in men and in the plane of uterocervical region/cul-de-sac in women (see **Fig. 4**).[42] In the axial plane, the peritoneal reflection has a V-shaped appearance (seagull sign) (**Fig. 7**).[41]

○ Best sequence to be evaluated: sagittal T2WI (midsagittal plane) and oblique axial high-resolution T2WI.

• The *retrorectal space* is defined by a virtual space between the posterior aspect of the MRF and the presacral fascia, which is a thin linear structure covering the presacral vessels (see **Fig. 4**). The retrorectal space is the posterior plane of dissection in TME surgeries and is divided into superior and inferior by the rectosacral fascia. The rectosacral fascia is a fascial band with variable thickness and inconstantly visible on MR imaging, which extends from the S4 level to the posteroinferior aspect of the MRF, bordering the anal sphincter.[43]

○ Best sequence to be evaluated: sagittal T2WI.

A   **B**

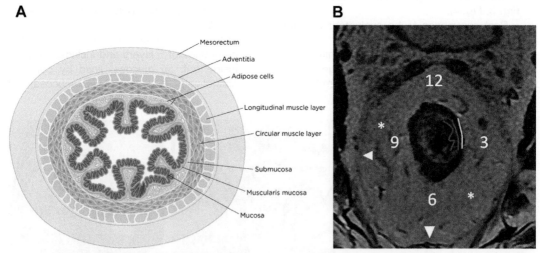

Fig. 5. Axial view anatomy. (*A*) Illustration and (*B*) high-resolution axial oblique T2WI demonstrate the MRF (*arrowheads*), mesorectum (*asterisks*), and rectal wall layers. The illustration shows the 5 intestinal layers: mucosa, muscularis mucosa, submucosa, muscularis propria (consisting of inner circular and outer longitudinal layers), and serosa. On MR imaging, 3 layers are mostly visible: mucosa, as the innermost thin hypointense layer (*red line*), submucosa, as a middle hyperintense layer (*blue line*), and muscularis propria, as the outer hypointense layer (*yellow line*). (*B*) The o'clock view is also demonstrated.

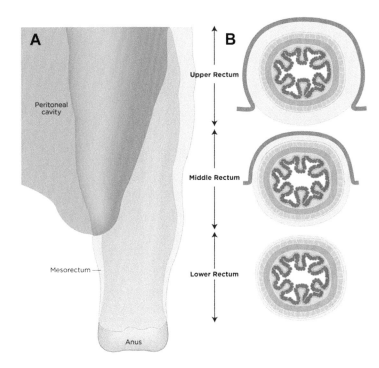

Fig. 6. The peritoneal and MRF coverage of the rectum. (*A*) Lateral view of the rectum and (*B*) axial sections demonstrating peritoneal coverage in the upper, middle, and low rectum. Note that the potential CRM described on the radiological report corresponds to the distance between the tumor and the MRF and do not include the portions of the rectum surrounded by peritoneum.

MR IMAGING FOR PRIMARY STAGING

In primary staging, rectal MR imaging adds value in the following aspects: (a) tumor location and morphology, (b) T category, (c) sphincter complex status, (d) CRM status, (e) EMVI, (f) pelvic sidewall status, and (g) N category. The report template in the primary staging setting used in the authors' institution is demonstrated in Box 1.

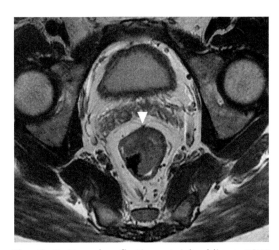

Fig. 7. Peritoneal reflection. Axial oblique T2WI shows the peritoneal reflection (*arrowhead*) as a thin line attaching to the anterior wall of the rectum in a V-shaped appearance (seagull sign).

Tumor Location and Morphology

For surgical planning, it is essential to describe the tumor location in the craniocaudal direction (lower, middle, or upper rectum) and circumferential plane (o'clock position), as well as its length, relationship to the anterior peritoneal reflection (above, below, or at), and distance from the inferior border of the tumor to AV and to the ARJ. The measurements should be along the anorectal angulation to avoid errors.[16]

The morphologic pattern of tumor growth (polypoid, ulcerating, circumferential, or partially circumferential) and tumor appearance (nonmucinous vs mucinous) can also be described. Nonmucinous tumors are more frequent and appear with an intermediate SI on T2WI (Fig. 8A), whereas mucinous tumors present with high SI on T2WI (Fig. 8B) and have a different biological behavior and poor prognosis.[44,45]

T Category

The T category is one of the prognostic factors for LR, along with N categorization and CRM. It depends on the depth of tumor penetration into the rectal wall and extramural spread into the mesorectum and adjacent organs, as demonstrated in Fig. 9 (see Table 1). The T category is one of the prognostic factors for LR, along with N categorization and CRM. High-resolution rectal MR imaging

Box 1
Report template for primary staging of rectal cancer

Primary staging

Clinical information: [free text]

Technique: [free text]

Comparison: [free text]

Tumor location and morphology:

Tumor location from anal verge: □ low (0–5 cm) □ mid (5.1–10 cm) □ high (10.1–15 cm)

Distance of inferior border of the tumor to anal verge: [free text] cm

Distance of inferior border of the tumor to anorectal junction/top of sphincter complex: [free text] cm

Relationship to anterior peritoneal reflection: □ above □ straddles □ below

Craniocaudal length: [free text] cm

Circumferential location (o'clock position): [free text]

Morphology: □ polypoid □ ulcerating □ circumferential □ semi-circumferential

Mucinous: □ no □ yes

T category: □ Tx □ T1/T2 □ T2 □ T3a □ T3b □ T3c □ T3d □ T4a □ T4b

If T4b, describe structures with possible invasion:

Genitourinary: □ bladder □ left ureter □ right ureter □ cervix □ uterus □ vagina □ prostate □ seminal vesicle □ urethra

Vessels: □ [left/right] internal iliac vessels □ [left/right] external iliac vessels

Nerves: □ lumbosacral nerve roots

Pelvic muscles: □ obturator internus □ piriformis □ ischiococcygeus

Pelvic floor: □ pubococcygeus □ ileococcygeus □ puborectalis □ levator ani

Bones: □ sacrum □ coccyx □ ilium □ ischium □ pubis

[a] Low rectal tumors:

Invasion of sphincter complex: □ no □ yes

If yes:

□ Internal sphincter only

□ Internal sphincter and intersphincteric plane

□ External sphincter

Length of anal canal: [free text] cm

Extramural vascular invasion (EMVI): □ no □ yes

Circumferential resection margin (CRM), for T3 only:

Shortest distance of tumor to mesorectal fascia (MRF) (or anticipated CRM): [free text] cm [location]

□ Not applicable (peritonealized portion of the rectum)

Separate tumor deposit, suspicious lymph node, or EMVI threatening (≤2 mm) or invading (≤1 mm) the MRF:

□ no □ yes [if yes, location and distance]

Suspicious mesorectal lymph nodes and/or tumor deposits:

□ no □ yes

Malignant morphologic criteria (MMC): irregular borders, heterogeneous signal intensity, and round shape.

Suspicious lymph node: ≥9 mm in the short-axis or 5–9 mm with 2 MMC or <5 mm with 3 MMC

Extramesorectal lymph nodes:

☐ no ☐ yes [if yes, location]

Other findings/additional comments: [free text]

Impression:

- Stage: T [free text] N [free text]
- CRM: ☐ clear ☐ threatened ☐ involved
- Suspicious node/EMVI near CRM: ☐ yes ☐ no
- Sphincter involvement: ☐ absent ☐ present
- Suspicious extramesorectal nodes: ☐ yes ☐ no

   [a] Refers to a subtopic within T-category.

in assessing T staging has an accuracy, sensitivity, and specificity of 85%, 87%, and 75%, respectively.[46]

One important step in the evaluation of tumor penetration is the identification of the invasive portion of the tumor, which corresponds to the most worrisome area for deeper infiltration. First, it is essential to identify the tumor in the sagittal plane; the most invasive area is usually halfway in the craniocaudal direction. After finding this area in the sagittal plane, it is necessary to open its corresponding view in the oblique axial plane. The tumor typically appears in a C-shaped configuration on the oblique axial plane with 2 raised edges; the most invasive area is usually located around the center of the C-shaped curvature (Fig. 10).

T1 tumors infiltrate into the submucosa, whereas T2 extends into the muscularis propria without extension to the mesorectum. Rectal MR imaging is not reliable in differentiating T1 from T2 tumors, and ERUS is considered the modality of choice in this differentiation.[16] However, in some patients with T1 tumors, it is possible to identify on MR imaging a tenuous preservation of the submucosal layer (hyperintense) beneath the tumor.[47,48]

T3 tumors are transmural and extend beyond the muscularis propria into the mesorectum, but do not infiltrate the serosal surfaces (MRF) or adjacent organs. On MR imaging, it is characterized by a discontinuity of the muscularis propria with extension of the tumor into the mesorectum with a broad-based bulging or nodular configuration.[34] T3 tumors are subclassified into 4 categories depending on the distance between the outermost edge of the muscularis propria and the maximum extramural spread of the tumor: T3a <1 mm, T3b = 1 to 5 mm, T3c = 5 to 15 mm, and T4d >15 mm (see Fig. 10; Fig. 11). It is of key importance to detect the continuity of the tumor into the mesorectal fat, because the outer longitudinal muscular layers can appear discontinuous because of penetration by small vessels.[34] Another pitfall that can lead to overstaging T2 as T3 is the desmoplastic reaction; however, it is characterized by spiculations with low SI on T2WI compared with the broad-based or nodular appearance of the T3 lesions with intermediate SI.[34] Despite this, differentiating T2 versus early

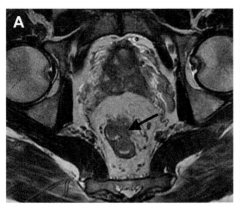 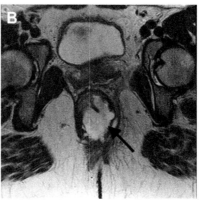

Fig. 8. Tumor appearance. Axial oblique T2WI shows (A) nonmucinous tumor, which appears with an intermediate SI (arrow), and (B) mucinous tumor, which, characteristically, has very high SI on T2WI (arrow).

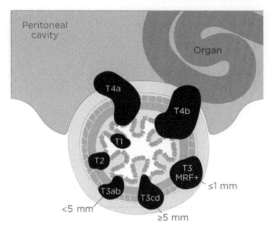

Fig. 9. The T category.

T3 can be difficult,[49] and a multidisciplinary team approach is indicated in order to choose the best treatment for the patient, especially in centers that apply the US guidelines.

Finally, T4 tumors are those that infiltrate the peritoneal reflection (T4a) or other pelvic organs and structures (T4b) (Fig. 12).

Sphincter Complex Status

Patients with low RC (lower edge of the tumor <5 cm above the AV) require special attention regarding the sphincter complex involvement. Given the tapering of mesorectum in the lower rectum, tumors in this location easily invade the MRF and adjacent organs, resulting in positive surgical margins in around 30% of cases.[50] As such, aggressive surgery requires careful consideration, given the significant impairment in quality of life of patients after APR.

In this scenario, radiologists play a pivotal role in the preoperative evaluation of the sphincter complex. Besides the distance to the AV and the ARJ, the report should describe whether the tumor invades (a) the internal sphincter, (b) intersphincteric plane, (c) external sphincter, and (d) levator ani (Fig. 13). Sphincter complex status will guide the surgeon in treatment planning as well as the type of surgery. The coronal oblique T2WI is the best plane to evaluate those structures; however, correlation with the other planes can be useful.

Circumferential Resection Margin Status

CRM is defined by the surgically dissected surface of the nonperitonealized part of the rectum and is obtained by measuring the shortest distance between the outmost edge of the primary tumor and the MRF.[51] CRM is not a synonym for MRF; the first one is determined by how the surgery was performed, whereas MRF is an anatomic parameter. MR imaging is the most trustworthy imaging modality to determine potential CRM involvement[46] and the cutoffs measurements are[16] as follows:

- Tumor-MRF distance less than 1 mm: potentially positive CRM (see Fig. 11B)
- Tumor-MRF distance 1 to 2 mm: threatened CRM

Using the cutoff of less than 1 mm, Oberholzer and colleagues[52] demonstrated sensitivity, specificity, positive predictive value (PPV), and negative predictive value (NPV) of 89%, 96%, 80%, and 89%, respectively, with a substantial interobserver agreement. The positivity of the CRM is the most important predictor of LR and poor

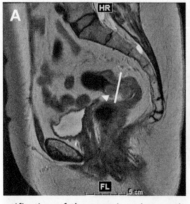
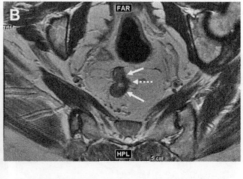

Fig. 10. Identification of the most invasive portion of the tumor, which is the most worrisome area for deeper infiltration. (A) Sagittal T2WI shows the tumor in the upper rectum below the peritoneal reflection (arrowhead). Its most invasive area is usually halfway (white line) in the craniocaudal direction. (B) High-resolution axial oblique T2 at this level demonstrates the tumor with a typical C-shape configuration. The most invasive area is classically located around the center of the C curvature (arrows). Inside that invasive portion, an area of deeper infiltration at 3 o'clock extends 4 mm beyond the muscularis propria into the mesorectum, T3b (dashed arrow).

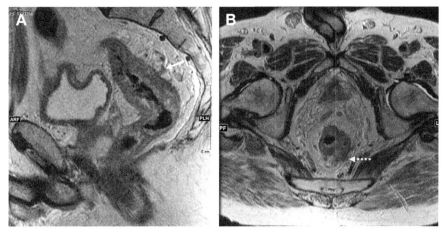

Fig. 11. Staging rectal MR imaging. (*A*) Sagittal T2WI shows the tumor in the upper/middle rectum with a posterior EMVI (*arrow*). (*B*) High-resolution axial oblique T2WI demonstrates the most invasive portion of the tumor, which extends 11 cm beyond the muscularis propria (T3c) at 4 o'clock and infiltrates the medially retracted MRF, resulting in a potentially positive CRM (*dashed arrow*).

survival[53]; thus, every report needs to describe the CRM status and the location where it is potentially positive or threatened based on the o'clock method.

Extramural Vascular Invasion

EMVI is an important predictor of metastatic disease and an important prognostic factor[54,55] that can be assessed on MR imaging with moderate sensitivity and high specificity.[56] It is defined by the presence of tumor within the vessels in the mesorectum. EMVI is characterized by an extension of the tumor resulting in (a) irregularity of the vessels and/or (b) SI of the tumor (intermediate) within the vessel, replacing the flow void, and/or (c) focal enlargement of the vessel[56] (**Fig. 14**).

Pelvic Organs and Pelvic Sidewall

In invasive tumors, it is also important to describe if the adjacent structures are involved, including the uterus, vagina, prostate gland, seminal vesicles, presacral fascia, sacral nerve roots, and

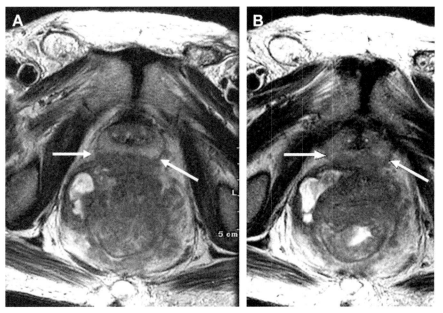

Fig. 12. Staging rectal MR imaging. (*A, B*) Axial oblique T2WI shows a tumor in the lower rectum infiltrating the Denonvilliers' fascia and the posterior peripheral prostate zone (*arrows*), T4b.

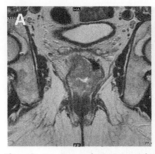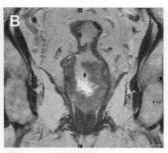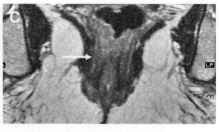

Fig. 13. Low rectal tumor without and with involvement of intersphincteric plane. (*A, B*) Coronal T2WI in a patient with low rectal tumor demonstrates a clean intersphincteric plane. (*C*) Coronal T2WI of a different patient shows infiltration of intersphincteric plane (*arrow*).

sacrum. Other structures along the pelvic sidewall are also important to be evaluated, such as the iliac vessels, ureters, and pelvic muscles, including the pyriform and internal obturator. This information provides a roadmap for the surgeon.

N Category

The MR imaging report should describe the following aspects of the LNs: (a) presence of nodes suspected for malignancy, (b) number and location of suspicious LNs, and (c) proximity between the suspicious LNs and the MRF. Although the proximity between LNs and MRF is important for surgical planning, it has not been shown to confer poor prognosis in the same manner that has been shown for primary tumor.[18]

On the other hand, metastatic LNs are an important prognostic factor and are considered an indication for neoadjuvant CRT. However, MR imaging is less accurate for assessing them compared with T categorization.[46]

Size criteria are not reliable for determining N category, because a large proportion of metastatic LNs in RC measure less than 5 mm,[57,58] but some studies have demonstrated that LNs greater than 8 mm in the short axis are highly specific for metastatic involvement.[59,60] For example, Kim and colleagues[59] demonstrated accuracy of 84% for LNs >8 mm in the short-axis diameter, with sensitivity of 45%, specificity of 100%, and PPV of 100%. Other well-known criteria for malignant LNs rely on morphologic characteristics, including the presence of either irregular borders or heterogeneous SI,[57] and this is used in various institutions. Brown and colleagues[57] prospectively demonstrated that the presence of both irregular borders and mixed SI resulted in a sensitivity of 85% and a specificity of 98%. Kim and colleagues[59] retrospectively showed sensitivity of 45% and specificity of 100% for spiculated borders, whereas for mottled heterogeneous pattern the sensitivity was 50% and specificity was 100%.

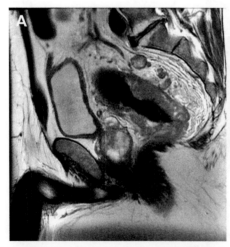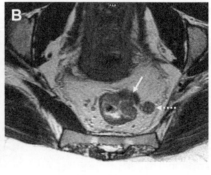

Fig. 14. Two different patients with RC with EMVI (*arrow*) and positive LNs (*dashed arrow*). (*A*) Mesorectal LN measuring 1.0 cm in the short axis and heterogeneous SI. (*B*) Mesorectal LN measuring 0.7 cm with round shape and heterogeneous SI.

The 2012 European Society of Gastrointestinal and Abdominal Radiology consensus meeting suggested for nodal assessment the use of both size and morphologic criteria.[16] However, there is no consensus in the literature regarding the best imaging criteria to diagnose malignant nodes. LN MR contrast agents, such as ultrasmall superparamagnetic iron oxide and Gadofosveset, are promising for differentiating benign from metastatic LN, but availability and safety concerns have mostly prevented their use.[61,62]

At the authors' institution, they consider both size and morphologic criteria to deem the LN as malignant. The malignant morphologic criteria (MMC) that the authors consider are (a) irregular borders, (b) heterogeneous SI, and (c) round shape (see **Fig. 14**). Depending on the size in the short axis, the number of morphologic features changes as follows:

- Less than 5 mm: needs 3 MMC
- 5 to 9 mm: needs 2 MMC
- Greater than 9 mm: suspicious regardless of the number of MMC[63]

The most important LN chains to be assessed in RC are mesorectal, superior rectal, inferior mesenteric, iliac (common, internal, and external), retroperitoneal, and inguinal.[36] Extramesorectal LNs, including those along the pelvic sidewall, are very important to identify, because they are not routinely resected. Furthermore, the presence of metastatic extramesorectal LNs is also a negative prognostic predictor.[64]

The number of metastatic regional LN is also crucial once it changes the N category (see **Table 1**). According to AJCC, *regional LNs* in RC are mesorectal, sigmoid mesenteric, inferior mesenteric, lateral sacral, presacral, internal iliac, sacral promontory, superior rectal, middle rectal, and inferior rectal. LNs out of these chains are considered M1, so the precise location of the LNs is also essential in the staging. Tumor deposits, defined as group of tumor cells not associated with lymphoid or vascular tissues, are characterized as N1c.

As mentioned before, the relationship between malignant LNs and the MRF is important to comment upon in the report. However, tumor-bearing LN adjacent to the MRF has no adverse prognostic significance compared with non-tumor-bearing LN in this location. The issue is simply one of planning a safe surgical margin.[18]

MR IMAGING FOR RESTAGING AFTER NEOADJUVANT THERAPY

Currently, neoadjuvant therapy is considered the standard of care for patients with locally advanced tumors. It has been shown to improve local control; induce tumor downstaging in approximately 50% to 60% of the patients, which can allow sphincter preservation; and result in pCR in 15% to 38% of cases.[12,65–68] This nonoperative approach has been emerging for patients with pCR as an alternative to resection. In this sense, the assessment of tumor response after neoadjuvant CRT has become more significant.

DRE and endoscopy have been used as the main tool to evaluate pCR with accuracies around 71% to 88%.[69,70] However, the clinical assessment is limited to the luminal view, and residual tumors can be observed in any layer of the bowel wall.[71] Rectal MR imaging has been used to assess treatment response using either morphologic[72,73] or functional sequences,[70,74] with variable diagnostic performances among different sequences and institutions.

The key steps before interpretation of a restaging rectal MR scan are to (1) verify the neoadjuvant modalities that the patients received and their time intervals, (2) evaluate the results of DREs and endoscopies, and (3) correlate with the pretreatment MR imaging in order to document the prior tumor location and morphology, including the most invasive area within the rectal wall circumference. The last step is of utmost importance to guide the correct location of the treated area and avoid a common pitfall after CRT. The rectal wall not previously involved by the tumor can present post-CRT changes and be misinterpreted as residual tumor. For example, the unaffected submucosa may become edematous, thickened, and intermediate to high in T2 SI, whereas the tumor after treatment may appear fibrotic low in T2 SI and atrophic, resulting in a pseudotumor appearance of the normal rectal wall (**Fig. 15**).[75]

After neoadjuvant treatment, rectal MR adds value in similar ways to primary staging with a few differences and exceptions. The following aspects are important.

Tumor Location and Morphology

Evaluation is similar to primary staging and includes the mucinous component. After CRT, the evaluation of mucin within the tumor is challenging and can present in 3 different scenarios:

- *Mucin (or colloid) degeneration.* Nonmucinous tumors can present necrosis after neoadjuvant therapy, resulting in mucinous degeneration, which appears as high SI on T2WI within the previous area of intermediate SI.[75] This degeneration can be interpreted as evidence of treatment response because these patients demonstrate better prognosis compared with

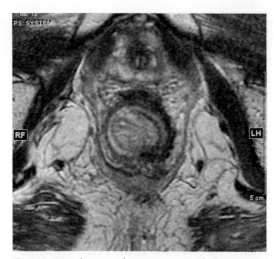

Fig. 15. Pseudotumoral appearance of the normal rectal wall after CRT. High-resolution axial oblique T2WI shows posttreated area in the left rectal wall with low SI. In contrast, the remaining wall appears thickened and higher in T2 SI due to submucosal edema from radiation therapy.

patients with preexisting mucinous carcinoma.[76]

- *Acellular mucin.* Mucinous tumors after treatment can present on pathology with cellular or acellular mucin, which is considered treatment response with no impact on recurrence-free survival.[77] However, there is no reliable imaging modality able to differentiate cellular form acellular mucin (**Fig. 16**).
- *Mucinous tumor without response.* These are associated with poor outcomes, including increased risk of LR.[75,76]

Presence or Absence of Residual Tumor and/or Fibrosis

Residual tumor has intermediate SI on T2WI, whereas fibrosis shows low SI. However, this visual differentiation is challenging. In order to improve the accuracy of T2WI, functional MR imaging sequences have been studied, including DWI (**Fig. 17**),[70,78] DCE-MR imaging,[74] and magnetization transfer imaging.[79] However,

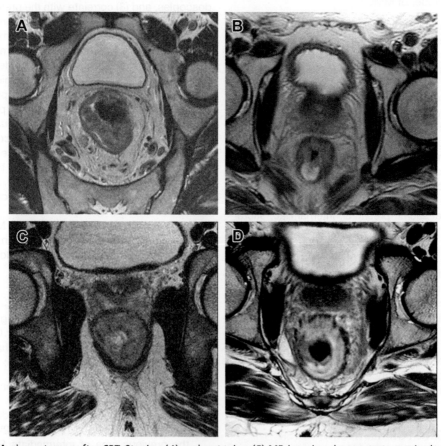

Fig. 16. Mucinous tumor after CRT. Staging (*A*) and restaging (*B*) MR imaging demonstrate mucin degeneration after the neoadjuvant treatment. The histopathological analysis after TME demonstrated residual tumor. Staging (*C*) and restaging (*D*) MR imaging in a different patient show a similar event; however, there was no tumor in the surgical specimen.

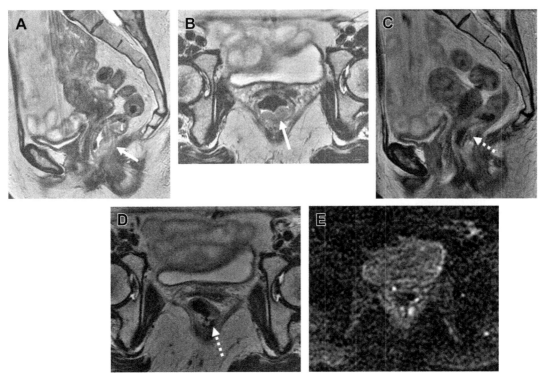

Fig. 17. Restaging MR imaging. Staging (A, B) and restaging (C, D, E) show the primary tumor in the lower rectum with intermediate SI on T2WI (A, B) (arrows). After CRT, the tumor reduced in size and became hypointense on T2WI (C, D); however, foci of restricted diffusion were observed (E). Patient underwent surgery, and residual tumor was detected.

consistent results and standardized techniques are still needed in order to implement them in the clinical practice.

Tumor Regression Grade

TRG was first described in 1994 for esophageal carcinomas[80] and is a measure of histopathological response to neoadjuvant treatment. Several TRG systems are used, and the vast majority correlate with clinical outcome.[81] MR imaging TRG has been proposed and demonstrates a correlation with survival outcomes[73] (Table 3).

Volumetric Analysis

Tumor volumetry has been reported to correlate with tumor response.[74,82] However, there is no consensus regarding which sequence to use to outline the tumor and which measurement is more reliable and applicable in clinical practice. In addition, it is a time-consuming process not well suited to daily clinical practice.

yT Stage and Any Remaining Tumor Deposit Within the Mesorectum

The accuracy of rectal MR imaging after neoadjuvant treatment is lower than in primary staging,

approximately 50%.[83] A systematic review demonstrated a mean sensitivity of 55% and specificity of 90% for MR imaging in differentiating T0-T2 versus T3-T4.[79]

Although consensus is growing but not yet established, DWI is recommended to be added

Table 3 MR imaging tumor regression grade	
	Response
TRG 1	Complete radiologic response: no evidence of ever treated tumor
TRG 2	Good response: dense fibrosis; no obvious residual tumor, signifying minimal residual disease; or no tumor
TRG 3	Moderate response: >50% fibrosis or mucin and visible intermediate signal
TRG 4	Slight response: little areas of fibrosis or mucin, but mostly tumor
TRG 5	No response: intermediate SI, same appearances as original tumor

Data from Taylor FG, Swift RI, Blomqvist L, et al. A systematic approach to the interpretation of preoperative staging MRI for rectal cancer. AJR Am J Roentgenol 2008;191(6):1827–35.

for restaging MR imaging, because recent studies have showed that it is beneficial for the evaluation of yT staging. Fibrosis demonstrates low SI on high-*b*-value DWI, whereas residual tumor shows high SI; therefore, the tumor stands out against the surrounding fibrotic background.[84] The mean specificity of DWI in a systematic review was 84.8%, whereas the mean sensitivity was 83.6%. Diagnostic performance of DWI was significantly better in studies published between 2009 and 2013, probably as a result of technical improvements. Maas and colleagues[70] demonstrated that T2WI and DWI together showed an accuracy of 79% in the diagnosis of complete response, and that incorporating clinical assessment in the evaluation led to an accuracy of 89%, with a positive posttest probability of 98%. Those results emphasize the value of a close cooperation of a multidisciplinary team using a combination of modalities in the assessment of tumor response as well as the growing importance of functional MR sequences in evaluation of the tumor environment.

Sphincter Complex Status

Evaluation is similar to primary staging.

Pelvic Sidewall Status

Evaluation is similar to primary staging.

yCRM Status

In the report, it is important to describe the smallest distance between the remaining tumor and the MRF as well as its location. Considering the potential difficulty in differentiating scar and viable tumor after neoadjuvant therapy, determining CRM status can be more challenging and less reproducible during restaging. Oberholzer and colleagues[52] demonstrated sensitivity, specificity, PPV, and NPV of 92%, 79%, 42%, and 98%, respectively, with a moderate interobserver agreement. Van der Paardt and colleagues[78] showed in a systematic review a mean sensitivity of 76% and mean specificity of 86%.

Extramural Vascular Invasion

EMVI can disappear after treatment and be replaced by fibrotic cords or strands.[75] Although EMVI is recommended to be described at primary staging MR imaging, it is not clear whether it should be reported (and its importance) at restaging.[16]

yN Stage

After CRT, it is important to describe the number of remaining suspicious LNs within and outside the mesorectum as well as whether some of them involve the MRF.

Although still challenging, the N categorization after CRT has been shown to be more accurate than at primary staging, possibly because of low prevalence of positive LNs after treatment and the fact that most of them become smaller or disappear.[85] Nodal size in the short axis is more reliable, whereas borders and shape are less reliable to assess residual malignancy.[16] Heijnen and colleagues[85] demonstrated that use of a cutoff size of 2.5 mm in the short axis resulted in an area under the curve of 0.78, and a decrease in size of at least 70% demonstrated ypN0 status in 100% of the cases. Another study evaluated the DWI for assessment node status after CRT and concluded that, although it is not a frequent finding, the absence of LNs on DWI can be a reliable predictor of negative node status after surgery.[86]

MR IMAGING IN LOCAL RECURRENCE

The definition of LR is controversial among different groups and organizations. According to NCCN, LR is defined by isolated pelvic/anastomotic recurrence of disease.[87] After the introduction of TME and neoadjuvant treatment, the reported rates of LR are less than 10%, and some groups describe rates lower than 5%.[88] Despite improvements in treatment, LR remains an important issue in the management of the patients with RC in terms of incidence, morbidity, and mortality. Early diagnosis is of vital importance to avoid disease progression and enable surgical resection, which is the only possibility of cure.

Most LR occurs in the first 3 years after the primary surgery, and synchronous metastatic disease is present in about 50% of patients.[22] The risk factors for LR are related to tumor biology, tumor location, and surgical technique, along with the experience of the surgical team. The most important risk factors are pathologic TNM stage, T substage, tumor differentiation, CRM status, distance from AV, lymphovascular invasion, surgical technique, anastomotic leak, and perforation at the time of surgery.[7]

Increase of carcinoembryonic antigen and development of symptoms should raise the suspicion of LR; however, up to 30% of LR occurs in asymptomatic patients. LR can be classified in compartments as the following: (a) *axial* (anastomotic, residual mesorectum, or perirectal soft tissue in the center of the pelvis or perineum including the pelvic floor); (b) *anterior* (bladder, vagina, uterus, seminal vesicles, or prostate); (c) *posterior* (presacral fascia, sacrum, coccyx, and sacral root sheaths); or (d) *lateral* (pelvic ureters, iliac vessels, lateral LNs, pelvic nerves, sidewall muscles, mainly piriformis and elevator and lateral bony pelvis). Most LR are anastomotic and easily identified by the surgeon and endoscopists on clinical evaluation and/or endoscopy. However, the other recurrence sites can be clinically challenging to detect and imaging may be helpful.

The role of imaging is (1) to identify LR, mainly in asymptomatic patients; (2) to verify if the disease is limited to the pelvis or has metastasized; and (3) to assess the local distribution of the disease in order to help the multidisciplinary team decide if the patient is eligible for curative or palliative approaches, and if indicated, to guide the surgical plan.

CT and PET/CT are useful to investigate local and distant recurrence; however, MR imaging is considered the most accurate imaging modality for local staging. For all imaging modalities, the distinction between postsurgical and postradiation changes from LR is challenging, considering they both can share similar imaging findings and may appear fludeoxyglucose-avid on PET-CT.

The following imaging features may raise the suspicion from LR[22,48,89]:

- Interval increase in size. Comparison with the first postoperative scan is suggested because small increases may be overlooked
- Asymmetric and/or round appearance
- Marked contrast enhancement, particularly if heterogeneous and/or early
- Invasive behavior
- Rim enhancement, which may be present but lacks accuracy in the recent postoperative period because abscesses can present the same pattern of enhancement

The radiological report should describe in detail the location of LR focused on the compartments and structures previously described. Furthermore, it is important to describe if the tumor invades S1 or S2 nerve roots and sciatic nerves; if the sacral infiltration is above the S2 level; if there is encasement of the iliac vessels; and nodal staging, mainly inguinal, pelvic, and retroperitoneal. Tumors that infiltrate the presacral space can directly access the retroperitoneal space; therefore, those LNs are important to evaluate. Distant staging is also of key importance and includes evaluation of peritoneal infiltration and presence of distant metastases as well as its resectability.

The most important contraindications for pelvic exenteration are (a) unresectable distant metastasis; (b) infiltration of the proximal sacrum (S2 or higher), because if resected it could result in pelvic instability; (c) invasion of the proximal lumbosacral plexus and sciatic nerves; (d) encasement of the

external or common iliac vessels, due to potential damage of the lower limbs; and (e) incapacitating medical comorbidities.[90,91]

SUMMARY

In the current era of RC management, the multidisciplinary approach is of utmost importance for improving patient outcome. The emergence of rectal MR imaging has played a key role in local staging and identifying risk factors for local and distant recurrence, which helps tailor treatment and improve patient outcome.

ACKNOWLEDGMENTS

The authors would like to thank Joanne Chin for editorial assistance.

REFERENCES

1. Ferlay J, Soerjomataram I, Dikshit R, et al. Cancer incidence and mortality worldwide: sources, methods and major patterns in GLOBOCAN 2012. Int J Cancer 2015;136(5):E359–86.
2. American Cancer Society. Cancer facts & figures 2017. Available at: https://www.cancer.org/content/dam/cancer-org/research/cancer-facts-and-statistics/annual-cancer-facts-and-figures/2017/cancer-facts-and-figures-2017.pdf. Accessed October 12, 2017.
3. Ferrari L, Fichera A. Neoadjuvant chemoradiation therapy and pathological complete response in rectal cancer. Gastroenterol Rep (Oxf) 2015;3(4):277–88.
4. MERCURY Study Group. Diagnostic accuracy of preoperative magnetic resonance imaging in predicting curative resection of rectal cancer: prospective observational study. BMJ 2006;333(7572):779.
5. Bailey CE, Hu CY, You YN, et al. Increasing disparities in the age-related incidences of colon and rectal cancers in the United States, 1975-2010. JAMA Surg 2015;150(1):17–22.
6. Nagtegaal ID, Quirke P. What is the role for the circumferential margin in the modern treatment of rectal cancer? J Clin Oncol 2008;26(2):303–12.
7. Heald RJ, Ryall RD. Recurrence and survival after total mesorectal excision for rectal cancer. Lancet 1986;1(8496):1479–82.
8. Krook JE, Moertel CG, Gunderson LL, et al. Effective surgical adjuvant therapy for high-risk rectal carcinoma. N Engl J Med 1991;324(11):709–15.
9. Gastrointestinal Tumor Study Group. Prolongation of the disease-free interval in surgically treated rectal carcinoma. N Engl J Med 1985;312(23):1465–72.
10. NIH consensus conference. Adjuvant therapy for patients with colon and rectum cancer. Consens Statement 1990;8(4):1–25.

11. Sauer R, Becker H, Hohenberger W, et al. Preoperative versus postoperative chemoradiotherapy for rectal cancer. N Engl J Med 2004;351(17):1731–40.

12. Maas M, Nelemans PJ, Valentini V, et al. Long-term outcome in patients with a pathological complete response after chemoradiation for rectal cancer: a pooled analysis of individual patient data. Lancet Oncol 2010;11(9):835–44.

13. Habr-Gama A, Perez RO, Bocchini SF, et al. Operative vs. nonoperative treatment for stage 0 distal rectal cancer following chemoradiation therapy: long-term results. Dis Colon Rectum 2004;47(6): 1005–6.

14. Garcia-Aguilar J, Shi Q, Thomas CR Jr, et al. A phase II trial of neoadjuvant chemoradiation and local excision for T2N0 rectal cancer: preliminary results of the ACOSOG Z6041 trial. Ann Surg Oncol 2012;19(2):384–91.

15. Weiss DL, Langlotz CP. Structured reporting: patient care enhancement or productivity nightmare? Radiology 2008;249(3):739–47.

16. Beets-Tan RG, Lambregts DM, Maas M, et al. Magnetic resonance imaging for the clinical management of rectal cancer patients: recommendations from the 2012 European Society of Gastrointestinal and Abdominal Radiology (ESGAR) consensus meeting. Eur Radiol 2013;23(9):2522–31.

17. Glimelius B, Tiret E, Cervantes A, et al. Rectal cancer: ESMO Clinical Practice Guidelines for diagnosis, treatment and follow-up. Ann Oncol 2013; 24(Suppl 6):vi81–8.

18. NCCN. NCCN guidelines version 2.2017 rectal cancer. Available at: https://www.nccn.org/professionals/physician_gls/pdf/rectal.pdf. Accessed September 10, 2017.

19. Bipat S, Glas AS, Slors FJ, et al. Rectal cancer: local staging and assessment of lymph node involvement with endoluminal US, CT, and MR imaging–a meta-analysis. Radiology 2004;232(3):773–83.

20. Balyasnikova S, Brown G. Optimal imaging strategies for rectal cancer staging and ongoing management. Curr Treat Options Oncol 2016;17(6):32.

21. Fernandez-Esparrach G, Ayuso-Colella JR, Sendino O, et al. EUS and magnetic resonance imaging in the staging of rectal cancer: a prospective and comparative study. Gastrointest Endosc 2011; 74(2):347–54.

22. Sinaei M, Swallow C, Milot L, et al. Patterns and signal intensity characteristics of pelvic recurrence of rectal cancer at MR imaging. Radiographics 2013;33(5):E171–87.

23. Memon S, Lynch AC, Akhurst T, et al. Systematic review of FDG-PET prediction of complete pathological response and survival in rectal cancer. Ann Surg Oncol 2014;21(11):3598–607.

24. Paspulati RM, Partovi S, Herrmann KA, et al. Comparison of hybrid FDG PET/MRI compared with PET/CT in colorectal cancer staging and restaging: a pilot study. Abdom Imaging 2015;40(6):1415–25.

25. Blomqvist L, Glimelius B. The 'good', the 'bad', and the 'ugly' rectal cancers. Acta Oncol 2008;47(1):5–8.

26. Willett CG, Compton CC, Shellito PC, et al. Selection factors for local excision or abdominoperineal resection of early stage rectal cancer. Cancer 1994; 73(11):2716–20.

27. Phang PT. Total mesorectal excision: technical aspects. Can J Surg 2004;47(2):130–7.

28. Bordeianou L, Maguire LH, Alavi K, et al. Sphincter-sparing surgery in patients with low-lying rectal cancer: techniques, oncologic outcomes, and functional results. J Gastrointest Surg 2014;18(7):1358–72.

29. Huang A, Zhao H, Ling T, et al. Oncological superiority of extralevator abdominoperineal resection over conventional abdominoperineal resection: a meta-analysis. Int J Colorectal Dis 2014;29(3):321–7.

30. Sasikumar A, Bhan C, Jenkins JT, et al. Systematic review of pelvic exenteration with en bloc sacrectomy for recurrent rectal adenocarcinoma: R0 resection predicts disease-free survival. Dis Colon Rectum 2017;60(3):346–52.

31. van der Pas MH, Haglind E, Cuesta MA, et al. Laparoscopic versus open surgery for rectal cancer (COLOR II): short-term outcomes of a randomised, phase 3 trial. Lancet Oncol 2013;14(3):210–8.

32. Stevenson AR, Solomon MJ, Lumley JW, et al. Effect of laparoscopic-assisted resection vs open resection on pathological outcomes in rectal cancer: the ALaCaRT randomized clinical trial. JAMA 2015; 314(13):1356–63.

33. Fleshman J, Branda M, Sargent DJ, et al. Effect of laparoscopic-assisted resection vs open resection of stage II or III rectal cancer on pathologic outcomes: the ACOSOG Z6051 randomized clinical trial. JAMA 2015;314(13):1346–55.

34. Taylor FG, Swift RI, Blomqvist L, et al. A systematic approach to the interpretation of preoperative staging MRI for rectal cancer. AJR Am J Roentgenol 2008;191(6):1827–35.

35. Vliegen RF, Beets GL, von Meyenfeldt MF, et al. Rectal cancer: MR imaging in local staging–is gadolinium-based contrast material helpful? Radiology 2005;234(1):179–88.

36. Kaur H, Choi H, You YN, et al. MR imaging for preoperative evaluation of primary rectal cancer: practical considerations. Radiographics 2012;32(2):389–409.

37. Torkzad MR, Pahlman L, Glimelius B. Magnetic resonance imaging (MRI) in rectal cancer: a comprehensive review. Insights Imaging 2010;1(4):245–67.

38. Salerno G, Sinnatamby C, Branagan G, et al. Defining the rectum: surgically, radiologically and anatomically. Colorectal Dis 2006;8:5–9.

39. Wasserman MA, McGee MF, Helenowski IB, et al. The anthropometric definition of the rectum is highly variable. Int J colorectal Dis 2016;31(2):189–95.

40. Kenig J, Richter P. Definition of the rectum and level of the peritoneal reflection - still a matter of debate? Wideochir Inne Tech Maloinwazyjne 2013;8(3):183–6.

41. Brown G, Kirkham A, Williams GT, et al. High-resolution MRI of the anatomy important in total mesorectal excision of the rectum. AJR Am J Roentgenol 2004; 182(2):431–9.

42. Gollub MJ, Maas M, Weiser M, et al. Recognition of the anterior peritoneal reflection at rectal MRI. AJR Am J Roentgenol 2013;200(1):97–101.

43. Beets-Tan RG, Beets GL. Rectal cancer: review with emphasis on MR imaging. Radiology 2004;232(2): 335–46.

44. Consorti F, Lorenzotti A, Midiri G, et al. Prognostic significance of mucinous carcinoma of colon and rectum: a prospective case-control study. J Surg Oncol 2000;73(2):70–4.

45. Symonds DA, Vickery AL. Mucinous carcinoma of the colon and rectum. Cancer 1976;37(4):1891–900.

46. Al-Sukhni E, Milot L, Fruitman M, et al. Diagnostic accuracy of MRI for assessment of T category, lymph node metastases, and circumferential resection margin involvement in patients with rectal cancer: a systematic review and meta-analysis. Ann Surg Oncol 2012;19(7):2212–23.

47. Costa-Silva L, Brown G. Magnetic resonance imaging of rectal cancer. Magn Reson Imaging Clin N Am 2013;21(2):385–408.

48. Furey E, Jhaveri KS. Magnetic resonance imaging in rectal cancer. Magn Reson Imaging Clin N Am 2014; 22(2):165–90, v–vi.

49. Beets-Tan RG, Beets GL, Vliegen RF, et al. Accuracy of magnetic resonance imaging in prediction of tumour-free resection margin in rectal cancer surgery. Lancet 2001;357(9255):497–504.

50. Shihab OC, Brown G, Daniels IR, et al. Patients with low rectal cancer treated by abdominoperineal excision have worse tumors and higher involved margin rates compared with patients treated by anterior resection. Dis Colon Rectum 2010;53(1):53–6.

51. Hermanek P, Junginger T. The circumferential resection margin in rectal carcinoma surgery. Tech Coloproctol 2005;9(3):193–9 [discussion: 199–200].

52. Oberholzer K, Junginger T, Heintz A, et al. Rectal cancer: MR imaging of the mesorectal fascia and effect of chemoradiation on assessment of tumor involvement. J Magn Reson Imaging 2012;36(3): 658–63.

53. Taylor FG, Quirke P, Heald RJ, et al. Preoperative high-resolution magnetic resonance imaging can identify good prognosis stage I, II, and III rectal cancer best managed by surgery alone: a prospective, multicenter, European study. Ann Surg 2011;253(4): 711–9.

54. Horn A, Dahl O, Morild I. Venous and neural invasion as predictors of recurrence in rectal adenocarcinoma. Dis Colon Rectum 1991;34(9):798–804.

55. Bugg WG, Andreou AK, Biswas D, et al. The prognostic significance of MRI-detected extramural venous invasion in rectal carcinoma. Clin Radiol 2014;69(6):619–23.

56. Smith NJ, Barbachano Y, Norman AR, et al. Prognostic significance of magnetic resonance imaging-detected extramural vascular invasion in rectal cancer. Br J Surg 2008;95(2):229–36.

57. Brown G, Richards CJ, Bourne MW, et al. Morphologic predictors of lymph node status in rectal cancer with use of high-spatial-resolution MR imaging with histopathologic comparison. Radiology 2003; 227(2):371–7.

58. Kotanagi H, Fukuoka T, Shibata Y, et al. The size of regional lymph nodes does not correlate with the presence or absence of metastasis in lymph nodes in rectal cancer. J Surg Oncol 1993;54(4):252–4.

59. Kim JH, Beets GL, Kim MJ, et al. High-resolution MR imaging for nodal staging in rectal cancer: are there any criteria in addition to the size? Eur J Radiol 2004; 52(1):78–83.

60. Beets-Tan RG. Pretreatment MRI of lymph nodes in rectal cancer: an opinion-based review. Colorectal Dis 2013;15(7):781–4.

61. Choi SH, Moon WK. Contrast-enhanced MR imaging of lymph nodes in cancer patients. Korean J Radiol 2010;11(4):383–94.

62. Lambregts DM, Heijnen LA, Maas M, et al. Gadofosveset-enhanced MRI for the assessment of rectal cancer lymph nodes: predictive criteria. Abdom Imaging 2013;38(4):720–7.

63. Beets-Tan RGH, Lambregts DMJ, Maas M, et al. Magnetic resonance imaging for clinical management of rectal cancer: updated recommendations from the 2016 European Society of Gastrointestinal and Abdominal Radiology (ESGAR) consensus meeting. Eur Radiol 2018;28(4):1465–75.

64. Sugihara K, Kobayashi H, Kato T, et al. Indication and benefit of pelvic sidewall dissection for rectal cancer. Dis Colon Rectum 2006;49(11):1663–72.

65. Habr-Gama A, Perez RO, Nadalin W, et al. Operative versus nonoperative treatment for stage 0 distal rectal cancer following chemoradiation therapy: long-term results. Ann Surg 2004;240(4):711–7 [discussion: 717–8].

66. Pahlman L, Bohe M, Cedermark B, et al. The Swedish rectal cancer registry. Br J Surg 2007;94(10): 1285–92.

67. Tulchinsky H, Shmueli E, Figer A, et al. An interval > 7 weeks between neoadjuvant therapy and surgery improves pathologic complete response and disease-free survival in patients with locally advanced rectal cancer. Ann Surg Oncol 2008; 15(10):2661–7.

68. Garcia-Aguilar J, Marcet J, Coutsoftides T, et al. Impact of neoadjuvant chemotherapy following chemoradiation on tumor response, adverse events,

and surgical complications in patients with advanced rectal cancer treated with TME. J Clin Oncol 2011;29(15):3514.

69. Perez RO, Habr-Gama A, Pereira GV, et al. Role of biopsies in patients with residual rectal cancer following neoadjuvant chemoradiation after downsizing: can they rule out persisting cancer? Colorectal Dis 2012;14(6):714–20.

70. Maas M, Lambregts DM, Nelemans PJ, et al. Assessment of clinical complete response after chemoradiation for rectal cancer with digital rectal examination, endoscopy, and MRI: selection for organ-saving treatment. Ann Surg Oncol 2015; 22(12):3873–80.

71. Duldulao MP, Lee W, Streja L, et al. Distribution of residual cancer cells in the bowel wall after neoadjuvant chemoradiation in patients with rectal cancer. Dis Colon Rectum 2013;56(2):142–9.

72. Patel UB, Brown G, Rutten H, et al. Comparison of magnetic resonance imaging and histopathological response to chemoradiotherapy in locally advanced rectal cancer. Ann Surg Oncol 2012;19(9):2842–52.

73. Patel UB, Taylor F, Blomqvist L, et al. Magnetic resonance imaging-detected tumor response for locally advanced rectal cancer predicts survival outcomes: MERCURY experience. J Clin Oncol 2011;29(28): 3753–60.

74. Hotker AM, Tarlinton L, Mazaheri Y, et al. Multiparametric MRI in the assessment of response of rectal cancer to neoadjuvant chemoradiotherapy: a comparison of morphological, volumetric and functional MRI parameters. Eur Radiol 2016;26(12):4303–12.

75. Patel UB, Blomqvist LK, Taylor F, et al. MRI after treatment of locally advanced rectal cancer: how to report tumor response–the MERCURY experience. AJR Am J Roentgenol 2012;199(4):W486–95.

76. Nagtegaal I, Gaspar C, Marijnen C, et al. Morphological changes in tumour type after radiotherapy are accompanied by changes in gene expression profile but not in clinical behaviour. J Pathol 2004; 204(2):183–92.

77. Shia J, McManus M, Guillem JG, et al. Significance of acellular mucin pools in rectal carcinoma after neoadjuvant chemoradiotherapy. Am J Surg Pathol 2011;35(1):127–34.

78. van der Paardt MP, Zagers MB, Beets-Tan RG, et al. Patients who undergo preoperative chemoradiotherapy for locally advanced rectal cancer restaged by using diagnostic MR imaging: a systematic review and meta-analysis. Radiology 2013;269(1):101–12.

79. Martens MH, Lambregts DM, Papanikolaou N, et al. Magnetization transfer imaging to assess tumour

response after chemoradiotherapy in rectal cancer. Eur Radiol 2016;26(2):390–7.

80. Mandard AM, Dalibard F, Mandard JC, et al. Pathologic assessment of tumor regression after preoperative chemoradiotherapy of esophageal carcinoma. Clinicopathologic correlations. Cancer 1994;73(11): 2680–6.

81. Trakarnsanga A, Gonen M, Shia J, et al. Comparison of tumor regression grade systems for locally advanced rectal cancer after multimodality treatment. J Natl Cancer Inst 2014;106(10) [pii:dju248].

82. Yeo SG, Kim DY, Kim TH, et al. Tumor volume reduction rate measured by magnetic resonance volumetry correlated with pathologic tumor response of preoperative chemoradiotherapy for rectal cancer. Int J Radiat Oncol Biol Phys 2010;78(1):164–71.

83. Chen CC, Lee RC, Lin JK, et al. How accurate is magnetic resonance imaging in restaging rectal cancer in patients receiving preoperative combined chemoradiotherapy? Dis Colon Rectum 2005;48(4): 722–8.

84. Lambregts DM, Vandecaveye V, Barbaro B, et al. Diffusion-weighted MRI for selection of complete responders after chemoradiation for locally advanced rectal cancer: a multicenter study. Ann Surg Oncol 2011;18(8):2224–31.

85. Heijnen LA, Maas M, Beets-Tan RG, et al. Nodal staging in rectal cancer: why is restaging after chemoradiation more accurate than primary nodal staging? Int J colorectal Dis 2016;31(6):1157–62.

86. van Heeswijk MM, Lambregts DMJ, Palm WM, et al. DWI for assessment of rectal cancer nodes after chemoradiotherapy: is the absence of nodes at DWI proof of a negative nodal status? AJR Am J Roentgenol 2017;208(3):W79–84.

87. NCCN. NCCN guidelines version 3.2017 pancreatic adenocarcinoma. 2017. Available at: https://www.nccn.org/professionals/physician_gls/pdf/pancreatic.pdf. Accessed June 15, 2017.

88. Syk E, Torkzad MR, Blomqvist L, et al. Local recurrence in rectal cancer: anatomic localization and effect on radiation target. Int J Radiat Oncol Biol Phys 2008;72(3):658–64.

89. Torkzad MR, Kamel I, Halappa VG, et al. Magnetic resonance imaging of rectal and anal cancer. Magn Reson Imaging Clin N Am 2014;22(1):85–112.

90. Moore HG, Shoup M, Riedel E, et al. Colorectal cancer pelvic recurrences: determinants of resectability. Dis Colon Rectum 2004;47(10):1599–606.

91. Sagebiel TL, Viswanathan C, Patnana M, et al. Overview of the role of imaging in pelvic exenteration. Radiographics 2015;35(4):1286–94.

MR Imaging of Perianal Fistulas

Kartik S. Jhaveri, MD[a],*, Seng Thipphavong, MD[a], Lijun Guo, MD[b],
Mukesh G. Harisinghani, MD[c]

KEYWORDS

• Perianal fistulas • MR imaging • Classification • Treatment

KEY POINTS

• MR imaging is considered a gold standard imaging technique for the evaluation of perianal fistulas.
• The 2 widely used classification systems for perianal fistulas include the Parks Classification system and the St James's University Hospital Classification system.
• Radiologists should evaluate for the presence of fistula, the relation to the anal sphincter complex, identify secondary tracks or abscesses, and report associated complications.
• MR imaging can be used to monitor treatment effects with the Van Assche MR imaging–based scoring system.
• Crohn disease–related fistulas often require medical treatment to achieve and maintain disease remission, rather than surgery.

INTRODUCTION

Perianal fistula, which is defined as an abnormal connection between the anal canal and the skin of the perineum, is an uncommon process but causes significant morbidity and predominantly affects young male adults.[1] Perianal fistula can be caused by several diseases, like Crohn disease (CD) and pelvic inflammation, whereas some of the cases are thought to be idiopathic. Patients with perianal fistula may be completely asymptomatic or present with symptoms of local pain and discharge.[2] Effective treatment and reduction in recurrence rates depend on an accurate detection and characterization of the perianal fistula.

Before the introduction of MR imaging, several imaging techniques have been used for perianal fistula evaluation, including fistulography, computed tomography (CT) with rectal and intravenous contrast agent, and endosonography. However, these techniques have several drawbacks: the inability of fistulography to visualize the anal sphincters and to determine their relationship to the fistula[3]; poor soft tissue resolution of CT to define subtle fistulas and abscesses[4]; limited field of view of endosonography preventing the detection of suprasphincteric or secondary tracts.[5]

With advances in techniques, MR imaging has been proven to play an important role in perianal fistula evaluation and is currently considered to be the gold standard method.[6] A prospective study conducted by Buchanan and colleagues[7] in 104 patients who were suspected of having perianal fistulas showed that the proportion of fistula tracts correctly classified with digital examination, endosonography, and MR imaging was 61%, 81%, and 90%, respectively; the internal openings of fistula tracts were correctly identified in 91% of

Disclosure Statement: There is no conflict of interest.
a Joint Department of Medical Imaging, University Health Network, Mount Sinai Hospital, Women's College Hospital, University of Toronto, 610 University Avenue, 3-957, Toronto, ON M5G 2M9, Canada; b Joint Department of Medical Imaging, University Health Network, 700 University Avenue, 2-84, Toronto, Ontario M5G 2M9, Canada; c Department of Abdominal Imaging, Massachusetts General Hospital, 55 Fruit Street, Boston, MA 02114, USA
* Corresponding author.
E-mail address: kartik.jhaveri@uhn.ca

Radiol Clin N Am 56 (2018) 775–789
https://doi.org/10.1016/j.rcl.2018.04.005
0033-8389/18/© 2018 Elsevier Inc. All rights reserved.

radiologic.theclinics.com

patients with endosonography and 97% of patients with MR imaging.

Treatment strategies of perianal fistula, including medical and surgical treatment, must be individualized according to the classification of fistula and the degree of surrounding pelvic structures involvement, especially the detection of secondary fistula tracts and abscesses in surrounding tissues. In the study by Buchanan and colleagues,[8] further recurrences arose in 16% of operations when surgeries were acted according to MR imaging findings, whereas recurrences arose in 57% of operations when MR imaging findings were ignored. The investigators concluded that surgery guided by MR imaging reduces further recurrence of perianal fistulas by 75% and should be performed in all patients with recurrent fistula.

In this review, we begin with an introduction of the perianal region anatomy, then review the definition, etiology, epidemiology, and 2 major classification systems of perianal fistulas. The role of MR imaging for assessment of perianal fistulas is mainly discussed. Finally, the medical and surgical treatment principles are reviewed.

ANATOMY OF THE ANAL CANAL

The anal canal is surrounded by the anal sphincter complex, which primarily consists of 2 muscular layers: the inner layer is the internal sphincter and the outer layer is the external sphincter. The internal sphincter is composed of involuntary smooth muscle, which is contiguous with the circular smooth muscle of the lower rectum.[9] The external sphincter is composed of striated muscle with strong voluntary contractions. Disruption of the external sphincter has high risk to cause fecal incontinence, whereas disruption of the internal sphincter will not lead to loss of continence.[10] The internal and external sphincters are separated by the intersphincteric space (also known as intersphincteric plane), which mainly contains fat, as well as connective tissue and the longitudinal muscle. Infection can easily spread in this space because of its natural low resistance[11] (Fig. 1).

In terms of the endoluminal anatomy of the anal canal, the dentate line (pectinate line), which is located at the base of the columns of Morgagni and the base of the crypts of Morgagni (between the columns),[5] is an important anatomic landmark for dividing the rectum and anal canal. At the level of the dentate line, the anal glands distributed along the anal canal wall (mainly in the intersphincteric space) drain into the anal canal via ducts opening into the crypts of Morgagni. When the draining duct is obstructed, intersphincteric anal

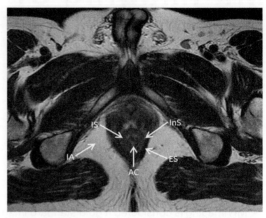

Fig. 1. Oblique axial T2-weighted MR image shows the normal anal sphincter anatomy in a 41-year-old man. AC, anal canal; ES, external sphincter; IA, ischioanal; InS, intersphincteric space; IS, internal sphincter.

gland infection may pass the internal sphincter to enter the intersphincteric space or penetrate both the internal and external sphincters toward the ischiorectal space and then lead to formation of a fistula tract or abscess in the corresponding location. This is the most widespread theory about the pathogenesis of perianal fistula, which is known as the cryptoglandular hypothesis.[11]

DEFINITION, ETIOLOGY, AND EPIDEMIOLOGY OF PERIANAL FISTULAS

Perianal fistula is defined as an abnormal connection between the anal canal and the skin of the perineum.

Most perianal fistula cases are thought to be idiopathic. Several inflammatory conditions, including pelvic infection, tuberculosis, diverticulitis, trauma during childbirth, pelvic malignancy, and radiation therapy can be etiologic factors for perianal fistulas.[5] CD is also a very common cause of perianal fistulas. It is reported that perianal fistulas occur in 30% to 50% of patients with CD at some stage during their lifetime.[12] Population-based studies in patients with CD demonstrated the cumulative risk for developing a perianal fistula is 21% after 10 years and 26% to 28% after 20 years.[13,14] It is worth mentioning that perianal fistulas in patients with CD are often more complex than those occurring in patients without CD and will not spontaneously close.[15]

Perianal fistula is an uncommon process with a prevalence of approximately 0.01% and predominantly affects young male adults.[1] Patients with perianal fistula may experience symptoms like local pain and discharge, whereas some patients with perianal fistula may be completely asymptomatic.[2]

CLASSIFICATION SYSTEMS

Two classification systems are often used for perianal fistulas: the Parks classification and the St James's University Hospital classification.

Parks Classification

In 1976, Parks and colleagues[16] proposed an anatomic-based classification system for perianal fistulas using the external sphincter as a central point of reference. This classification was especially important for patients treated surgically, as it was developed primarily from the surgical findings of 400 patients referred to the St Mark's Hospital surgery department in London. Our institution uses the Parks classification system in radiologic reports.

In this classification system, 4 types of perianal fistulas were described in the coronal plane according to the perianal fistula relationship to the anal sphincter complex.

Intersphincteric fistulas

This is the most common type in the study by Parks and colleagues[16] (accounted for 45% of the cases). The fistula opens at the anal canal (internal opening) and passes through the internal sphincter and the intersphincteric space to reach the perianal skin (external opening). This fistula does not traverse the external sphincter, which serves as a barrier to confine the spread of infection (Fig. 2).

Transsphincteric fistulas

The fistula passes through the internal sphincter, the intersphincteric space, and the external sphincter to enter ischiorectal and ischioanal fossae (Fig. 3).

Suprasphincteric fistulas

The fistula progresses upward into the intersphincteric space, passes over the top of the puborectalis muscle, then descends through the levator plate to the ischiorectal fossa and finally to the skin (Fig. 4).[16]

Extrasphincteric fistulas

This is a relatively rare type. The fistula opens at the rectum (internal opening) and passes through the levator muscles and ischiorectal fossa to reach the perianal skin (external opening). This fistula lies completely outside the anal sphincter complex and the anal canal is not involved. This type of

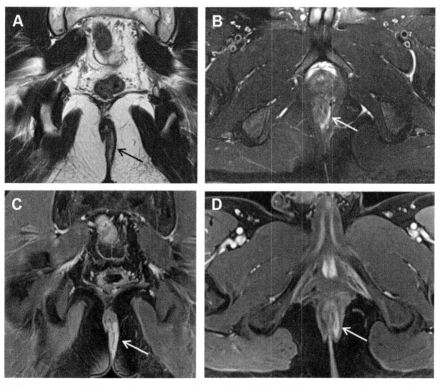

Fig. 2. (A) Oblique coronal (without fat suppression) and (B) axial (with fat suppression) T2-weighted MR images show an intersphincteric fistula (arrow) in a 24-year-old man. Postcontrast coronal (C) and axial (D) images with fat suppression show the fistula wall was significantly enhanced, whereas the fluid within the tract did not enhance (arrow). The relationship of fistula to the external sphincter was clearly defined on the contrast-enhanced image.

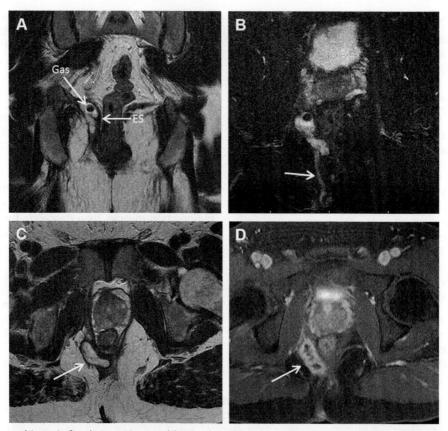

Fig. 3. Transsphincteric fistula in a 32-year-old man. (*A*) Oblique coronal (without fat suppression) T2-weighted MR image shows a signal intensity void of gas within a fistula tract that crossed the external sphincter (ES). (*B*) Oblique coronal (with fat suppression) T2-weighted MR image shows the course of the fistula tract (*arrow*): through the ischioanal fossa to skin surface. Both oblique axial T2-weighted MR image (without fat suppression) (*C*) and postcontrast image (*D*) clearly define the fistula tract (*arrow*).

fistula cannot be explained by the cryptoglandular hypothesis for its pathogenesis (**Fig. 5**).

Superficial fistulas, which were not included in the original publication of fistula classifications by Parks and colleagues,[16] have been added to describe fistulas that do not involve the anal sphincter complex (**Fig. 6**).

Complex fistulas, which were not included in the classification by Parks and colleagues[16] either, are composed of a primary fistula and associated secondary tracts (also known as extensions) and/or abscesses (**Fig. 7**). The secondary tracts are branches that can arise anywhere along the primary tract and develop most commonly in the ischioanal fossa or intersphincteric space. Secondary tracts that extend bidirectionally and wrap the internal sphincter either within the intersphincteric space or along the puborectalis muscles are known as "horseshoeing" branches or abscesses,[3,16] which require careful surgery to ensure proper drainage (**Fig. 8**).

St James's University Hospital Classification

In 2000, Morris and colleagues[10] proposed an MR imaging–based classification system for perianal fistulas. Compared with the Parks classification, this classification includes relevant findings at MR imaging and describes the primary fistulous tract as well as the secondary extensions and associated abscesses. This classification uses the reproducible anatomic landmarks and can be easily understood by radiologists who can then provide accurate information to surgeons.

This classification system is composed of 5 grades according to the anatomy seen on MR imaging using the axial and the coronal planes.

Grade 1 simple linear intersphincteric fistula
The fistulous tract extends from the anal canal through the intersphincteric space to reach the perianal skin. No secondary tracts or abscesses are found in the intersphincteric space or ischiorectal and ischioanal fossae. The fistula is entirely confined by the external sphincter, which is not involved.

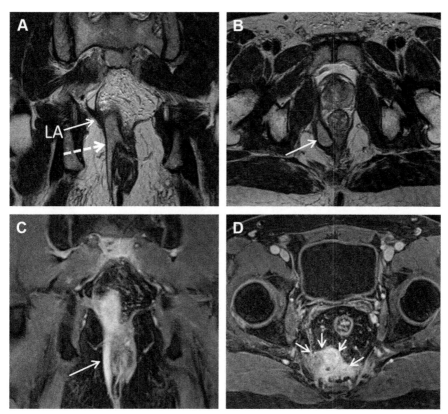

Fig. 4. Suprasphincteric fistulas in a 47-year-old man with CD. (*A*) Oblique coronal and (*B*) axial (without fat suppression) T2-weighted MR images show a wide right-sided extrasphincteric tract (*dash arrow*) that courses through the level of the levator ani (LA) to the ischiorectal fossa (*arrow*) and finally to the skin. (*C*) Postcontrast coronal and (*D*) axial images show the enhanced fistula tract (*arrow*), which is contiguous with an abscess in the presacral space (*arrows*).

Grade 2 intersphincteric fistula with an abscess or secondary tract

A primary tract and any numbers of secondary tracts or abscesses occur in the intersphincteric space. The secondary tracts or abscesses may manifest as "horseshoeing" type.[10] They are confined by the external sphincter, which is not crossed.

Grade 3 transsphincteric fistula

The transsphincteric fistula pierces both layers of the sphincter complex and then arcs down to the perineal skin through the ischiorectal and ischioanal fossae. The fistula is distinguished by the site of the internal opening, which is often located at level of dentate.[10] Surgical treatment of this fistula type has high risk to cause fecal incontinence, as the fistulas disrupt the integrity of both the internal and external sphincters.

Grade 4 transsphincteric fistula with an abscess or secondary tract within the ischiorectal fossa

As with grade 3, grade 4 fistulas also cross the external sphincter, and then are complicated by abscesses in the ischiorectal or ischioanal fossa, which may manifest as an expansion along the primary tract or as a collection distorting or filling the ischiorectal fossa.

Grade 5 supralevator and translevator disease

In rare cases, perianal fistulous disease extends above the insertion of the levator ani muscle. Supralevator fistulas extend upward in the intersphincteric space and pass over the top of the levator ani to pierce downward through the ischiorectal fossa.[10] These fistulas often indicate the existence of primary pelvic disease.

MR IMAGING ASSESSMENT OF PERIANAL FISTULAS

The role of MR imaging techniques in the evaluation of perianal fistulas has been addressed by many authors and is now "considered the gold standard method for evaluation of perianal fistula."[6]

Endoanal coils were initially used for perianal fistula evaluation, as they provided excellent

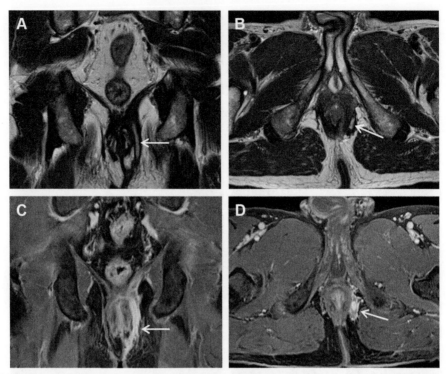

Fig. 5. (*A*) Oblique coronal (without fat suppression) and (*B*) axial (without fat suppression) T2-weighted MR images show an extrasphincteric fistula (*arrow*) in a 45-year old man. Postcontrast coronal (*C*) and axial (*D*) images show the fistula tract (*arrow*) was totally outside the sphincters without involving the anal canal.

anatomic resolution of the anal sphincter complex[17]; however, 2 substantial disadvantages limited the application of endoanal MR imaging: poorly tolerated in symptomatic patients and limited field of view.[5] In contrast, external phased array coils, which require no patient preparation, are well tolerated. Furthermore, these surface coils provide a larger field of view, which is especially important for visualization of supralevator disease that can be missed using endoanal coils.[18]

MR Imaging Protocol

With advances in MR imaging technique and high signal-to-noise ratio provided by high field strength, perianal fistula MR imaging examinations can be performed using either 1.5-T or 3.0-T scanners. The MR imaging protocol and parameters of all sequences used in our institution are listed in **Tables 1** (1.5-T) and **2** (3.0-T).

Multiplanar assessment of MR imaging is critical for studying perianal fistulas. However, the commonly used straight axial and coronal images cannot allow correct evaluation of the anal canal anatomy, as it is tilted forward from the vertical by approximately 45° in the sagittal plane.[5] After 3-plane locating views, oblique axial and coronal images oriented perpendicular and parallel to the long axis of the anal canal are obtained, respectively, by using the sagittal locating images (**Fig. 9**).

MR Imaging Appearance of Perianal Fistulas

On T2-weighted images, the normal sphincters and muscles show low signal intensity, whereas active primary fistulous tracts, secondary tracts, and abscesses have high signal intensity, and the fibrous walls of the fistulas are hypointense. Chronic fistulous tracts show low signal intensity on T2-weighted images.

On precontrast T1-weighted images, the anatomy of the sphincter complex, levator plate, and ischiorectal fossa are displayed well with low signal intensity, whereas fistulous tracts and abscesses also appear as areas of low to intermediate signal intensity, which may be difficult to distinguish from these normal muscle structures.

On gadolinium-enhanced T1-weighted images, primary fistulous tracts, secondary tracts, and abscesses, as well as the fistula's relationship to the anal sphincters can be clearly defined: the internal and external sphincters show mild or no enhancement, whereas active fistulous tracts and granulation tissue show significant enhancement, and fluid within the tracts does not enhance; abscesses show ring enhancement around a central

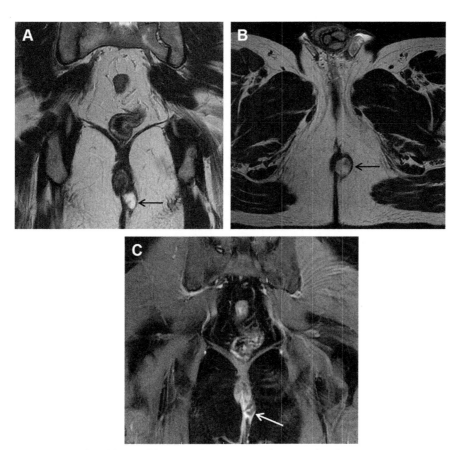

Fig. 6. (A) Oblique coronal and (B) axial (without fat suppression) T2-weighted MR images show a superficial fistula (*arrow*) in a 41-year-old man. (C) Postcontrast image clearly shows the course of the fistula tract (*arrow*), which did not involve the sphincter complex.

fluid collection (pus). Chronic fistula tracts can demonstrate mild enhancement, often progressive on dynamic imaging, indicating underlying fibrosis. High signal intensity within the fistulous tract on both precontrast and enhanced T1-weighted images may suggest hemorrhagic material.

After treatment, on T2-weighted images, inactive and healing fistulas gradually lose hyperintensity to become hypointense tracts. On enhanced T1-weighted images, the healing fistulas gradually lose enhancement, which generally parallel the loss of T2 signal intensity.

With the emergence of functional MR imaging techniques, some new sequences have been proposed to be added to conventional MR imaging protocols in the evaluation of perianal fistulas. Diffusion-weighted imaging (DWI) has been reported to provide significant added value for perianal fistula diagnosis when compared with T2-weighted imaging alone, and may improve diagnostic confidence when patients are unable to receive contrast agent administration due to poor renal function.[19] Furthermore,

Yoshizako and colleagues[20] reported that DWI was a feasible method for evaluating perianal fistula activity after conservative treatment with antibiotics, which showed the apparent diffusion coefficient of the positive inflammation activity group was significantly lower than the negative inflammation activity group. A pilot study conducted by Ziech and colleagues[21] showed dynamic contrast-enhanced MR imaging parameters, such as maximum enhancement and initial slope of increase, correlate with disease activity in perianal fistulizing CD. The investigators also proposed K (trans) might be an indicator of the fistula healing.

WHAT DOES THE CLINICIAN WANT TO KNOW FROM A PERIANAL MR IMAGING EXAMINATION?

When a patient who is suspected of having perianal fistulas undergoes pelvic MR imaging examination, the clinician wants to know the following detailed information.

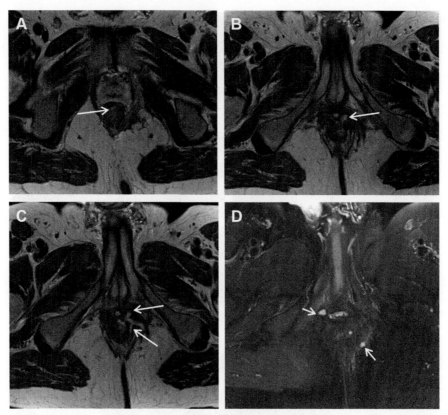

Fig. 7. Complex fistulas with multiple tracts in a 56-year-old man. Oblique axial T2-weighted MR images (without fat suppression) show the first (*arrow*) (*A*) and second internal openings (*B*), respectively. (*C*) At the lower level of the anal canal, several secondary tracts (*arrows*) communicated with the primary fistula tract at different points. (*D*) Multiple small abscesses (*arrows*) were also found in ischioanal fossa in axial T2-weighted image with fat suppression.

Whether the Perianal Fistula Does Exist (Detection of Perianal Fistulas)

The oblique axial fat-suppressed T2-weighted images are often initially interpreted to answer this question. Once a perianal fistula is detected, the internal opening (the origin of the fistula, which can be located in the anus or low rectum) and external opening should be identified as well. An anatomic "anal clock" can be used to locate the point of origin and describe the direction of the fistulous tract[5,10] (**Fig. 10**).

The Fistula Relationship to the Anal Sphincter Complex (Classification of Perianal Fistulas)

The oblique axial T2-weighted images without fat suppression can be used to classify the fistula as its relationships to the anal sphincters are better seen with this sequence. To enhance communication between the radiologist and surgeon, the radiologist's report should use the same classification system that the clinician uses.

Identification of Secondary Tracts and/or Abscesses

If a fistulous tract exists, the radiologist should identify whether it is a single fistula or a complex fistula and describe the primary tract, secondary tract, and/or abscess. Both T2-weighted and enhanced T1-weighted images can be used to determine the secondary tract at the point of communication with the primary fistula. Enhanced T1-weighted images can be used for identifying abscesses that show rim enhancement around a central fluid collection.

Other Complications

Anogenital or rectovaginal fistulation, which is difficult to treat and often requires surgery,[22] should be inspected carefully on MR images to avoid misdiagnosis (**Fig. 11**). Endoanal coil or endosonography, which can provide high-resolution images, may be required for detection of some small lesions.[23] *Anorectal strictures,* which include inflammatory strictures occurring in the acute

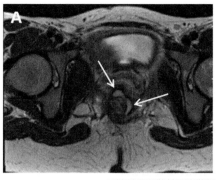
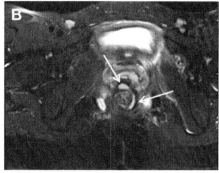
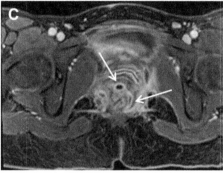

Fig. 8. "Horseshoeing" abscesses in a 43-year-old woman who is a CD patient. (A) Oblique axial T2-weighted MR image (without fat suppression) and (B) oblique axial T2-weighted MR image (with fat suppression) shows "horseshoeing" abscesses tracking from approximately 10 o'clock to 5 o'clock (arrows). (C) Postcontrast axal images show clearly the enhancement of the horseshoe branch within the intersphincteric space (arrows).

phase and fibrostenotic stricture occurring in the chronic phase, can occur anywhere from the anus to the midrectum and often are difficult to identify with MR imaging.[15,24] *Malignant transformation*, which is a consequence of chronic fistula inflammation,[25,26] is uncommon, and biopsy directed by the imaging appearance of suspected malignancy is required to confirm the diagnosis (**Fig. 12**). *Avascular necrosis* of the femoral head is often caused by steroid treatment in patients with CD and can be detected by MR imaging at an early stage.[15]

Bowel Disease

Perianal fistulas can be caused by underlying bowel disease, such as CD, tuberculosis, and diverticulitis. When a fistula exists, the real pathogenic cause should not be ignored.

Monitor the Treatment Effect

Van Assche and colleagues[27] developed an MR imaging–based scoring system to evaluate the response of fistulous tracts to medical treatment in patients with CD and makes comment on whether the fistula tract remains active or at the healing process. In their study, the results demonstrated that despite closure of draining external

orifices after infliximab therapy, fistula tracts persist with varying degrees of residual inflammation, which may cause recurrent fistulas and pelvic abscesses.

Understanding what the clinician needs to know, the radiologist can provide an accurate and time-efficient interpretation of perianal MR imaging examinations that are maximally useful for optimizing patient care.

TREATMENT

The goal of management of perianal fistulas is to control infection and subsequently to heal the fistula tract and maintain continence. Several factors have been regarded as independent risk factors associated with a poor outcome after surgery and a higher risk of recurrence, including previous fistula surgery, complex fistulas, lack of identification of the internal fistulous opening, wrongly diagnosed primary tracts, and missed secondary tracts.[28,29]

Accurately identifying and classifying perianal fistulas from MR imaging findings is critical for determining individualized treatment strategies and achieving successful results. Generally, simple submucosal, intersphincteric, or low transsphincteric tracts located in the distal third of the

Table 1
Parameters of all MR sequences (1.5-T) used for evaluation of perianal fistulas in patients at our institution

MR Imaging Pulse Sequences	TR, ms	TE, ms	Flip Angle	Acceleration Factor	Voxel Size, mm	FOV, mm	Slice Thickness, mm	Slice Numbers	Acquisition Time
Axial TSE T2-weighted imaging without fat suppression	6180	102	160	2	0.7 × 0.7 × 3.0	220	3	46	6 min
Axial TSE T2-weighted imaging with fat suppression	8650	102	160	2	0.7 × 0.7 × 3.0	220	3	46	8 min 41 s
Coronal TSE T2-weighted imaging without fat suppression	5600	102	160	2	0.7 × 0.7 × 3.0	220	3	38	5 min 4 s
Axial VIBE T1-weighted imaging with fat suppression, precontrast and postcontrast	3.69	1.51	10	2	0.7 × 0.7 × 4.0	220	4	40	43 s (precontrast) 2 min 10 s (postcontrast)
Coronal VIBE T1-weighted imaging with fat suppression, delay	5.41	1.93	10	2	0.7 × 0.7 × 3.0	220	3	48	2 min 30 s
Sagittal VIBE T1-weighted imaging with fat suppression, delay	3.94	1.51	10	2	0.7 × 0.7 × 3.0	220	3	48	2 min

Abbreviations: FOV, field of view; TE, echo time; TR, repetition time; TSE, turbo spin echo; VIBE, volumetric interpolated breath-hold examination.

Table 2
Parameters of all MR sequences (3.0-T) used for evaluation of perianal fistulas in patients at our institution

MR Imaging Pulse Sequences	TR, ms	TE, ms	Flip Angle	Acceleration Factor	Voxel Size, mm	FOV, mm	Slice Thickness, mm	Slice Numbers	Acquisition Time
Axial TSE T2-weighted imaging without fat suppression	3560	91	140	2	0.7 × 0.7 × 3.0	220	3	45	5 min 54 s
Axial TSE T2-weighted imaging with fat suppression	3790	91	140	2	0.7 × 0.7 × 3.0	220	3	45	6 min 17 s
Coronal TSE T2-weighted imaging without fat suppression	5620	108	140	2	0.7 × 0.7 × 3.0	220	3	40	3 min 35 s
Axial VIBE T1-weighted imaging with fat suppression, precontrast and postcontrast	4.44	1.57	10	2	0.8 × 0.8 × 4.0	240	4	48	1 min 12 s (precontrast) 3 min 35 s (postcontrast)
Coronal VIBE T1-weighted imaging with fat suppression, delay	4.44	1.57	10	2	0.8 × 0.8 × 4.0	240	4	40	2 min 7 s

Abbreviations: FOV, field of view; TE, echo time; TR, repetition time; TSE, turbo spin echo; VIBE, volumetric interpolated breath-hold examination.

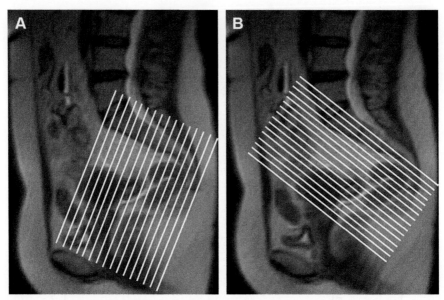

Fig. 9. Perpendicular (*A*) and parallel (*B*) to the long axis of the anal canal to obtain the oblique axial and coronal images, which can be used for better showing the anal sphincter anatomy.

anal canal can be treated with fistulotomy without a significant impact on continence, whereas for higher (two-thirds upper part of the anal sphincter) or complex fistulas, retention of continence is problematic.[5,30]

Medical Treatment

Unlike non–CD-related fistulas, in which surgery is often used to cure the fistula, CD-related patients

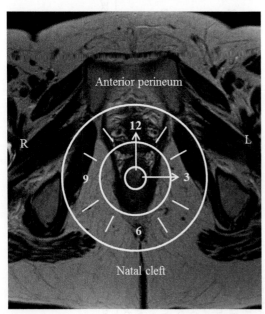

Fig. 10. "Anal clock" used to locate the point of origin and describe the direction of the fistulous tract.

are often treated medically, and the main goal of therapy is to achieve and maintain disease remission.

Antibiotics

Using antibiotics (metronidazole, ciprofloxacin) is the usual first step of therapy. Although treatment with oral metronidazole results in improved symptoms in 50% of patients,[31] the clinical fistula healing rates from antibiotic therapy alone are less than 50%, and symptoms for most cases will recur if antibiotics are withdrawn.[32] So, antibiotic therapy often acts as an effective bridge to immunosuppressive therapy.[33]

Immunosuppression

Azathioprine and 6-mercaptopurine (6-MP) are the commonly used immunosuppressants for induction and maintenance of remission in fistulizing disease. A meta-analysis of 5 randomized controlled trials demonstrated a 54% healing rate in patients who received 6-MP and azathioprine, compared with 21% of the control group, in which patients received only placebo.[34]

Tumor necrosis factor antagonists

Tumor necrosis factor (TNF) antagonists are effective in achieving remission in fistulizing disease. Infliximab, a chimeric monoclonal antibody to TNF-α, is the most commonly used anti-TNF antibody for treatment of CD perianal fistulizing disease. It has been reported that treatment with infliximab prevented additional surgeries and hospitalizations.[35] When compared with perianal

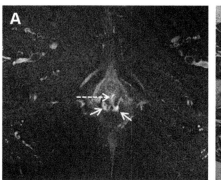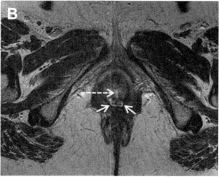

Fig. 11. Anogenital fistulation in a 55-year-old woman who is a CD patient. Oblique axial T2-weighted MR images with (A) and without (B) fat suppression show the anal vaginal fistula that is located at the 12 o'clock position (*dashed arrow*). There are also intersphincteric branches noted in both right and left intersphincteric spaces (*arrows*).

fistula healing, rectovaginal fistula healing had a poor response to infliximab therapy.[36]

Adalimumab and certolizumab pegol, the other 2 TNF antagonist antibodies, also have been shown to be effective for CD perianal fistulizing disease.[37] However, head-to-head comparisons among the 3 major TNF antagonist antibodies have not yet been performed.

Surgical Treatment

When to do surgery

Surgical treatment is indicated for patients with non–CD-related perianal fistulas. Surgical options are dependent on the type of fistula tract.[38] Accurate preoperative classification is essential, as inadequate assessment of the fistula may result

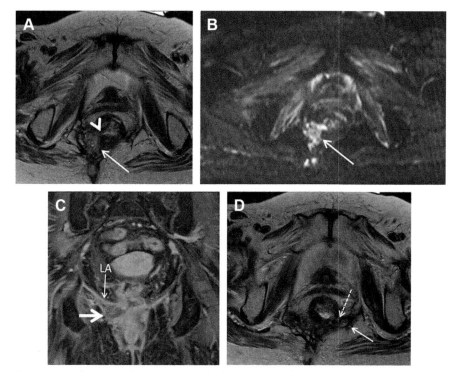

Fig. 12. Malignant transformation (mucinous rectal adenocarcinoma) in a 59-year-old woman. (A) Oblique axial T2-weighted MR image (without fat suppression) shows a mass (*arrow*) with intermediate T2 signal intensity extending through a defect (*arrowhead*) of low rectal/high anal canal. (B) DWI (b value = 800) shows diffusion restriction of the mass (*arrow*). (C) Postcontrast coronal image shows heterogeneous enhancement of the mass (*thick arrow*) and the levator ani (LA) was involved. (D) Oblique axial T2-weighted MR image (without fat suppression) shows a fistulous tract (*dashed arrow*) at 4 o'clock and small ischiorectal abscess formation (*arrow*).

in a simple fistula developing into a complex fistula, and failure to recognize secondary extensions can result in recurrent sepsis.

For CD-related fistulas, surgical intervention is used only as a palliative treatment when medical therapy fails in many patients. Because of poor wound-healing capability, major sphincter involvement, and underlying mucosal inflammation, only a few surgical options can be used for CD-related fistulas.[15]

The commonly used surgical options for patients with perianal fistulas patients are listed in the following sections.

Setons

A seton, which is made of silk suture, silastic cord, or surgical rubber bands, is often inserted to drain the tract and improve symptoms like discharge and exacerbations of abscess formation where other treatments are difficult to initiate. The insertion of a seton can be used as a temporary or bridging therapy.[15]

Fistulotomy

Fistulotomy, which is performed by excision of the fistula tract and surrounding involved tissue, is a commonly used treatment for curing a fistula.[39] Preoperative assessment of the involved sphincter is critical for avoiding fecal incontinence. This curative surgery is often used for low superficial, intersphincteric, or transsphincteric fistulas.[15]

Fibrin glue

Fibrin glue is injected along the tract and subsequent fibrin clot closes the fistula. This approach has been reported with high recurrence rates in CD-related patients and those with complex fistulas.[40]

Plugs

Fistula plug made of lyophilized porcine intestinal submucosa is a widely used bioabsorbable xenograft. However, this treatment was also reported with high rates of recurrence of 50% to 70%.[41]

Advancement flap

Following surgical excision of a fistula from the external to the internal opening, a flap of rectal wall is mobilized and brought down into the anal canal to close the internal opening. This is a challenging surgical technique, and therefore it is not widely used.[15]

Ligation of intersphincteric track

This technique was described in the early 1990s and has recently been revised for treatment of transphincteric fistulas.[39] This procedure is performed via the intersphincteric space to ligate the intersphincteric component of the tract at both the internal and external sphincter margins and remove the intersphincteric tract.

Video-assisted anal fistula treatment

This is a minimally invasive sphincter-sparing technique in which the complex fistula tract is irrigated with fluid via an endoscope introduced through the external opening and the necrotic material is removed. The internal opening is subsequently closed.[39]

Fecal diversion

A diverting loop ileostomy is required when other treatments fail to control the condition.

SUMMARY

MR imaging allows accurate identification and classification of perianal fistulas. Detection of secondary fistulas or abscesses by MR imaging is of particular importance for determining appropriate treatment and decreasing the incidence of recurrence and avoiding side effects, such as fecal incontinence.

Familiarity with the St James's University Hospital MR imaging–based grading system is critical for the radiologist to provide accurate interpretation and reporting of perianal MR imaging studies.

REFERENCES

1. Sainio P. Fistula-in-ano in a defined population: incidence and epidemiological aspects. Ann Chir Gynaecol 1984;73:219–24.
2. Practice parameters for treatment of fistula-in-ano: supporting documentation. The standards practice task force. The American Society of Colon and Rectal Surgeons. Dis Colon Rectum 1996;39:1363–72.
3. Halligan S, Stoker J. Imaging of fistula in ano. Radiology 2006;239:18–33.
4. Yousem DM, Fishman EK, Jones B. Crohn disease; perirectal and perianal findings at CT. Radiology 1988;167:331–4.
5. de Miguel Criado J, del Salto LG, Rivas PF, et al. MR imaging of perianal fistulas: spectrum of imaging features. Radiographics 2012;32:175–94.
6. Gecse KB, Bemelman W, Kamm MA, et al. A global consensus on the classification, diagnosis and multidisciplinary treatment of perianal fistulising Crohn's disease. Gut 2014;63:1381–92.
7. Buchanan GN, Halligan S, Bartram CI, et al. Clinical examination, endosonography, and MR imaging in preoperative assessment of fistula in ano: comparison with outcome-based reference standard. Radiology 2004;233:674–81.
8. Buchanan G, Halligan S, Williams A, et al. Effect of MRI on clinical outcome of recurrent fistula-in-ano. Lancet 2002;360:1661–2.
9. Milligan ET, Morgan CN. Surgical anatomy of the anal canal: with special reference to anorectal fistula. Lancet 1934;224:1150–6.

10. Morris J, Spencer JA, Ambrose NS. MR imaging classification of perianal fistulas and its implications for patient management. Radiographics 2000;20:623–35.

11. Eisenhammer S. A new approach to the anorectal fistulous abscess based on the high intermuscular lesion. Surg Gynecol Obstet 1958;106:595–9.

12. Szurowska E, Wypych J, Izycka-Swieszewska E. Perianal fistulas in Crohn's disease: MRI diagnosis and surgical planning. Abdom Imaging 2007;32:705–18.

13. Schwartz DA, Loftus EV Jr, Tremaine WJ, et al. The natural history of fistulizing Crohn's disease in Olmsted County, Minnesota. Gastroenterology 2002; 122:875–80.

14. Eglinton TW, Barclay ML, Gearry RB, et al. The spectrum of perianal Crohn's disease in a population-based cohort. Dis Colon Rectum 2012;55:773–7.

15. Sheedy SP, Bruining DH, Dozois EJ, et al. MR imaging of perianal Crohn disease. Radiology 2017;282:628–45.

16. Parks AG, Gordon PH, Hardcastle JD. A classification of fistula-in-ano. Br J Surg 1976;63:1–12.

17. deSouza NM, Hall AS, Puni R, et al. High resolution magnetic resonance imaging of the anal sphincter using a dedicated endoanal coil: comparison of magnetic resonance imaging with surgical findings. Dis Colon Rectum 1996;39:926–34.

18. deSouza NM, Gilderdale DJ, Coutts GA, et al. MRI of fistula-in-ano: a comparison of endoanal coil with external phased array coil techniques. J Comput Assist Tomogr 1998;22:357–63.

19. Cavusoglu M, Duran S, Sözmen Cılız D, et al. Added value of diffusion-weighted magnetic resonance imaging for the diagnosis of perianal fistula. Diagn Interv Imaging 2016. https://doi.org/10.1016/j.diii.2016.11.002.

20. Yoshizako T, Wada A, Takahara T, et al. Diffusion-weighted MRI for evaluating perianal fistula activity: feasibility study. Eur J Radiol 2012;81:2049–53.

21. Ziech ML, Lavini C, Bipat S, et al. Dynamic contrast-enhanced MRI in determining disease activity in perianal fistulizing Crohn disease: a pilot study. AJR Am J Roentgenol 2013;200:W170–7.

22. Andreani SM, Dang HH, Grondona P, et al. Rectovaginal fistula in Crohn's disease. Dis Colon Rectum 2007;50:2215–22.

23. Dwarkasing S, Hussain SM, Hop WC, et al. Anovaginal fistulas: evaluation with endoanal MR imaging. Radiology 2004;231:123–8.

24. de Zoeten EF, Pasternak BA, Mattei P, et al. Diagnosis and treatment of perianal Crohn disease: NASPGHAN clinical report and consensus statement. J Pediatr Gastroenterol Nutr 2013;57:401–12.

25. Thomas M, Bienkowski R, Vandermeer TJ, et al. Malignant transformation in perianal fistulas of Crohn's disease: a systematic review of literature. J Gastrointest Surg 2010;14:66–73.

26. Hongo K, Kazama S, Sunami E, et al. Perianal adenocarcinoma associated with anal fistula: a report of 11 cases in a single institution focusing on treatment and literature review. Hepatogastroenterology 2013;60:720–6.

27. Van Assche G, Vanbeckevoort D, Bielen D, et al. Magnetic resonance imaging of the effects of infliximab on perianal fistulizing Crohn's disease. Am J Gastroenterol 2003;98:332–9.

28. Garcia-Aguilar J, Belmonte C, Wong WD, et al. Anal fistula surgery. Factors associated with recurrence and incontinence. Dis Colon Rectum 1996;39: 723–9.

29. Chapple KS, Spencer JA, Windsor AC, et al. Prognostic value of magnetic resonance imaging in the management of fistula-in-ano. Dis Colon Rectum 2000;43:511–6.

30. Whiteford MH, Kilkenny J III, Hyman N, et al. Practice parameters for the treatment of perianal abscess and fistula-in-ano (revised). Dis Colon Rectum 2005;48:1337–42.

31. Turunen UM, Farkkila MA, Hakala K, et al. Long-term treatment of ulcerative colitis with ciprofloxacin: a prospective, double-blind, placebo-controlled study. Gastroenterology 1998;115:1072–8.

32. Brandt LJ, Bernstein LH, Boley SJ, et al. Metronidazole therapy for perineal Crohn's disease: a follow-up study. Gastroenterology 1982;83:383–7.

33. Dejaco C, Harrer M, Waldhoer T, et al. Antibiotics and azathioprine for the treatment of perianal fistulas in Crohn's disease. Aliment Pharmacol Ther 2003; 18:1113–20.

34. Pearson DC, May GR, Fick GH, et al. Azathioprine and 6-mercaptopurine in Crohn disease: a meta-analysis. Ann Intern Med 1995;123:132–42.

35. Feagan BG, Rochon J, Fedorak RN, et al. Methotrexate for the treatment of Crohn's disease. The North American Crohn's Study Group Investigators. N Engl J Med 1995;332:292–7.

36. Sandborn WJ, Present DH, Isaacs KL, et al. Tacrolimus for the treatment of fistulas in patients with Crohn's disease: a randomized, placebo-controlled trial. Gastroenterology 2003;125:380–8.

37. Kelley KA, Kaur T, Tsikitis VL. Perianal Crohn's disease: challenges and solutions. Clin Exp Gastroenterol 2017;10:39–46.

38. Spencer JA, Chapple K, Wilson D, et al. Outcome after surgery for perianal fistula: predictive value of MR imaging. AJR Am J Roentgenol 1998;171:403–6.

39. Nicholls RJ. Fistula in ano: an overview. Acta Chir Iugosl 2012;59:9–13.

40. Grimaud JC, Munoz-Bongrand N, Siproudhis L, et al. Fibrin glue is effective healing perianal fistulas in patients with Crohn's disease. Gastroenterology 2010;138:2275–81.

41. Sordo-Mejia R, Gaertner WB. Multidisciplinary and evidence-based management of fistulizing perianal Crohn's disease. World J Gastrointest Pathophysiol 2014;5:239–51.

Imaging Workup of Acute and Occult Lower Gastrointestinal Bleeding

Trevor C. Morrison, MD[a], Michael Wells, MD[b],
Jeff L. Fidler, MD[b], Jorge A. Soto, MD, PhD[a],*

KEYWORDS

- Gastrointestinal • Bleed • Acute • Occult • Lower • Radiology • Angiography • Enterography

KEY POINTS

- Lower gastrointestinal bleeding is defined as occurring distal to the ligament of Treitz and presents as hematochezia, melena, or with anemia and positive fecal occult blood test.
- Imaging tests in the workup of acute lower gastrointestinal bleeding include computed tomography (CT) angiography, nuclear medicine scintigraphy, and conventional catheter angiography.
- Imaging tests in the workup of occult lower gastrointestinal bleeding include CT enterography and nuclear medicine Meckel scan.

INTRODUCTION

Lower gastrointestinal (GI) bleeding is a frequent cause for hospital admissions with an annual incidence of approximately 20 to 27 cases per 100,000 persons in the United States.[1] Morbidity and mortality vary according to the underlying cause of the GI bleed, with reported mortality rates of 2% to 20% for lower GI bleeding and as high as 40% for hemodynamically unstable patients.[2]

Lower GI bleeding is defined as bleeding that occurs distal to the ligament of Treitz, with upper GI bleeding occurring proximally. Clinical presentations vary based on the source of the bleed and cause; however, acute lower GI bleeds typically present with hematochezia, noting that secondary to the cathartic effects of blood, a brisk upper GI bleed may present in a similar manner.[3] Causes of lower GI bleeding may be anatomic, such as diverticulosis (33.5%); vascular, such as hemorrhoids (22.5%), angioectasia, or

ischemia; neoplastic (12.7%); inflammatory as with inflammatory bowel disease; or infectious.[4] If the workup of the large bowel is negative, then patients are suspected of having a small bowel bleed.

There are several classification schemes used to describe lower GI bleeding related to the duration and severity of the bleed as well as the results of upper and lower endoscopy/imaging. When correlating with the amount of bleeding, lower GI bleeds can be categorized as massive, moderate, or occult. Massive bleeding is defined by the passage of profuse hematochezia with hemodynamic instability. Moderate bleeding reflects hematochezia in hemodynamically stable patients. Occult bleeding refers to the presence of a positive fecal-occult blood test or iron deficiency anemia without another identifiable source and without frank hematochezia.[5] Obscure bleeding refers to patients who have recurrent bleeding after negative endoscopic evaluation and advanced

Disclosure Statement: Nothing to disclose.
[a] Boston University Medical Center, 830 Harrison Avenue, FGH 3rd Floor, Boston, MA 02118, USA;
[b] Department of Radiology, Mayo Clinic, 200 First Street Southwest, Rochester, MN 55905, USA
* Corresponding author.
E-mail address: Jorge.Soto@bmc.org

Radiol Clin N Am 56 (2018) 791–804
https://doi.org/10.1016/j.rcl.2018.04.009

radiologic assessment of the small bowel and can be either acute or occult.[2]

WORKUP RECOMMENDATIONS FOR ACUTE LOWER GASTROINTESTINAL BLEEDING

The workup of patients presenting with acute lower GI bleeding involves resuscitation, localizing the site of bleeding, and intervention to stop the source of the bleeding, as appropriate. The main tools of the workup include direct visualization with proctoscopy/colonoscopy and imaging with computed tomography angiography (CTA), nuclear scintigraphy, or angiography. Although surgery was once a necessity for patients with ongoing lower GI bleed, advanced techniques in endoscopy and angiography have improved detection and treatment, with surgery now reserved for cases in which more conservative management has failed.[6]

The clinical presentation of patients during the triaging process as well as the services available at a hospital dictate the order and priority in which tests are used in the workup of an active lower GI bleed.[1] Any patient with hemodynamic instability must first be resuscitated. If endoscopy is available, it is generally the first test preformed; however, there are significant limitations. The colon must first be prepped in order to clear enteric contents and blood, which could obscure the source of bleeding. Even rapid bowel preparations take at least several hours, which may not be possible in patients with ongoing bleeding. Additionally, in some series, colonoscopy detects the source of bleeding in only 13% to 40%.[2] In cases whereby emergent endoscopy is not indicated, patients will typically be sent for an imaging study, such as CTA, nuclear scintigraphy, or catheter angiography, depending on the local availability and clinical expertise. In patients who are clinically stable at presentation, more conservative management is generally indicated, with many patients being worked up with elective endoscopy.[7]

COMPUTED TOMOGRAPHY ANGIOGRAPHY

CTA has excellent sensitivity and specificity for the identification and localization of acute GI bleeds. A meta-analysis by Garcia-Blazquez and colleagues[8] reported a sensitivity of 85.2% and specificity of 92.1% for the detection of acute, active GI bleeds. Yoon and colleagues[9] used arterial phase CTA in 26 patients with massive GI bleeding and reported an overall accuracy of 89%. CTA can detect bleeding rates as low as 0.3 mL/s in in vitro studies.[10] Advantages of CTA include that it is widely available, noninvasive, provides excellent localization, and additionally can provide the cause of the GI bleed. CTA can diagnose diverticular disease, vascular abnormalities (such as angioectasia), tumors, colitis/enteritis, bowel ischemia, and postoperative/iatrogenic causes. Additionally, the arterial phase imaging demonstrates vascular anatomy and any vascular variants. This information can be observed on the source images and reformatted using maximum intensity projections (MIPs) to provide valuable information for the subsequent mesenteric angiography.[2]

Disadvantages of CTA include radiation dose, as it is usually done in 3 phases; however, improvements in CT dose reduction have made this less of an issue than in the past.[11] CTA also requires an intravenous (IV) contrast dose, which is relatively contraindicated in patients with acute renal failure. As with all imaging tests, patients must be actively bleeding at the time of the scan.

CTA for acute GI bleeding is typically preformed as a triphasic study. Enteric contrast is not given as is critical to acquire the examination as quickly as possible in patients with active hemorrhage. A precontrast examination is first acquired using low radiation dose settings. The purpose of the precontrast portion of the examination is to identify any hyperdense enteric contents, such as pills, residual oral contrast, hyperdense stool, and so forth, so they are not confused for contrast extravasation on later phases. Next, at least 100 mL noniodinated contrast is administered intravenously by a power injector at a rate of 4 to 5 mL/s. Automated bolus technique is preferred, with arterial phase obtained 8 to 10 seconds after the attenuation coefficient in the proximal abdominal aorta reaches a threshold of 150 Hounsfield units (HU). Portal venous phase is then acquired approximately 50 seconds after start of the arterial phase.[12]

Computed Tomography Angiography: Findings

Active GI bleeding is manifest by contrast extravasation into the bowel lumen on CTA. The contrast extravasation appears as a blush on arterial phase imaging, which propagates further down the bowel on the portal venous phase due to peristalsis[11] (Figs. 1 and 2). If bleeding is arterial, a jet of contrast may be seen. Lower intensity bleeds are often better seen on the portal venous phase, as more time has been allowed for the contrast to accumulate.[13] It is important to look at the precontrast and contrast-enhanced images side by side, as inherently hyperdense intraluminal

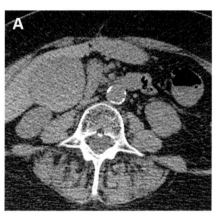
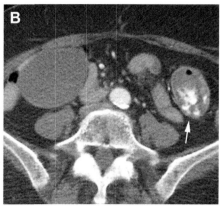

Fig. 1. CTA of active GI bleed. A 76-year-old woman with history of diverticulosis and recurrent lower GI bleeds presents with hematochezia. Axial precontrast (*A*) and arterial phase (*B*) images from a CTA examination demonstrate contrast extravasation into bowel lumen in the descending colon (*white arrow*), consistent with active GI bleeding. Precontrast images are critical to ensure that contrast extravasation is not confused for hyperdense enteric contents. Subsequent colonoscopy revealed a diverticular bleed.

contents can mimic contrast extravasation. In some cases, active bleeding with contrast extravasation is not identified, but there is visualization of a clot at the site of bleeding. The clot should be hyperdense compared with the enteric contents on precontrast images. HU should measure approximately 30 to 45 HU for unclotted blood and 40 to 70 HU for clotted blood.[13] The area of highest HU should be at the origin of the bleed, which is called the sentinel clot.[14]

NUCLEAR SCINTIGRAPHY

Nuclear scintigraphy is most commonly performed combining the patients' own red blood cells tagged with a radiotracer technetium 99-m (Tc-99m). Autologous red blood cells are tagged in vitro with 20 to 30 mCi Tc-99m and then administered as an IV bolus. Patients are placed supine under the gamma camera and scanned from the xiphoid process through the pubic symphysis. Initial dynamic flow images are obtained at 3 seconds each, for 1 minute, to show flow in the abdominal viscera. This imaging is followed by static images every minute continued for 90 minutes. If patients have an episode of rebleeding, additional static images can then be obtained up to 24 hours after the initial injection. Although patients can be reimaged up to 24 hours after injection without rebleeding, it is often not useful, as

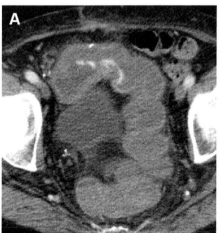
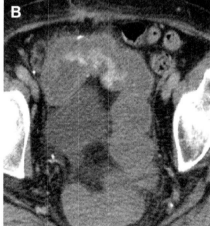

Fig. 2. CTA of active GI bleed. An 87-year-old woman with history of hemicolectomy due to colon cancer presents with hematochezia. Axial arterial phase (*A*) and portal venous phase (*B*) images demonstrate contrast extravasation into the sigmoid colon adjacent to the anastomosis. Note that there is increasing extravasation on delayed images. A subsequent sigmoidoscopy revealed ischemic colitis at the surgical anastomosis.

peristalsis can provide false localization of the site of the bleed. When positive findings are seen, the examination can be discontinued once the clinician is confident of the origin of the bleed.[15]

Nuclear scintigraphy is the most sensitive test to image GI bleeding, as it can detect bleeding rates as low as 0.05 mL/min.[16] Other advantages include that the test is noninvasive and that no patient preparation is needed other than obtaining a blood sample.

The main disadvantage of nuclear scintigraphy is that it generally relies on 2-dimensiona (2D) planar imaging, and localization of the bleed can be a significant limited factor. For example, a redundant transverse colonic loop in the pelvis could be confused for a small bowel loop or more distal colonic bleed. Also, because of intermittent bleeding and noncontinuous imaging, the radiolabeled blood may have already moved downstream from the bleeding site at the time the image is acquired, thus, giving false localization of the origin of the bleed. Single-photon emission CT/CT fusion imaging has shown promise to improve localization by pairing a CT scan with 3-dimensional radiotracer imaging; however, this is not widely available.[17]

In many institutions, nuclear scintigraphy is performed before angiography, because of the higher sensitivity for detection of active bleeding, with a negative examination potentially eliminating the need for the more invasive angiographic procedure.[18] When the study is positive, studies have shown improved bleed detection in subsequent angiography.[19] However, although nuclear scintigraphy is the most sensitive imaging study to detect GI bleeds, CT is far more widely available, with faster acquisition, and improved localization, making it the test of choice at many institutions.

Nuclear Scintigraphy: Findings

A positive nuclear bleeding study will show focal increased activity and radiotracer uptake at the site of the bleeding (**Fig. 3**). Over time, with bowel peristalsis, the radiolabeled blood will continue to move along the GI tract, which aids in localization. Observing the course the blood takes over time enables the clinician to determine if the blood is following a large or small bowel pathway. Imaging should be continued until the clinician is confident that they can identify the source of the bleed.

MESENTERIC ANGIOGRAPHY

Mesenteric angiography is typically reserved for treatment of bleeding that was first diagnosed

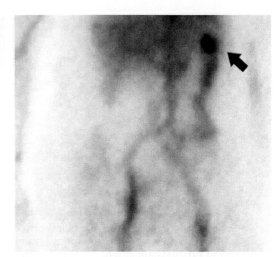

Fig. 3. Nuclear scintigraphy of active GI bleed. A 76-year-old woman with history of diverticulosis and recurrent lower GI bleeds presents with hematochezia (same patient as in **Fig. 1**A, B). A 2D planar image demonstrates increased radiotracer uptake in the region of the splenic flexure of the colon (*black arrow*), consistent with active GI bleeding.

on a previous CTA or nuclear scintigraphy. Selective mesenteric angiography can detect bleeding at a rate of 0.5 mL/min, an approximately 10-fold higher rate than that detected by nuclear scintigraphy.[20] The main advantage of angiography is that it can be used to deliver treatment if a focus of active bleeding is identified, such as embolization or vasopressin drip. Angiography also does not require bowel preparation and provides excellent localization of the site of bleeding.

There are significant disadvantages of using angiography as a first-line diagnostic method in GI bleeding. Angiography is invasive, may require a large load of iodinated contrast, and the radiation dose can be high in complicated cases. Angiography is not as widely available as CT, and many hospitals lack expertise. An associated complication of angiography is embolization causing bowel ischemia.

For diagnosis, angiography is reserved for patients with life-threatening, ongoing lower GI bleeding, when there may be no time for a CTA or nuclear study. In these cases, emergent angiography is often performed as a last remaining option before laparotomy. Typically, the superior mesenteric artery is cannulated first, as most significant lower GI bleeds occur from the right colon. If no bleed is identified, the inferior mesenteric artery is cannulated followed by the celiac axis. Digital subtraction angiography (DSA) is a technique that uses a computer algorithm to subtract a

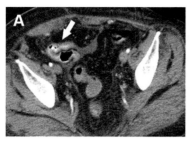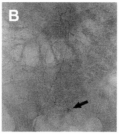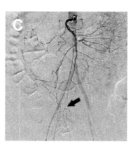

Fig. 4. CTA and DSA of active GI bleed. A 65-year-old woman with recurrent lower GI bleeds, without identifiable source despite extensive workup, presents with hematochezia. Axial image from a CTA (*A*) demonstrates active GI bleeding within the small bowel (*white arrow*). DSA of the superior mesenteric artery (SMA) (*B*) demonstrates small focus of extravasation in the pelvis (*black arrow*). Note the embolization clips from prior treatment. DSA of the SMA (*C*) after embolization demonstrates no evidence of contrast extravasation (*black arrow*).

precontrast image from a postcontrast image, so that only the blood vessels are visualized. This technique should be used if available, as it is generally thought to be more sensitive than angiography alone in the detection of GI bleeds.[21]

Mesenteric Angiography: Findings

On DSA, a lower GI bleed is identified as an area of contrast extravasation outside of the normal confines of a blood vessel, which typically increases over time (**Fig. 4**). After successful embolization, an additional angiogram can be done to show that the bleeding has stopped. Angiography also has characteristic findings in angiodysplasia, which often appears as a vascular blush with early and persistent visualization of a draining vein[21] (**Fig. 5**).

WORKUP RECOMMENDATIONS FOR OCCULT GASTROINTESTINAL BLEEDING

Occult GI bleeding is diagnosed when patients have a positive fecal occult test or iron deficiency anemia without another source and the absence of visible enteric blood. Upper endoscopy and colonoscopy identify an upper GI source of occult GI bleeding in 29% to 56% and a lower GI source in 20% to 30% of patients; synchronous lesions in

the upper and lower tract are discovered in 1% to 17%.[22]

Patients with negative esophagogastroduodenoscopy and colonoscopy by definition have suspected small bowel bleeding (SBB). Small bowel lesions are responsible for 5% to 10% of all patients presenting with GI bleeding.[23] Video capsule endoscopy (VCE), CT enterography (CTE), and double balloon endoscopy (DBE) can all be used to assess the small bowel. VCE is recommended by gastroenterology societies as the first-line test because of its high yield (40%–60%) of positive findings after negative endoscopy; however, the test is limited by low specificity, the potential for obstruction/capsule retention, incomplete small bowel visualization, limited visualization of submucosal masses, and limited evaluation of the duodenum and proximal jejunum.[23]

Because of the limitations of VCE, CTE may be considered the first-line evaluation in patients with SBB who have suspicion of stricture (inflammatory bowel disease, prior surgery, nonsteroidal antiinflammatory drug [NSAID] use, radiation), obstruction, or a small bowel mass (young patients or known malignancy).[24,25] A meta-analysis showed a diagnostic yield of 40% for CTE compared with 53% for VCE in patients with SBB.[26] CTE and VCE are considered

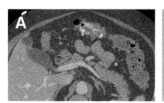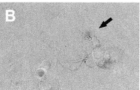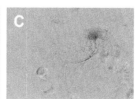

Fig. 5. CTA and DSA of active GI bleed. A 58-year-old woman presents with dark red bowel movements and dizziness. Axial CT in portal venous phase (*A*) demonstrates contrast extravasation into the transverse colon. Superselective DSA of the middle colic artery in the early (*B*) and more delayed (*C*) phase demonstrates a persistent blush of contrast (*black arrow*). Patient was treated with coil embolization. Patient had known angiodysplasia on the colon diagnosed on previous colonoscopy.

complementary modalities; when one study is negative, evaluation with the other should be considered before proceeding with DBE.[25]

DBE affords detailed examination of the small bowel but is costly and time consuming. Therefore, the test is typically used in a targeted fashion after the small bowel has been evaluated with VCE or CTE. Patients who do not receive a diagnosis or who have recurrent bleeding after full diagnostic evaluation of the bowel (obscure GI bleeding) may benefit from repeated capsule endoscopy, Meckel scan, surgical evaluation, or observation/iron supplements.[25]

COMPUTED TOMOGRAPHY ENTEROGRAPHY

CTE has been used successfully for the evaluation of occult obscure GI bleeding for more than a decade.[27] CTE is advantageous in the workup of occult GI bleeding because of its wide availability, relatively rapid examination performance, and consistent good examination quality. CTE has benefits over endoscopic techniques for evaluating the entirety of the intra-abdominal GI tract, delineating postoperative GI tract anatomy and evaluating extraenteric structures.

Limitations of CTE include exposure to ionizing radiation, iodinated IV contrast exposure, and need for large-volume oral contrast administration. Improvements in dose reduction techniques have allowed CTE radiation doses to decline substantially from 15 to 20 mGy to less than 10 mGy per phase.[28] Exposure to iodinated IV contrast is associated with a low risk of severe allergic reaction (0.04%) and contrast-induced nephropathy (minimal risk with renal function >30 mL/min/1.73 m^2).[29] Large-volume

oral contrast administration may not be tolerated by patients, particularly those who are acutely ill; for some patients, placement of a nasogastric catheter may be necessary for contrast administration.

Studies have consistently demonstrated the ability of CTE to identify vascular, inflammatory, structural, and neoplastic conditions in the bowel responsible for GI bleeding.[27,30] Although the diagnostic yield for vascular and inflammatory lesions may be lower than that of VCE, the technique is superior for the detection of small bowel masses and has been shown to identify inflammation and vascular malformations not seen using VCE.[24,27,30] As with all imaging studies performed for the evaluation of GI bleeding, the diagnostic yield of CTE is higher in patients with overt bleeding than in those with occult bleeding.[23,27]

CTE requires distention of the small bowel by ingestion of 900 to 1350 mL of neutral oral contrast over 30 to 60 minutes. (Please see Shannon P. Sheedy and colleagues' article, "CT Enterography," in this issue for a detailed discussion of CTE.) A variation of enterography, enteroclysis may be used to increase distention of the small bowel. Enteroclysis involves the placement of a naso-enteric catheter and active infusion of contrast agent to increase small bowel distention. Enteroclysis may have an advantage in detecting subtle strictures and pathologic conditions of small bowel, but it is poorly tolerated by patients and rarely performed outside of referral centers (Fig. 6).

IV contrast administration for CTE is typically performed using 300 to 350 mg of iodine per milliliter contrast agents and infusion rates between 3 and 5 mL/s. CTE performed for the

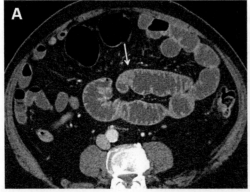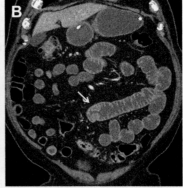

Fig. 6. Jejunal lymphoma. A 77-year-old man with history of occult GI bleeding. Capsule endoscopy suggested a possible small bowel mass. Axial (A) and coronal (B) images from a CT enteroclysis demonstrate a subtle mass (arrows) in the jejunum that was subsequently shown to be a lymphoma. Note the isodense appearance that potentially could have been missed with poor bowel distention with enterography.

evaluation of suspected small bowel bleeding requires acquisition of multiple phases of contrast enhancement, although the specific phases acquired vary between institutions. The examination typically includes the arterial phase timed using bolus tracking techniques and an enteric phase acquired at 50 to 60 seconds after injection. A precontrast phase and/or a delayed phase may also be acquired depending on the preferences of the radiologist. Precontrast images are helpful for identifying high-attenuation ingested material, which can mimic pathology. Data demonstrating the added benefit of additional contrast-enhanced phases are lacking; however, limited evidence suggests an improvement in sensitivity and reader confidence when increasing an examination from 2 to 3 contrast-enhanced phases.[31] The use of dual-energy data acquisition and postprocessing can be helpful for improving lesion detection and limiting the radiation dose. The generation of iodine maps and low kiloelectron volt monoenergetic series can be helpful for making enhancing pathology more conspicuous. The generation of virtual noncontrast series may negate the need for acquiring precontrast data sets.

Occult Gastrointestinal Bleeding: Causes and Findings

There are many potential causes of occult GI bleeding, which are listed in **Table 1**.[32,33] In the next section, the authors review some of the more frequently seen causes and their imaging findings. They highlight unique or subtle findings that may not be well known. The discussion focuses on CTE, which is the most commonly performed imaging test for occult bleeding. Although CTE can detect lesions in the stomach and colon missed by endoscopy, the authors focus their discussion on small bowel pathology.

Vascular lesions

Vascular lesions can be classified as high-flow lesions (arteriovenous malformation [AVM], Dieulafoy lesion) (**Fig. 7**), angioectasia (**Fig. 8**), and venous lesions (varix, venous angioma) (**Fig. 9**).[32] High-flow lesions are best seen on the arterial phase and may only be seen on this phase. The presence of an enlarged draining vein is more suggestive of an AVM. Angioectasias are usually best seen on the enteric phase and appear as nodular or discoid areas of enlargement of the intramural veins. Venous angiomas show slow progressive enhancement and may have associated phleboliths.

CTE has potential benefits for the evaluation of bowel vascular malformations in addition to evaluation with VCE. CTE has been shown to identify vascular lesions missed by endoscopy.[27,30] Dieulafoy lesions may be particularly conspicuous at arterial phase enterography and can be difficult to visualize at endoscopy.

Visualization at endoscopy is limited to the mucosal surface; therefore, intramural malformations may only be detected at cross-sectional imaging (**Fig. 10**). In addition, imaging is able to better localize lesions, provide a better overview of the extent of the malformation, and reliably survey the entire GI tract.

Polyps

Polyps can have variable enhancement. In a poorly distended bowel, a polyp that enhances similar to the adjacent bowel wall may be obscured. Examinations performed with positive oral contrast may perform better for identifying masses that enhance similar to the bowel wall; this should be considered when evaluating patients with polyposis syndromes, such as Peutz-Jeghers syndrome.

A unique enhancement characteristic with central lower density and surrounding hyperenhancement is suggestive of inflammatory fibroid polyps

---

Table 1
Common causes of occult small bowel gastrointestinal bleeding

Inflammatory	Neoplastic	Vascular	Miscellaneous
Celiac sprue	Metastasis	Angioectasia	Meckel diverticulum
Ulcerative colitis	Neuroendocrine tumor	AVM	
Crohn disease	Adenocarcinoma	Dieulafoy lesion	
NSAID	Lymphoma	Venous angioma	
	GIST		
	Pancreatic heterotopia		
	Polyp		

Abbreviations: AVM, arteriovenous malformation; GIST, gastrointestinal stromal tumor.

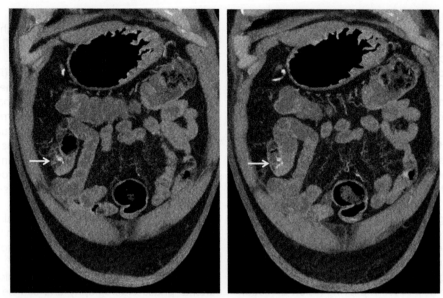

Fig. 7. High flow vascular lesion. A 71-year-old man with symptomatic anemia. Coronal MIP images from the arterial phase of a multiphasic CTE examination show a rapidly enhancing enlarged vessel in the ileum (*arrows*) suggestive of a high flow vascular lesion, such as a Dieulafoy lesion. The lesion was not seen on the enteric phase (not shown).

(**Fig. 11**). Inflammatory fibroid polyps are rare non-neoplastic lesions composed of blood vessels, connective tissue, and inflammatory cells. They originate within the submucosa, most commonly of the stomach, with the small bowel being the second most common site. These lesions frequently become several centimeters in size and may present with obstruction or intussusception.

Neoplasms

The most common primary malignancy of the small bowel is a neuroendocrine tumor (NET).[33] NETs most commonly develop in the ileum. With the more widespread use of CTE, small bowel NETs are being detected earlier and at a smaller size. These lesions are typically small with a flat or plaquelike morphology (**Fig. 12**). Desmoplastic reaction associated with the mass may cause bending/kinking of the bowel loop. The small size and shape of the lesion may make them difficult to detect. They are best seen on the arterial or enteric phases as a focus of mural hyperenhancement. When a small bowel NET is identified, it is important to carefully search the remaining bowel for additional lesions, as they can be multifocal.

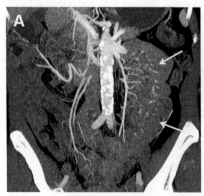
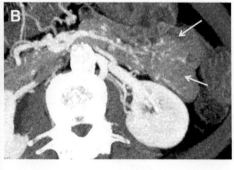

Fig. 8. Angioectasia. A 68-year-old man with iron deficiency anemia. Coronal (*A*) and axial (*B*) MIPs from the enteric phase of a multiphase CTE show enlarged and nodular vessels in the jejunum (*arrows*) suggestive of angioectasia.

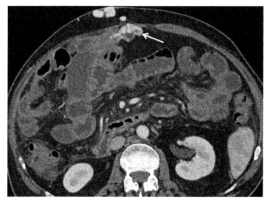

Fig. 9. Small bowel varix. A 68-year-old man with cirrhosis, portal hypertension, and recurrent GI bleeding. CTE demonstrates serpiginous enhancing structures in the small bowel consistent with varices (*arrow*). Also note the varices in the anterior abdominal wall.

Adenocarcinoma most commonly presents as a hypoenhancing polypoid mass or an annular constricting lesion (**Fig. 13**).[33] Lymphoma of the small bowel may have a similar appearance but also may result in aneurysmal dilation of the bowel (see **Fig. 6**). Lymphoma may also be

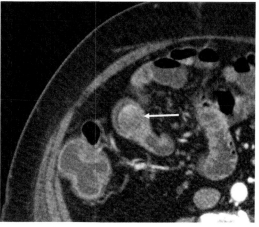

Fig. 11. Inflammatory fibroid polyp. A 56-year-old man with iron deficiency anemia. CTE demonstrates an intraluminal mass (*arrow*) in the ileum. The mass has unique enhancement characteristics with peripheral hyperenhancement and central low attenuation near water density.

multifocal, associated with lymphadenopathy or lymphomatous masses in other organs. Adenocarcinoma is more likely to obstruct than lymphoma.

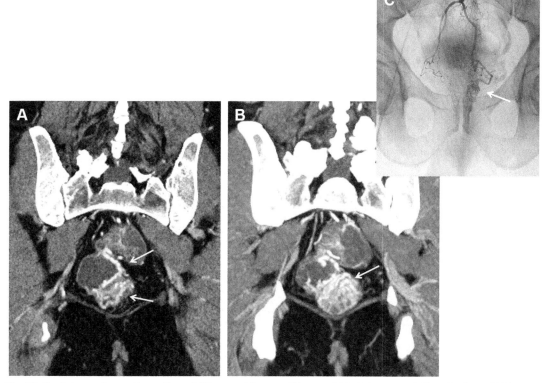

Fig. 10. Rectal vascular malformation. A 58-year-old man with recent black tarry stool. Enteric phase CTE images demonstrate a tangle of large vessels (*white arrows*) in the rectum on coronal reformats (A) and coronal MIPs (B) consistent with a rectal vascular malformation confirmed on subsequent angiography (C).

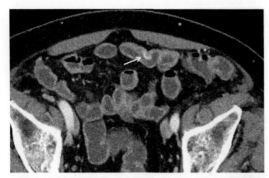

Fig. 12. NET. An 82-year-old man with iron deficiency anemia. CTE shows a small plaquelike hyperenhancing lesion (*arrow*) in the small bowel with puckering of the underlying wall consistent with a NET.

Gastrointestinal stromal tumors (GISTs) have varied appearances based on their size. When small, the masses are well circumscribed and hyperenhancing (Fig. 14). These masses originate from a mural position but typically become endoluminal or exophytic as they grow. As they grow, the enhancement becomes variable; necrosis, internal hemorrhage, and ulceration may be found. Large masses may also directly invade into adjacent structures.

Heterotopic pancreatic tissue

Pancreatic tissue with no anatomic continuity with the remaining pancreas is most commonly found in the stomach, duodenum, and proximal jejunum.[34] It can also be found within Meckel diverticula and the remainder of the ileum. Heterotopic pancreatic tissue typically has an intramural or serosal flat plaquelike appearance that can mimic a GIST or NET (Fig. 15).

Inflammation

Inflammatory bowel disease is discussed in greater detail elsewhere in this issue. Classic findings of small bowel Crohn disease include asymmetric mural hyperenhancement and bowel wall thickening in a skipping pattern. Penetrating (sinus tracts, fistula, abscess) and perianal disease may be present.

Nonsteroidal antiinflammatory enteropathy

Focal small bowel wall injury caused by NSAID exposure can result in thin circumferential regions of submucosal fibrous deposition and frequently have superimposed inflammation. The circumferential columns of fibrosis result in short (5–10 mm long) strictures or diaphragms with superimposed hyperenhancement, which are characteristic of NSAID exposure (Fig. 16). However, other causes, such as Crohn disease, may have similar findings. The strictures are often multiple and found in close proximity. They may be mistaken for peristaltic contractions or missed because of poor bowel distention, especially those without superimposed inflammation. Multiphase CT or MR imaging is helpful for identifying NSAID strictures by maximizing luminal distention in each segment of the bowel.

Meckel diverticulum

Meckel diverticulum occurs within 1% to 3% of the population and most (84%) are asymptomatic.[35,36] Of symptomatic diverticula occurring in adults, the most common presentation is bleeding (38%).[36] Fifty percent of diverticula contain ectopic tissue that is gastric in greater than 60% and pancreatic in 16%.[35]

Tc-99m pertechnetate scan (Meckel scan) is a useful test for detecting ectopic gastric mucosa within a diverticulum. The sensitivity of the test is 85% to 90% in the pediatric population and 62% in patients 16 years of age and older.[37] A Meckel scan may give false-positive results because of detection of ectopic mucosa, which may be in

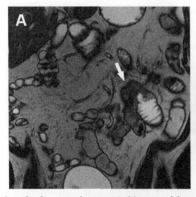
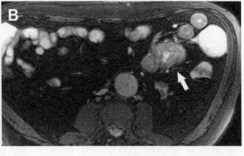

Fig. 13. Jejunal adenocarcinoma. A 64-year-old man with melena. Coronal (*A*) and axial (*B*) T2-weighted images from magnetic resonance enterography show a focal mass (*arrows*) in the jejunum with mild proximal dilatation suggestive of an adenocarcinoma. Most sites prefer using CTE for evaluating occult bleeding; however, magnetic resonance enterography can be used if there are contraindications to CT.

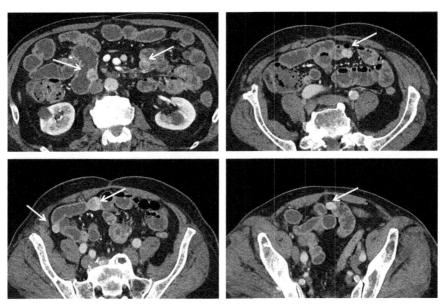

Fig. 14. Multifocal GIST. An 82-year-old man with melena requiring multiple transfusions. CTE shows multiple hyperenhancing lesions throughout the small bowel consistent with multiple GISTs (*arrows*).

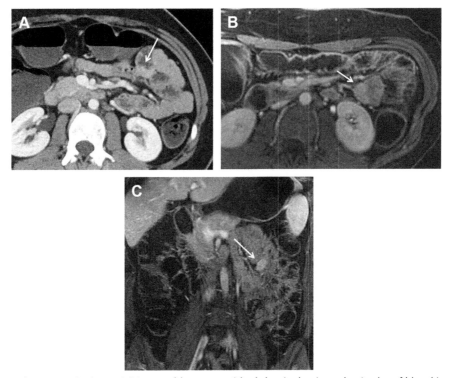

Fig. 15. Ectopic pancreatic tissue. A 21-year-old woman with abdominal pain and episodes of blood in stool. CTE (*A*) and magnetic resonance enterography (*B, C*) show a mural mass (*arrows*) in the jejunum near the ligament of Treitz. The lesion is somewhat flat in appearance and enhances similar to pancreatic tissue. Findings could represent a GIST or NET. However, heterotopic pancreatic tissue is also in the differential diagnosis which was confirmed at surgery.

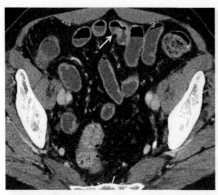
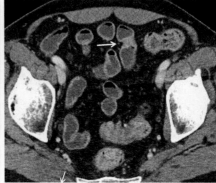

Fig. 16. NSAID diaphragms. A 64-year-old man with iron deficiency anemia. CTE demonstrates multiple focal inflammatory strictures (*arrows*) consistent with NSAID enteropathy.

another location, such as an enteric duplication cyst. Ectopic pancreatic tissue within the diverticulum can be a source of a false-negative Meckel scan.

To perform a Meckel scan, 1.85 MBq/kg Tc-99m pertechnetate is administered.[38] Pretreatment with pentagastrin and/or histamine receptor antagonists may increase the rate of positive examinations.[38] Dynamic planar images are typically acquired every 30 to 60 seconds for 30 minutes. Single positron emission CT can also be performed and may assist in better localization of tracer uptake. Positive examinations show a focal region of uptake in the right lower quadrant, which appears at the time the stomach is visualized (Fig. 17). Meckel diverticula can be identified by CTE. These diverticula appear as blind-ending pouches arising from the ileum. Superimposed

Fig. 17. Positive Meckel scan. A 4-year-old boy who presents with bloody stools. On the Meckel scan, there is a focal area of increased radiotracer uptake in the right lower quadrant (*arrow*) consistent with a Meckel diverticulum.

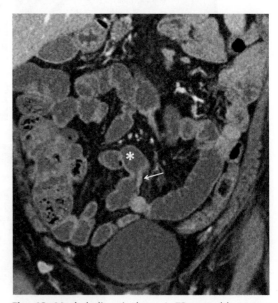

Fig. 18. Meckel diverticulum. A 73-year-old woman with melena and transfusion-dependent anemia. Coronal image from a CTE shows a blind ending loop arising in the distal small bowel (*asterisk*) consistent with a Meckel diverticulum. Associated wall thickening (*arrow*) consistent with superimposed inflammation.

hyperenhancement and wall thickening suggest superimposed inflammation (**Fig. 18**).

SUMMARY

Lower GI bleeding occurs distal to the ligament of Treitz and is an important clinical problem with a variety of causes. The bleeding can be acute, presenting with hematochezia, or occult, presenting with iron deficiency anemia and/or positive fecal occult blood test. Obscure bleeding refers to patients with rebleeding after a negative endoscopic and radiologic assessment of the bowel.

The workup of lower GI bleeding includes endoscopy, CTA, CTE, nuclear scintigraphy, conventional angiography, and surgery. The clinical presentation of patients dictates the order and urgency that the test/intervention is performed. Radiologic assessment of lower GI bleeding has come to the forefront of the workup, especially in patients with acute ongoing bleeding. Conventional angiography with embolization is now often the first-line treatment in patients who are unstable. CTE has become a first-line test for many patients with occult GI bleeding, especially in those whereby there is a contraindication to capsule endoscopy.

This article discusses the various imaging modalities used in the workup of lower GI bleeding and includes some of the common imaging findings using each modality.

REFERENCES

1. Manning-Dimmitt LL, Dimmitt SG, Wilson GR. Diagnosis of gastrointestinal bleeding in adults. Am Fam Physician 2005;71:1339–46.
2. Soto JA, Park SH, Fletcher JG, et al. Gastrointestinal hemorrhage: evaluation with MDCT. Abdom Imaging 2015;40:993–1009.
3. Zimmerman HM, Curfman K. Acute gastrointestinal bleeding. AACN Clin Issues 1997;8:449–58.
4. Gayer C, Chino A, Lucas C, et al. Acute lower gastrointestinal bleeding in 1,112 patients admitted to an urban emergency medical center. Surgery 2009;146(4):600–6 [discussion: 606–7].
5. Rockey DC. Gastrointestinal bleeding. In: Feldman M, Friedman LS, Brandt LJ, editors. Sleigenger and Fordtran's gastrointestinal and liver disease. 8th edition. Philadelphia: Saunders; 2006. p. 255–99.
6. Cirocchi R, Grassi V, Cavaliere D, et al. New trends in acute management of colonic diverticular bleeding: a systematic review. Medicine (Baltimore) 2015;94(44):e1710.
7. Saad WE, Lippert A, Saad NE, et al. Ectopic varices: anatomical classification, hemodynamic classification, and hemodynamic-based management. Tech Vasc Interv Radiol 2013;16:158–75.
8. Garcia-Blazquez V, Vicente-Bartulos A, Olavarria-Delgado A, et al. Accuracy of CT angiography in the diagnosis of acute gastrointestinal bleeding: systematic review and meta-analysis. Eur Radiol 2013;23(5):1181–90.
9. Yoon W, Jeong YY, Shin SS, et al. Acute massive gastrointestinal bleeding: detection and localization with arterial phase multi-detector row helical CT. Radiology 2006;239:160–7.
10. Kuhle WG, Sheiman RG. Detection of active colonic hemorrhage with use of helical CT: findings in a swine model. Radiology 2003;228:743–52.
11. Mayo-Smith WW, Hara AK, Mahesh M, et al. How I do it: managing radiation dose in CT. Radiology 2014;273(3):657–72.
12. Artigas JM, Martí M, Soto JA, et al. Multidetector CT angiography for acute gastrointestinal bleeding: technique and findings. Radiographics 2013;33:1453–70.
13. Kirchhof K, Welzel T, Mecke C, et al. Differentiation of white, mixed, and red thrombi: value of CT in estimation of the prognosis of thrombolysis—phantom study. Radiology 2003;228:126–30.
14. Hamilton JD, Kumaravel M, Censullo ML, et al. Multidetector CT evaluation of active extravasation in blunt abdominal and pelvic trauma patients. RadioGraphics 2008;28:1603–16.
15. Zuckier LS. Acute gastrointestinal bleeding. Semin Nucl Med 2003;33:297–311.
16. Howarth DM. The role of nuclear medicine in the detection of acute gastrointestinal bleeding. Semin Nucl Med 2006;36:133–46.
17. Wang ZG, Zhang GX, Hao SH, et al. Technological value of SPECT/CT fusion imaging for the diagnosis of lower gastrointestinal bleeding. Genet Mol Res 2015;14(4):14947–55.
18. Emslie JT, Zarnegar K, Siegel ME, et al. Technetium-99m-labeled red blood cell scans in the investigation of gastrointestinal bleeding. Dis Colon Rectum 1996;39(7):750–4.
19. Gunderman R, Leef J, Ong K, et al. Scintigraphic screening prior to visceral arteriography in acute lower gastrointestinal bleeding. J Nucl Med 1998;39(6):1081–3.
20. Laine L. Acute and chronic gastrointestinal bleeding. In: Feldman M, Scharschmidt BF, Sleisenger MH, editors. Gastrointestinal and liver disease. 6th edition. Philadelphia: Saunders; 1997. p. 198–219.
21. Walker TG, Salazar GM, Waltman AC. Angiographic evaluation and management of acute gastrointestinal hemorrhage. World J Gastroenterol 2012;18(11):1191–201.
22. Zuckerman GR, Prakash C, Askin MP, et al. AGA technical review on the evaluation and management of occult and obscure gastrointestinal bleeding. Gastroenterology 2000;118(1):201–21.

23. Gerson LB, Fidler JL, Cave DR, et al. ACG clinical guideline: diagnosis and management of small bowel bleeding. Am J Gastroenterol 2015;110(9): 1265–87 [quiz: 1288].

24. Hakim FA, Alexander JA, Huprich JE, et al. CT-enterography may identify small bowel tumors not detected by capsule endoscopy: eight years experience at Mayo Clinic Rochester. Dig Dis Sci 2011;56(10):2914–9.

25. Gerson LB. Small bowel bleeding: updated algorithm and outcomes. Gastrointest Endosc Clin N Am 2017;27(1):171–80.

26. Wang ZJ, Chen Q, Liu JL, et al. CT enterography in obscure gastrointestinal bleeding: a systematic review and meta-analysis. J Med Imaging Radiat Oncol 2013;57(3):263–73.

27. Huprich JE, Fletcher JG, Alexander JA, et al. Obscure gastrointestinal bleeding: evaluation with 64-section multiphase CT enterography–initial experience. Radiology 2008;246(2):562–71.

28. Baker ME, Hara AK, Platt JF, et al. CT enterography for Crohn's disease: optimal technique and imaging issues. Abdom Imaging 2015;40(5):938–52.

29. ACR. ACR manual on contrast media version 10.2. A. C. o. D. a. C. Media. 2016.

30. Huprich JE, Fletcher JG, Fidler JL, et al. Prospective blinded comparison of wireless capsule endoscopy and multiphase CT enterography in obscure gastrointestinal bleeding. Radiology 2011;260(3): 744–51.

31. Thacker P, Huprich J, Barlow JB, et al. The performance of triple-phase CT enterography compared to single-phase and double-phase enterography in the evaluation of obscure GI bleeding. Radiological Society of North America 2009 Scientific Assembly and Annual Meeting. Chicago (IL), November 29-December 4, 2009.

32. Huprich JE, Barlow JM, Hansel SL, et al. Multiphase CT enterography evaluation of small-bowel vascular lesions. AJR Am J Roentgenol 2013; 201(1):65–72.

33. McLaughlin PD, Maher MM. Primary malignant diseases of the small intestine. AJR Am J Roentgenol 2013;201(1):W9–14.

34. Rezvani M, Menias C, Sandrasegaran K, et al. Heterotopic pancreas: histopathologic features, imaging findings, and complications. Radiographics 2017;37(2):484–99.

35. Turgeon DK, Barnett JL. Meckel's diverticulum. Am J Gastroenterol 1990;85(7):777–81.

36. Park JJ, Wolff BG, Tollefson MK, et al. Meckel diverticulum: the Mayo Clinic experience with 1476 patients (1950-2002). Ann Surg 2005;241(3):529–33.

37. Lin S, Suhocki PV, Ludwig KA, et al. Gastrointestinal bleeding in adult patients with Meckel's diverticulum: the role of technetium 99m pertechnetate scan. South Med J 2002;95(11):1338–41.

38. Grady E. Gastrointestinal bleeding scintigraphy in the early 21st century. J Nucl Med 2016;57(2): 252–9.

Dual Energy Computed Tomography Scans of the Bowel
Benefits, Pitfalls, and Future Directions

Benjamin M. Yeh, MD[a],*, Markus M. Obmann, MD[a],
Antonio C. Westphalen, MD, PhD[a], Michael A. Ohliger, MD, PhD[a],
Judy Yee, MD[b,c], Yuxin Sun, MS[a], Zhen J. Wang, MD[a]

KEYWORDS

- Dual energy CT • Multi-energy CT • Bowel • Computed tomography

KEY POINTS

- The evaluation of bowel may be dramatically improved by simple dual energy computed tomography image reconstructions, with attention to a few caveats.
- Iodine and water maps, viewed together, allow for the differentiation of iodinated contrast material, such as in gastrointestinal bleeding, from high attenuation pills.
- Owing to gas–tissue interface artifacts, iodine maps must always be viewed with virtual monoenergetic images to confirm the presence or absence of bowel wall enhancement abnormalities.
- Iodine maps may be used to minimize the severity of bowel peristalsis artifact on the bowel wall and adjacent structures.
- Future dual energy computed tomography contrast agents may increase the confidence in diagnosis of a range of disease involving the bowel and adjacent structures.

INTRODUCTION

The diagnostic evaluation of the gastrointestinal tract is one of the most challenging tasks in medicine. Direct endoscopic visualization is difficult owing to the long length of the intestines and the need for sedation. Cross-sectional imaging may be confounded by artifacts created by gas, particularly when MR imaging or ultrasound examination are used, and by the large physical size of the bowel. Furthermore, peristalsis continuously changes the location and distension of individual bowel segments, as well as bowel contents, creating additional pitfalls in all imaging modalities.

Dual energy computed tomography (DECT) of the bowel has not been as extensively studied as for solid abdominal organs. Nevertheless, many of the benefits of DECT are uniquely beneficial to imaging of the gastrointestinal tract. DECT provides the ability to distinguish between different materials that cause high density in and around the bowel, and to highlight areas of mural hypoenhancement or hyperenhancement. Furthermore, the decrease in beam hardening artifacts, for

Disclosure Statement: Grants: General Electric Healthcare, Philips Healthcare, Guerbet, NIH. Speaker: General Electric Healthcare. Shareholder: Nextrast, Inc. Book royalties: Oxford University Press (B.M. Yeh). Grants: Philips Healthcare, Echopixel (J. Yee). Employee: Nextrast, Inc (Y. Sun). Shareholder: Nextrast, Inc (Z.J. Wang).
[a] UCSF Department of Radiology, 505 Parnassus Avenue Box 0628, San Francisco, CA 94143-0628, USA;
[b] Montefiore Department of Radiology, New York, NY, USA; [c] Montefiore Department of Radiology, Montefiore Hospital, 111 East 210th Street, Bronx, NY 10467, USA
* Corresponding author.
E-mail address: Ben.yeh@ucsf.edu

Radiol Clin N Am 56 (2018) 805–819
https://doi.org/10.1016/j.rcl.2018.05.002

example, from hip arthroplasty, spinal hardware, and abdominal surgical implants, is beneficial for the evaluation of the intestines. Relatively unexplored aspects of DECT include material decomposition and the impact of potential additional artifacts that may be introduced by DECT. This review describes the basic technical aspects of DECT image reconstruction and its benefits and potential pitfalls for the evaluation of several individual clinical scenarios involving the bowel.

BASIC CONCEPTS OF DUAL ENERGY COMPUTED TOMOGRAPHY IMAGING

Although an in-depth review of DECT physics is beyond the scope of our article, we provide an overview of concepts that are relevant to bowel imaging. DECT is based on the knowledge that (1) any given material will attenuate low versus high-energy spectra x-rays to a predictable material-specific degree, and (2) different materials will attenuate low versus high-energy spectra x-rays in distinctly different and predictable degrees. In this way, DECT images can be used to distinguish different materials, even if they have the same Hounsfield unit (HU) value at conventional CT, which employs a single polychromatic X-ray beam and detector array to generate images.

Five different DECT platforms are available, each with its own theoretic advantages and limitations. A brief description of these options is given below.

The dual-source DECT scanner uses 2 orthogonally mounted x-ray source/detector arrays that operate at different tube potentials, one at a low and the other at a high kVp. A drawback of this configuration is that one of the tubes is located closer to the patient, and, therefore, has a slightly smaller field of view. A benefit of this arrangement is the ability to filter the high kVp x-ray source with tin to improve the x-ray spectral separation between the 2 sources (Fig. 1).

The rapid kV-switching DECT scanner uses a single x-ray source that switches between a high and a low kVp hundreds of times per gantry rotation. This arrangement grants full field-of-view imaging and near perfect co-registration of the low- and high-energy projection data, which allows for projection-based, rather than image-based, material decomposition, which reduces noise.

The split filter DECT scanner uses a single x-ray source and gold and tin filters that block high and low keV photons of one-half of the x-ray beam, respectively, thereby creating 2 different photon energy spectra in the z-axis. This arrangement

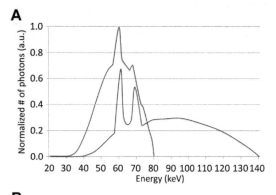

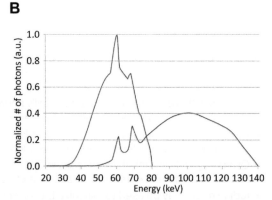

Fig. 1. X-ray energy spectra at low and high kVp. (*A*) X-ray energy spectra produced by a commercial CT scanner at 80 kVp (*red*) and 140 kVp (*blue*). The difference in x-ray spectra, and the fact that individual materials show different and predictable characteristic attenuation x-rays of different energies, allows imaged materials to be differentiated on dual energy computed tomography (DECT). (*B*) Tin filtration of the 140 kVp x-ray beam results in reduced overall flux of x-rays, and a harder x-ray beam with a higher mean x-ray energy. The resultant greater difference in x-ray spectra between the 80-kVp and the tin-filtered 140-kVp beams allows for better material separation at DECT.

provides full field of view imaging, but generally requires a slow table speed and gives less robust spectral separation than other dual energy implementations.

The sandwich detector DECT scanner (spectral detector or dual/double layer DECT scanner) achieves spectral separation of the x-ray beam at the detector level. The thin top layer of the detector, which is closer to the patient, detects the low-energy photons and the thicker deeper layer of the detector detects the remainder of the photons, which are largely higher in energy. As with the rapid kV-switching system, this arrangement provides full field-of-view imaging and outstanding co-registration of the low- and high-energy data, allowing for projection-based, rather than image-based, material decomposition and noise reduction.

The sequential acquisition DECT scanners (rotate–rotate, dual spin, or dual spiral dual energy) switches kVp after each revolution of the CT gantry. This type of DECT can be performed on any CT scanner, but may be optimized in some scanners to minimize time between low- and high-kVp image acquisitions.

The relative benefits and drawbacks of the existing DECT platforms for bowel imaging have not been determined, but one theoretic advantage of better co-registration of the low- and high-energy projection data is a decrease of the effect of bowel peristaltic motion on image co-registration. Also, improved spectral separation and better material decomposition may allow for superior differentiation of bowel contents and be particularly valuable when novel DECT contrast agents are used.

Regardless of how the DECT data are acquired, the reconstructed DECT images show similar properties across scanner platforms. The main types of image reformations are iodine density maps, virtual unenhanced (water density maps), virtual monoenergetic images, and effective Z images. The iodine density maps and their mirror image water density maps are best viewed as a pair. These images can be thought of as a reassignment of voxel values from the original low- and high-energy CT data. The iodine map reflects voxels with a dramatic relative decrease in HU between the low- and high-kVp images, as occurs with iodine and barium; conversely, the water density map reflects voxels that show little to no decrease in HU. Voxels with intermediate relative change in HU are assigned proportionally to the iodine and water density maps. For example, the values of voxels representing calcium (eg, bone) are divided into both the iodine and water density maps.

The virtual monoenergetic image is a reverse extrapolation of what a CT image might look like had it been obtained at a given monoenergetic x-ray photon energy. The x-ray photon energy may be selected to be between 40 and 140 keV, or even up to 200 keV in some platforms. Low-keV monoenergetic images show higher image contrast and higher iodine attenuation, but are generally more affected by metal and other artifacts. These low-keV images are used to emphasize iodine enhancement to improve lesion detection. Conversely, high keV virtual monoenergetic images are often used to improve the evaluation of anatomic detail because artifacts are generally less prominent, and may be used as a virtual unenhanced image, because the attenuation of iodine and barium are minimized. Virtual monoenergetic images are less prone to gas–tissue interface artifacts than are iodine maps (see **Fig. 1**).

General Concerns for Dual Energy Computed Tomography

A common misconception is that DECT requires higher radiation doses than needed for conventional single-energy CT because the patient is scanned at 2 different energies. In reality, in most cases, DECT scans may be obtained with similar radiation dose as a conventional scan because the overall dose is split between both energy levels.[1] Furthermore, overall dose savings may be achieved when virtual noncontrast scans are used in place of additional true noncontrast scans. Radiation dose levels have in general decreased for CT since 2009 with the routine use of iterative and model-based image reconstructions, which are incorporated into DECT scans.

Another concern for the use of DECT is the potential for difficulty in comparing HU values with conventional abdominal CT, which has typically been performed at 120 kVp. Because the Hounsfield values of materials vary depending on the kVp, DECT scans may not produce identical Hounsfield numbers as conventional 120-kVp CT scans. To bridge this issue, virtual monoenergetic images of about 65 to 70 keV, or mixed low- and high-kVp images, are used by different DECT platforms to provide roughly equivalent HU values as 120 kVp CT images.

Artifact Reduction

The gastrointestinal tract is unique among abdominal organs because of its dynamic and variable appearance. Unlike all other organs, the bowel is highly mobile, may be collapsed or distended, and may contain a wide variety of materials, including food and fluid at various stages of digestion, gas, and nonorganic foreign materials. DECT may be useful for reducing image artifacts that are common at CT imaging of the abdomen. Marked reduction of peristaltic motion artifact is seen in most patients on iodine density images compared with 120-kVp–equivalent images of single-source DECT scanners[2] (**Fig. 2**). Beam hardening artifact from radiodense catheters, metallic shrapnel, surgical implants, and dense contrast material can be minimized using high-keV virtual monoenergetic images[3] (**Fig. 3**). Bright truncation artifacts, which occur at the periphery of the abdomen of obese patients when tissues extend beyond the maximum field of view, are also minimized on iodine density maps.[4]

However, dual energy may introduce its own artifacts to CT imaging of the bowel. Several of these

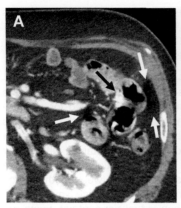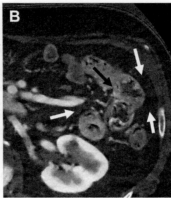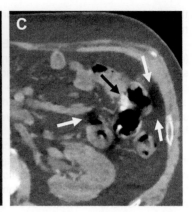

Fig. 2. Gas peristalsis artifact reduction at single source dual energy computed tomography. (*A*) Scanner 120 kVp equivalent image shows bright (*black arrow*) and dark streaks (*white arrows*) owing to peristalsis that obscures the bowel and adjacent anatomy. (*B*) Iodine density image shows much less artifact and a clear depiction of the bowel and adjacent anatomy because motion artifacts are non–kVp-dependent. (*C*) Water density image shows the motion artifact; the artifact is present to similar extent at both the low and high kVp source computed tomography data.

artifacts occur predominantly in the material decomposition images rather than virtual monoenergetic images. Iodine and water density images, which are calculated based on x-ray data from 2 different relatively photon-starved kVp datasets, generally have greater noise than blended low and high kVp images or virtual monochromatic images. Furthermore, edge artifacts that simulate pneumatosis intestinalis (**Fig. 4**) or bowel wall hyperemia may be seen at gas–tissue interfaces on iodine density map images.[5] As such, low-keV virtual monoenergetic images may be more reliable than iodine density maps for the assessment of derangements in bowel wall enhancement.

CLINICAL APPLICATIONS
Bowel Tumors

The detection of intestinal tumors is notoriously challenging on conventional CT scans and several measures are used to improve tumor visualization. Prone positioning in conjunction with multiplanar reformations is a simple approach that may improve the visualization of bowel and adjacent tissues on coronal reformations. Further emphasis has been placed on obtaining adequate bowel preparation through cleansing by fasting or the use of cathartics, distension with contrast material such as positive or neutral agents, and reduction of bowel peristalsis with glucagon (in the United States) or butylscopalamin (in Europe).

More recently, DECT low-keV virtual monoenergetic images and iodine density maps have been used to accentuate subtle focal hypervascular or hypovascular intramural bowel tumors, such as carcinoid[6] or metastatic disease (**Figs. 5 and 6**), and to improve the detection of tumors adjacent to bowel, such as peritoneal metastases.[7] Iodine density maps may improve the detection and delineation of colorectal carcinomas, even in the unprepped colon by separating it from stool and other enteric contents (**Figs. 7–9**).[8] Once tumors are identified, colorectal carcinomas may be further characterized as well-differentiated or poorly differentiated based on iodine and normalized iodine contents (**Fig. 10**).[9,10] A preliminary study of patients with rectal carcinoma further suggests that DECT iodine content may also be

Fig. 3. Metal artifact reduction. Conventional computed tomography (*left image*) is highly limited by excessive streak artifact from bilateral hip prosthesis, which prevents meaningful evaluation of the rectosigmoid colon (*arrows*) and the associated fat planes (*arrowhead*) with other viscera such as the bladder and pelvic side wall. The 120 keV virtual monochromatic image (*right image*) shows a reduction in streak artifact and marked improvement in the delineation of the viscera and fat planes.

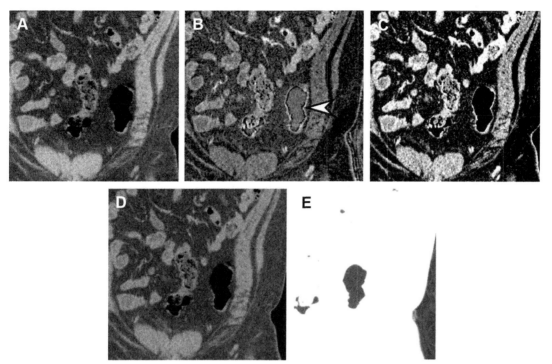

Fig. 4. Conventional image (*A*) shows unremarkable gas-filled descending colon. On the iodine density image (*B*) pseudopneumatosis is seen with linear low attenuation seen on the lumen-side of the bowel wall (*arrowhead*). A 40-keV monoenergetic image (*C*) and the water image (*D*) show no pneumatosis, which is further confirmed on the lung window (*E*).

useful to differentiate benign from malignant mesorectal lymph nodes in the excised surgical specimen[11] (**Fig. 11**). Similar results were seen in patients with gastric cancer, where metastatic lymph nodes tended to have higher relative enhancement on both the arterial and venous phases than benign lymph nodes.[12] The finding of an iodine concentration normalized to that of the aorta greater than 0.145 for the arterial phase and greater than 0.333 for the portal venous phase improved the sensitivity and specificity for nodes with metastatic disease, and such measures can be obtained at DECT without need for a corresponding unenhanced CT scan.[12] Iodine quantification also aided with staging of advanced gastric cancer by better assessing serosal

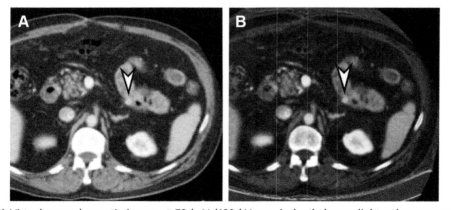

Fig. 5. (*A*) Virtual monochromatic image at 70 keV (120 kVp-equivalent) shows slight enhancement of small bowel intramural gastrointestinal stromal tumor (*arrowhead*). (*B*) Enhancement is more vivid in the corresponding iodine density image. (*Courtesy of* Bhavik Patel, MD, Duke University Medical Center, Durham, NC; with permission.)

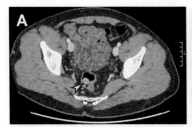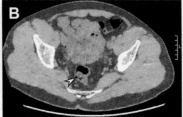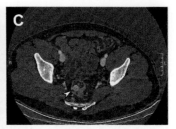

Fig. 6. Germ cell tumor (*arrowhead*) resembles dense stool on conventional image (*A*). Improved visibility of the brightly enhancing tumor is seen on the iodine density image (*C*) with corresponding low attenuation on the water density image (*B*). This pattern confirms that the mass represents iodine enhancement in a tumor rather than dense stool.

invasion.[13] Furthermore, the use of virtual noncontrast scans has shown promising results for the detection of gastric tumor calcifications.[14]

Gastrointestinal Bleeding

There are many different etiologies of bleeding, some of which are amenable to endoscopic treatment, for example, varices and other vascular anomalies. However, owing to the sheer length and challenging anatomy of bowel, a full endoscopic evaluation of the gastrointestinal tract is rarely possible. Upper endoscopy is generally limited to the evaluation of the esophagus, stomach, and duodenum, and colonoscopy is generally limited to the colon and distal-most ileum. Capsule endoscopy can be used for the diagnosis of causes of gastrointestinal bleeding, but it involves technical challenges that limit the accurate localization of findings. Furthermore, the endoscopic approaches cannot evaluate lesions deep to the intestinal mucosa and may be curtailed by difficult anatomy or obstructing masses that may prevent passage or manipulation of the endoscope, and may be associated with complications and patient morbidity.

Although imaging has several advantages over endoscopic evaluation, it is critical to recognize that the preparation of the bowel with positive,

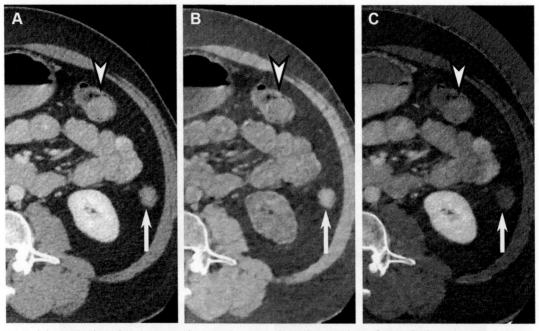

Fig. 7. (*A*) Standard 120-kVp image in the portal venous phase shows 2 dense foci in the bowel lumen (*white arrow* and *arrowhead*), which may be due to dense stool versus enhancing polyps. (*B*) Dual energy computed tomography water density image shows high computed tomography attenuation in the dense stool (*white arrow*) and low density in the polyp (*arrowhead*). (*C*) Iodine image shows iodine uptake in the polyp (*arrowhead*) and no iodine uptake in the dense stool (*white arrow*).

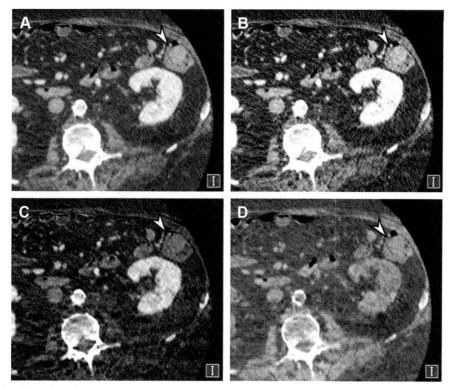

Fig. 8. Polyp (*arrowhead*) was missed on initial reading on the conventional computed tomography images (*A*). A low keV image (*B*) improves visualization of the polyp. Iodine (*C*) and water (*D*) density images show contrast enhancement of polyp with clear bright iodine density, which seems to be brighter than that of muscle, and no substantial increased water density of the focus compared with muscle.

neutral, or no oral contrast will each improve the sensitivity of CT for some types of findings, but will also decrease the accuracy of CT for other types of findings. The presence of positive oral iodinated or barium contrast material may mask the detection of active extravasation of intravenous contrast material into the bowel lumen. The proper technique for the detection of active extravasation, as opposed to a tumor or polyp, is to avoid the use of radiodense oral contrast material. With this caveat, intravenous contrast-enhanced CT scans with neutral or no

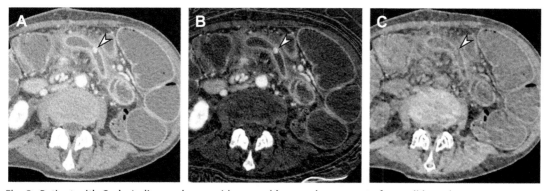

Fig. 9. Patient with Crohn's disease shows avid mucosal hyperenhancement of a small bowel segment on a conventional computed tomography image (*A*). A hyperdense focus (*arrowhead*) is seen in the affected small bowel and is ambiguous for a radiodense pill versus a polyp. Iodine density image (*B*) shows bright iodine density in the mass, whereas the water density image (*C*) shows no increased density, confirming that the focus is an enhancing polyp rather than an ingested pill.

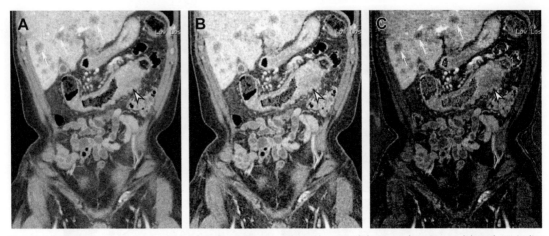

Fig. 10. Colonic adenocarcinoma (*arrowhead*) on the conventional image (*A*). a Low keV image (*B*) and AN iodine density image (*C*) shows heterogeneous iodine uptake in the mass. Hypodense liver metastases are also more vividly seen (*arrows*) in the low keV and iodine density map than on the conventional computed tomography image.

oral contrast are increasingly used for the detection of gastrointestinal bleeds that were missed by endoscopy or colonoscopy. CT can detect 0.1 mL of active contrast material extravasation into the bowel lumen. For conventional CT imaging, it is helpful to have an unenhanced and/or delayed scans in addition to images obtained during the arterial or venous phase of enhancement to confidently identify active bleeding. Bleeding is confirmed if a focus of intraluminal radiodensity is seen on the post–intravenous contrast scan, but not on the unenhanced images (**Fig. 12**). Alternatively, if unenhanced images are not available, intestinal bleeding can be confirmed by the finding of an increased volume of radiodense material in the bowel lumen on the delayed scan compared with the earlier intravenous contrast-enhanced scan.[15] These additional scans are necessary because of the high frequency of nonpathologic intraluminal radiodense materials, such as pharmaceuticals or food matter.[15]

DECT can streamline the process of identifying gastrointestinal bleeding because iodinated contrast material can be positively identified using the iodine map and virtual unenhanced images.[16] As such, a single phase DECT scan may be able to confirm whether a radiodense focus is due to gastrointestinal bleeding or ingested non–iodine-containing material such as a dissolving pill. In general, if a radiodense focus is seen as bright signal exclusively on the iodine map, then the focus is likely due to contrast material. If substantial signal is seen on the water or virtual nonenhanced image, then the high signal in the focus is likely related to ingested or surgically placed material (**Fig. 13**). Some materials, such as calcium, show up nearly equally on the iodine and virtual unenhanced images. In contrast with those radiodense substances, for example, nonsteroidal antiinflammatory drug pills, show little signal on iodine density map images, and show a predominant signal on virtual unenhanced images because the atomic composition of pills composed of

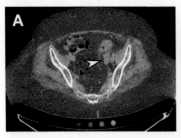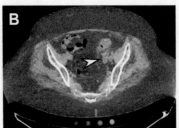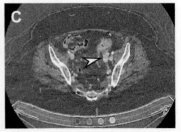

Fig. 11. Patient with colon carcinoma showing external iliac lymph node metastasis (*arrowhead*) poorly characterized on conventional CT 120 kVp image (*A*). Iodine uptake is clearly visible on the iodine density image (*C*) with a lack of dense signal on the water density image (*B*), confirming that the lesion is not calcified, but rather is enhancing.

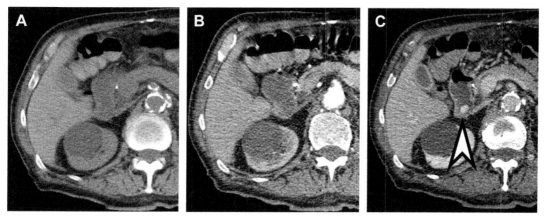

Fig. 12. Conventional computed tomography for gastrointestinal bleeding includes a noncontrast (*A*), arterial (*B*) and venous (*C*) phase scan that shows active bleeding (*arrowhead*) from a duodenal ulcer that was subsequently confirmed at endoscopy. Imperfect bowel anatomic co-registration between scans is due to bowel peristalsis and variability in the depth of breath holding. This example shows the importance of obtaining multiple phases of contrast by conventional imaging to confirm active bleeding. Unfortunately, such repeated imaging results in increased radiation exposure to the patient.

largely organic matter is close to that of soft tissue and water (**Fig. 14**).

Metastatic Peritoneal Implants

The detection of peritoneal implants poses a challenge to conventional imaging owing to the highly variable appearance of the bowel and metastatic peritoneal implants. DECT may improve the conspicuity of some peritoneal lesions by highlighting foci with increased or decreased enhancement relative to bowel, or with calcifications (**Fig. 15**).[7] Alternatively, nonenhancing radiodense materials such as a blood clot, which is relatively bright on water density images and not bright on iodine density images, may be readily differentiated from enhancing peritoneal tumors, which show similar density to muscle on water density

images and substantial iodine density on the iodine images.

Computed Tomography Colonography

The detection of colorectal polyps and cancers is the focus of CT colonography. Although current CT colonography protocols are highly effective, colonic preparation still impacts widespread use of the modality, because some patients do not obtain adequate colonic cleansing with the currently recommended protocols and others prefer not to undergo a thorough cathartic preparation. As a consequence, continued efforts are underway to simplify the colonic preparation to further improve screening compliance while maintaining a high likelihood for a diagnostic study.

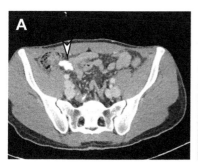
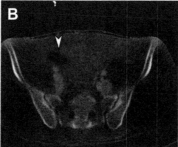
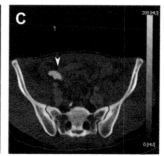

Fig. 13. A 23 year-old man with right lower quadrant pain. (*A*) Mixed image from a twin-beam dual energy computed tomography scanner shows radiodense material (*arrowhead*) in distal ileum, which was ambiguous for active extravasation versus radiodense ingested material. (*B*) Iodine density image and (*C*) iodine density overlay confirm that the radiodense material was neither iodine contrast or calcium, and hence was likely bismuth subsalicylate, a common over-the-counter drug.

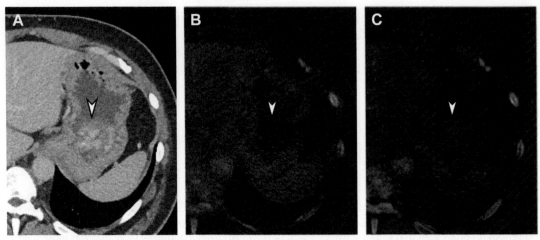

Fig. 14. A 52 year-old man with gastrointestinal bleeding. (*A*) Mixed image from a twin-beam dual energy computed tomography scanner shows radiodense material (*arrowhead*) in the stomach that was ambiguous for active extravasation. (*B*) Iodine density image and (*C*) iodine density overlay confirm that the radiodense material was not iodine contrast.

One suggested alternative to a thorough cathartic preparation is stool tagging with iodine or barium. Stool tagging provides diagnostic value by mixing with stool and intraluminal liquid to differentiate enhanced stool from soft tissue-density polyps, or may coat the surface of some cancers to draw attention to those lesions. However, suboptimal stool tagging may paradoxically lead to diagnostic ambiguity at conventional CT owing to inability to fully subtract the tagged stool from the images by thresholding. The use of DECT, however, may improve the differentiation of stool that has been tagged with contrast media from soft tissue polyps. DECT can detect miniscule amounts of contrast material and gas entrapped within stool and thereby differentiate poorly

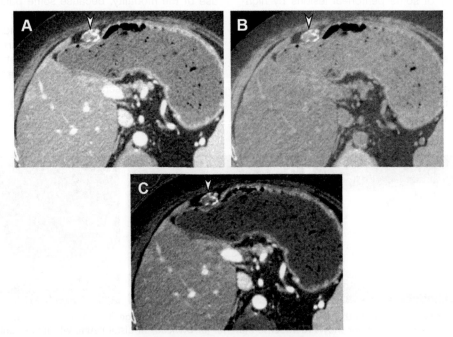

Fig. 15. Calcified peritoneal metastasis. A conventional computed tomography image (*A*) shows a radiodense focus (*arrowheads*) anterior to the stomach antrum. This focus showed high signal on both the water (*B*) and iodine (*C*) density images, which is a pattern typical for a calcified focus.

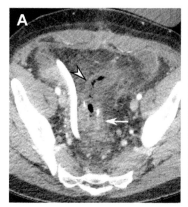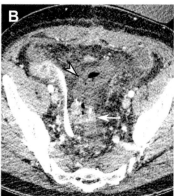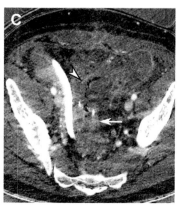

Fig. 16. Ischemic bowel. After sigmoidectomy, an elevation in serum lactic acid led to a dual energy computed tomography scan. On the 70-keV image (*A*), the colon proximal to the anastomosis (*arrowhead*) showed decreased computed tomography attenuation compared with the rectal remnant (*arrow*). The low keV image (*B*) and the iodine density image (*C*) confirmed the marked difference in enhancement and showed no identifiable iodine signal in the colon proximal to the anastomosis, indicating postoperative bowel ischemia.

tagged stool from true lesions when conventional electronic cleansing of tagged stool is suboptimal.[17–22] This approach to colon cancer screening remains an experimental technique and currently requires higher radiation dose than that of a low-dose conventional CT colonography examination.[19] Nevertheless, the potential benefits suggest that further research is warranted for effectiveness, optimization, and to identify the appropriate screening population that would benefit from this approach.

Bowel Ischemia and Hyperemia

DECT has been shown to improve the detection of hypovascular lesions in solid organs such as the pancreas and liver, and there is hope is that it will improve the detection of poorly enhancing, hypovascular, segments of bowel (**Fig. 16**). Initial preclinical studies in pigs showed promising ability of DECT to delineate intestinal infarction.[23] Subsequently, the first clinical results have shown increased diagnostic confidence when assessing ischemia in small bowel obstruction using low-keV virtual monoenergetic images.[24] Conversely, increased vascularization of the bowel wall in inflammatory change such as Crohn's disease (**Fig. 17**) may also be highlighted using low-keV virtual monoenergetic images. Iodine density images may also be used to identify artifactual causes of false bowel hyperemia, such as may be seen in and around bowel with active peristalsis at the moment of CT imaging (**Fig. 18**).

Oral Contrast Studies

Oral or rectal contrast studies are performed for a variety of reasons, but most often in postoperative

situations to answer questions of anastomotic leaks or fistulas. In these cases, DECT is valuable to differentiate between contrast material, calcification or other hyperdense material, particularly when a concurrent unenhanced CT scan was not obtained (**Figs. 19–21**).

FUTURE CONTRAST AGENTS

Our current DECT applications are constrained by our limited options of contrast materials, all of which are based on either iodine or barium. Because iodine and barium have very similar atomic numbers to each other (Z = 53 and 56,

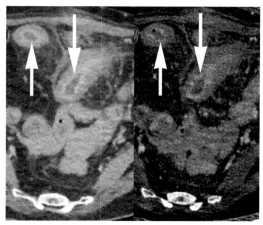

Fig. 17. Crohn's disease. Hyperenhancement of the mucosa (*arrows*) is more conspicuous on the iodine map (*right*) than on the 120-kVp image (*left*). Bowel wall hyperenhancement is the computed tomography finding most well-correlated with active inflammation at Crohn disease.

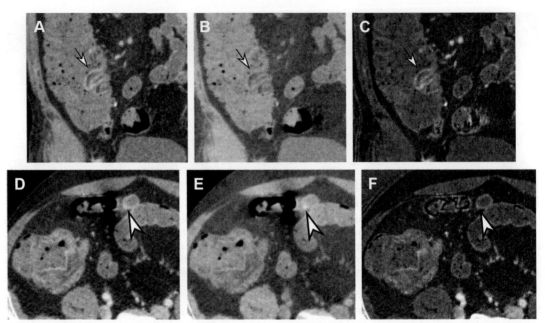

Fig. 18. A 70-keV (120-kVp equivalent) coronal image (*A*) shows a hyperattenuating ileocecal valve (*arrow*). In the water density image (*B*), no corresponding hyperdensity is seen, whereas hyperdensity is seen on the iodine density image (*C*), proving that the ileocecal valve demonstrates true hyperenhancement and inflammation. A different bowel segment (*arrowhead*) in the 70-keV axial image (*D*) also shows a hyperattenuating bowel wall. However, the water density image (*E*) showed marked increase density whereas the iodine density image (*F*) image does not show increased density compared with other bowel wall segments, revealing that the hyperdensity seen at 70 keV was not due to iodine enhancement. Rather, it was likely due to bowel wall peristaltic motion.

respectively), they are poorly differentiated from each other using either conventional CT or DECT scans. Bright barium or iodine enteric contrast material prevents accurate evaluation of bowel wall hyperenhancement or hypoenhancement. Novel contrast noniodinated contrast

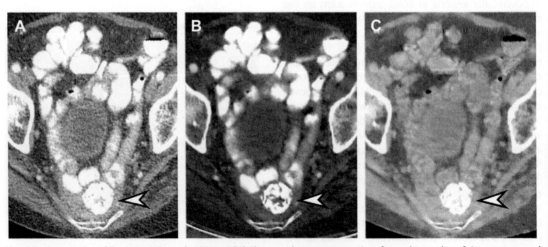

Fig. 19. Conventional image with oral contrast (*A*) shows a hyperattenuating focus (*arrowhead*) in a computed tomography of the pelvis that is ambiguous for being bowel contrast or a lesion. Iodine density image (*B*) also shows also high density of the focus. However, high density is also seen in the water density image (*C*), confirming that the bright signal was due to calcification rather than oral contrast material. This case illustrates the critical need to look at both the iodine and water density images as a pair to differentiate calcified structures from those with iodine contrast material enhancement.

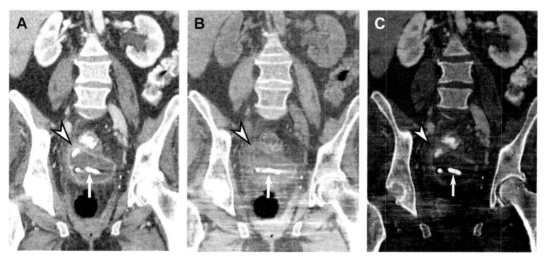

Fig. 20. Conventional image (*A*) in a study with rectal iodinated contrast shows 2 hyperattenuating foci in a perirectal abscess: A tubular structure (*arrow*), which is a known catheter, and another focus (*arrowhead*) close to a segment of colon containing rectal contrast material. The hyperdense focus is also seen on the iodine density image (*C*) but not the corresponding water density image (*B*), confirming that the bright focus was due to leakage of the rectal contrast agent into the abscess. A true unenhanced computed tomography scan was not required to confirm this active rectal contrast material leakage.

materials are under development and may be particularly useful for imaging of the abdomen (**Fig. 22**).[25–28] Use of paired complementary DECT contrast material for intravenous and oral contrast material allows for ready separation of bowel lumen contrast from bowel wall enhancement, and may allow substantial reduction in radiation dose and improved confidence in certain abdominal diagnoses, such as whether contrast leakage is from a bowel or vascular source.[27] Currently, no noniodine nonbarium contrast agents that have been approved by the US Food and Drug Administration are available for multicontrast DECT, but novel agents are under development.[28] Updates to current material decomposition software will also be needed to maximize the benefits of multicontrast enhanced DECT.[25]

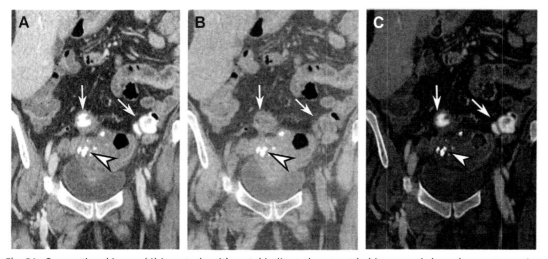

Fig. 21. Conventional image (*A*) in a study with rectal iodinated contrast (*white arrows*) shows hyperattenuating foci adjacent to the sigmoid colon (*arrowhead*). The intraluminal rectosigmoid contrast material is also seen on the iodine density image (*C*), but not the corresponding water density image (*B*). The hyperdensities adjacent to the colon remain hyperdense on both the water and iodine density images, confirming that they are calcifications rather than contrast material leakage.

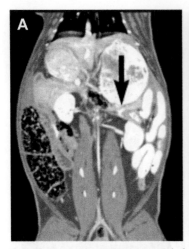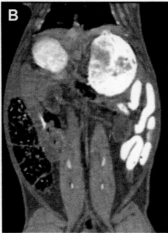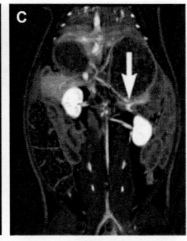

Fig. 22. Future contrast material for double contrast dual energy computed tomography. Conventional computed tomography image (*A*) in a rabbit model of sharp penetrating abdominal trauma, with iodinated intravenous and high-Z oral contrast media. Extraluminal contrast leakage (*black arrow*) is seen below the stomach. In the high-Z density image (*B*) no extraluminal contrast is seen, which confirms that the contrast leakage is not due to oral contrast leakage from bowel. In the iodine density image (*C*) extraluminal iodinated contrast agent is seen (*white arrow*), confirming that the contrast agent leakage was due to a vascular, rather than bowel, injury. Note the excellent visualization of the bowel wall enhancement in the iodine density image, which was difficult to appreciate on the conventional computed tomography image. High-Z dual energy computed tomography contrast agents are not currently clinically available.

SUMMARY

The advantages of DECT over conventional CT can provide substantial benefits for imaging of the bowel. The most promising scenarios described to date involve the decrease of artifacts, improved sensitivity for the detection of hypo and hypervascular lesions, and material decomposition to better characterize intraluminal contents. Further advances continue to be defined for this relatively nascent technology.

REFERENCES

1. Jepperson MA, Cernigliaro JG, Ibrahim E-SH, et al. In vivo comparison of radiation exposure of dual-energy CT versus low-dose CT versus standard CT for imaging urinary calculi. J Endourol 2015;29(2):141–6.
2. Winklhofer S, Lambert JW, Wang ZJ, et al. Reduction of peristalsis-related gastrointestinal streak artifacts with dual-energy CT: a patient and phantom study. Abdom Radiol (NY) 2016;41(8):1456–65.
3. Yu L, Leng S, McCollough CH. Dual-energy CT-based monochromatic imaging. AJR Am J Roentgenol 2012;199(5 Suppl):S9–15.
4. Dotson B, Lambert JW, Wang ZJ, et al. Benefit of iodine density images to reduce out-of-field image artifacts at rapid kVp switching dual-energy CT. Abdom Radiol 2017;42(3):735–41.
5. Wu E-H, Kim SY, Wang ZJ, et al. Appearance and frequency of gas interface artifacts involving small bowel on rapid-voltage-switching dual-energy CT iodine-density images. Am J Roentgenol 2016; 206(2):301–6.
6. Ganeshan D, Bhosale P, Yang T, et al. Imaging features of carcinoid tumors of the gastrointestinal tract. Am J Roentgenol 2013;201(4):773–86.
7. Benveniste AP, de Castro Faria S, Broering G, et al. Potential application of dual-energy CT in gynecologic cancer: initial experience. Am J Roentgenol 2017;208(3):695–705.
8. Ozdeniz I, Idilman IS, Koklu S, et al. Dual-energy CT characteristics of colon and rectal cancer allows differentiation from stool by dual-source CT. Diagn Interv Radiol 2017;23(4):251–6.
9. Gong HX, Zhang KB, Wu LM, et al. Dual energy spectral CT imaging for colorectal cancer grading: a preliminary study. Woloschak GE, editor. PLoS One 2016;11(2):e0147756.
10. Chuang-bo Y, Tai-ping H, Hai-feng D, et al. Quantitative assessment of the degree of differentiation in colon cancer with dual-energy spectral CT. Abdom Radiol 2017;42(11):2591–6.
11. Al-Najami I, Beets-Tan RGH, Madsen G, et al. Dual-energy CT of rectal cancer specimens: a CT-based method for mesorectal lymph node characterization. Dis Colon Rectum 2016;59(7):640–7.
12. Pan Z, Pang L, Ding B, et al. Gastric cancer staging with dual energy spectral CT imaging. PLoS One 2013;8(2):e53651.
13. Yang L, Shi G, Zhou T, et al. Quantification of the iodine content of perigastric adipose tissue by

dual-energy CT: a novel method for preoperative diagnosis of T4-stage gastric cancer. Wei Q-Y, editor. PLoS One 2015;10(9):e0136871.

14. Chai Y, Xing J, Gao J, et al. Feasibility of virtual non-enhanced images derived from single-source fast kVp-switching dual-energy CT in evaluating gastric tumors. Eur J Radiol 2016;85(2):366–72.

15. Barlow JM, Goss BC, Hansel SL, et al. CT enterography: technical and interpretive pitfalls. Abdom Imaging 2015;40(5):1081–96.

16. Fulwadhva UP, Wortman JR, Sodickson AD. Use of dual-energy CT and iodine maps in evaluation of bowel disease. Radiographics 2016;36(2):393–406.

17. Cai W, Lee J-G, Zhang D, et al. Electronic cleansing in fecal-tagging dual-energy CT colonography based on material decomposition and virtual colon tagging. IEEE Trans Biomed Eng 2015;62(2):754–65.

18. Cai W, Kim SH, Lee JG, et al. Virtual colon tagging for electronic cleansing in dual-energy fecal-tagging CT colonography. Conf Proc IEEE Eng Med Biol Soc 2012;2012:3736–9.

19. Karcaaltincaba M, Ozdeniz I, Cai W, et al. Dual-energy CT for diagnostic CT colonography. Radiographics 2014;34(3):847–8.

20. Cai W, Kim SH, Lee J-G, et al. Informatics in radiology: dual-energy electronic cleansing for fecal-tagging CT colonography. Radiographics 2013;33(3):891–912.

21. Karcaaltincaba M, Karaosmanoglu D, Akata D, et al. Dual energy virtual CT colonoscopy with dual source computed tomography: initial experience. Rofo 2009;181(9):859–62.

22. Eliahou R, Azraq Y, Carmi R, et al. Dual-energy based spectral electronic cleansing in non-cathartic computed tomography colonography: an emerging novel technique. Semin Ultrasound CT MR 2010;31(4):309–14.

23. Potretzke TA, Brace CL, Lubner MG, et al. Early small-bowel ischemia: dual-energy CT improves conspicuity compared with conventional CT in a swine model. Radiology 2014;275(1):119–26.

24. Darras KE, McLaughlin PD, Kang H, et al. Virtual monoenergetic reconstruction of contrast-enhanced dual energy CT at 70keV maximizes mural enhancement in acute small bowel obstruction. Eur J Radiol 2016;85(5):950–6.

25. Rathnayake S, Mongan J, Torres AS, et al. In vivo comparison of tantalum, tungsten, and bismuth enteric contrast agents to complement intravenous iodine for double-contrast dual-energy CT of the bowel: enteric contrast comparison for dual-energy CT of the bowel. Contrast Media Mol Imaging 2016;11(4):254–61.

26. Mongan J, Rathnayake S, Fu Y, et al. In vivo differentiation of complementary contrast media at dual-energy CT. Radiology 2012;265(1):267–72.

27. Mongan J, Rathnayake S, Fu Y, et al. Extravasated contrast material in penetrating abdominopelvic trauma: dual-contrast dual-energy CT for improved diagnosis–preliminary results in an animal model. Radiology 2013;268(3):738–42.

28. Yeh BM, FitzGerald PF, Edic PM, et al. Opportunities for new CT contrast agents to maximize the diagnostic potential of emerging spectral CT technologies. Adv Drug Deliv Rev 2016;113:201–22.

Lower Gastrointestinal Tract Applications of PET/ Computed Tomography and PET/MR Imaging

Onofrio Catalano, MD, PhD[a],*, Aoife Kilcoyne, MD[b],
Alberto Signore, MD, PhD[c], Umar Mahmood, MD, PhD[d],
Bruce Rosen, MD, PhD[e]

KEYWORDS

- PET/CT • PET/MR imaging • Small bowel • Large bowel

KEY POINTS

- Knowledge of the technical pitfalls, potential artifacts and limitations/strengths of PET/CT and PET/MR imaging is pivotal in the selection of the appropriate imaging modality.
- Patient preparation and protocol optimization are essential to ensure high-quality imaging.
- PET/MR imaging is of particular use in the long-term evaluation of inflammatory bowel disease, where serial imaging is required over the lifetime of these patients.

INTRODUCTION

PET/computed tomography (CT) is an established technique in the staging and assessment of disease response in multiple malignancies. The role of PET/CT in the evaluation of inflammatory disorders such as Crohn's disease (CD) is evolving. PET/MR imaging is a newer hybrid imaging technique that integrates the advantages related to MR imaging while optimizing the role of PET in lesion detection and diagnostic performance. The emerging role of PET/MR imaging in the evaluation of inflammatory and malignant diseases is discussed.

TECHNIQUE

Techniques for Imaging of the Small Bowel

PET computed tomography

To maximize tracer uptake at pathologic sites, it is essential to minimize tracer uptake at background or potentially confounding sites. Patients are advised to avoid strenuous activity and exercise on the day before the examination to reduce skeletal muscle uptake.[1] Patients fast for between 4 and 6 hours before [18]fluorodeoxyglucose (FDG) administration to ensure that serum glucose and insulin levels are low. Hydration with water is encouraged. Blood glucose is

Disclosure statement: The authors have no disclosures.
[a] Department of Radiology, Division of Abdominal Imaging, A. Martinos Center for Biomedical Imaging, Massachusetts General Hospital, Harvard University Medical School, 55 Fruit Street, Boston, MA 02114, USA;
[b] Department of Radiology, Division of Abdominal Imaging, Massachusetts General Hospital, Harvard University Medical School, 55 Fruit Street, Boston, MA 02114, USA; [c] Nuclear Medicine Unit, Department of Medical-Surgical Sciences and of Translational Medicine, Sapienza University, Via del policlinico 32, Roma 0023, Italy;
[d] Massachusetts General Hospital, A. Martinos Center for Biomedical Imaging, Harvard University Medical School, Building 149, Room 2301, 13th Street, Charlestown, MA 02129, USA; [e] Martinos Center for Biomedical Imaging, Harvard University Medical School, Massachusetts Institute of Technology, 149 Thirteenth Street, Room 2301, Charlestown, MA 02129, USA
* Corresponding author.
E-mail address: ocatalano@mgh.harvard.edu

Radiol Clin N Am 56 (2018) 821–834
https://doi.org/10.1016/j.rcl.2018.05.001

measured before FDG administration. If the blood glucose is greater than 200 mg/dL, the test is typically rescheduled. Patients are kept warm before and immediately after FDG administration to minimize brown fat activation and tracer uptake. Screening for pregnancy is performed in all women of childbearing age.

PET computed tomography protocol PET imaging is usually performed within 60 to 90 minutes of FDG injection. During this period patients are encouraged to rest. Talking, chewing, and walking are restricted. For studies that are tailored to evaluate the small bowel, patients are asked to drink 1350 mL of low-attenuating oral contrast over 45 minutes.[2]

The typical scan coverage extends from the skull base to the mid thighs for oncologic indications. In the case of inflammatory bowel disease (IBD), it extends from the mid-thighs to the diaphragm. The patients arms are raised to minimize scatter when imaging the chest and abdomen. Immediately before scanning, patients are asked to void, to reduce tracer activity in the bladder, which can be a source of artifact. The typical acquisition time for a whole body PET scan can vary between 15 and 45 minutes or 2 to 5 minutes per bed position, and depends on factors, including scan coverage, tracer dose, scanner technology, and patient body habitus.[3]

CT-based attenuation correction is the standard of modern-day PET-CT scanners. It permits rapid acquisition of low-noise transmission images and is required to allow semiquantitative calculation of tumor glucose metabolism using standardized uptake values (SUVs).[1] The CT performed with a PET can be an attenuation correction or a diagnostic study, or both. At our institution, a fully diagnostic, standard radiation dose contrast-enhanced study is performed.

Radiation dose considerations The total radiation dose from a PET-CT or PET study represents the sum of injected radiopharmaceutical activity (eg, FDG) and of the CT dose.[1] Low-dose CT scanning for attenuation correction only is consistent with an effective dose of between 1.5 and 5.0 mSv.[4] For diagnostic CT scanning, there is a wide range of reported doses in the literature, with 4 to 18 mSv in the thorax, 3.5 to 25 mSv in the abdomen, and 3.3 to 10 mSv for the pelvis.[5] The American College of Radiology practice guidelines suggest an effective dose of 370 to 740 MBq (10–20 mCi),[6] resulting in an effective dose from the PET component of 7 to 15 mSv.[3]

PET MR imaging
Patients fast for 6 hours before image acquisition to ensure blood glucose levels of less than 140 mg/mL.[7] For studies performed for the assessment of chronic IBD, patients drink 2 L of a diluted polyethylene glycol solution before image acquisition at a rate of 125 mL every 5 minutes. For other indications, including the assessment of rectal and colonic malignancy, oral contrast is not administered.

Five minutes before PET/MR imaging acquisition, 20 mg of hyoscine butylbromide or 0.5 to 1.0 mg of glucagon are injected intravenously. PET/MR images are acquired using body coils combined to form a multichannel coil. PET/MR imaging typically begins at a mean of 60 to 80 minutes after FDG injection.[7]

MR imaging Image acquisition commences from mid-thigh and extends to the diaphragm in the case of IBD, and it extends to the vertex when imaging bowel malignancy. The MR images are coacquired with PET, to ensure temporal and spatial matching of the respective data, which is a feature unique to PET/MR, specifically:

- Coronal T1 Dixon,
- Coronal short tau inversion recovery (STIR),
- Axial T2-weighted half-Fourier acquisition single shot turbo spin echo (HASTE), and
- Axial diffusion-weighted imaging (DWI).

For imaging of IBD, the following breath hold MR imaging sequences are also acquired:

- Coronal T2-weighted HASTE,
- Axial T1-weighted dual gradient echo, and
- Coronal and axial dynamic contrast enhanced T1-weighted volume interpolated breath hold (VIBE).

When imaging a case of rectal or sigmoid malignancy, high-resolution T2-weighted fast spin echo sequences are co-acquired with a second list-mode PET acquisition.

In the case of a bowel malignancy not arising from the rectum or sigmoid colon, and for follow-up of treated rectal/sigmoid cancers with a low level of suspicion for local recurrence, the following upper abdominal sequences are co-acquired with a second list-mode PET:

- Coronal T2-weighted HASTE,
- Axial T2-weighted fat-saturated respiratory gated fast spin echo,
- Axial in and out of phase T1-weighted dual gradient echo, and
- Axial dynamic contrast enhanced T1-weighted VIBE.

After this, whole body axial and coronal VIBE images are obtained. The MR images are co-registered and fused with PET on a dedicated multi-modality workstation.

Radiation dose considerations For an equivalent injected activity, PET/MR imaging permits a 20% decrease in radiation exposure compared with PET/CT when attenuation correction only is used and a 60% to 73% decrease when both attenuation correction and diagnostic quality CT studies are acquired with PET-CT scanners.[9,10]

Technical Pitfalls and Limitations

Oral contrast and PET computed tomography
The benefit of oral contrast administration in imaging of the bowel is in the distension of bowel, which can increase the conspicuity of bowel luminal, mural, and extraluminal disease.[2] It may also improve the visibility of the adjacent mesenteric and retroperitoneal metastatic deposits and allow for the identification of synchronous small bowel and colonic lesions. A potential disadvantage of using high-density oral contrast is the effect on attenuation correction. Barium can lead to reconstruction artifacts that cause apparent FDG uptake owing to differences in attenuation correction. A review of the non–attenuation-corrected images can resolve this pitfall, because these images should not demonstrate the artificially increased FDG accumulation. The artifact can also be reduced by using low or neutral density barium[11,12] or diatrizoate (Gastrografin).[11]

Patient motion
Patient motion and bowel peristalsis can lead to difficulty with lesion localization. This finding is particularly relevant in imaging of the bowel. PET/MR image acquisition is typically longer than PET/CT (with an average duration of approximately 50–80 minutes depending on the protocol), but the synchronous acquisition of PET and MR images mitigates this issue. To better account for this problem, hyoscine butylbromide or glucagon are administered to all of our patients undergoing PET/MR enterography and to patients with a pelvic malignancy. However, for patients who are unable to sustain the longer PET/MR imaging acquisition, PET/CT is preferred.

Hyoscine butylbromide or glucagon?
Glucagon has been demonstrated, in some cases, to affect PET images owing to a shift of FDG from the blood into skeletal muscle.[13] Hyoscine butyl-bromide has been demonstrated to cause smooth muscle relaxation, reducing the risk of misinterpreting focal muscular spasms as strictures, while not affecting PET image quality.[13] However, hyoscine butylbromide is not currently approved by the Food and Drug Administration for use in the United States. With the advancement of MR imaging technology, newer MR imaging sequences potentially could be acquired using shorter scan times, obviating the need for small bowel relaxants.

False-positive [18]fluorodeoxyglucose uptake
This phenomenon can occur secondary to bacterial overgrowth or to postoperative or postradiation change. In general, it is recommended to wait at least 6 weeks after radiation therapy or surgical treatment to avoid a false-positive interpretation.[14]

Elevated tracer metabolism can also be seen in small and large bowel in diabetic patients receiving metformin.[15] It has been demonstrated that cessation of metformin administration before PET can decrease bowel uptake.

Some benign tumors can demonstrate FDG uptake. Colonic polyps and adenomas, for example, can demonstrate variable uptake.[16] Typically, uptake in benign lesions is less than that of malignant lesions. However, there can be some overlap.

False-negative [18]fluorodeoxyglucose uptake
False-negative findings on PET can be due to small lesion size, malignancies that do not demonstrate hypermetabolism, and tumors that are obscured by increased radiotracer uptake locally.[1]

Modern PET CT scanners have a resolution limit of 4 mm. Structures measuring less than 0.7 to 10.0 mm cannot be sampled reliably.[17]

Tumors that do not demonstrate hypermetabolism can be difficult to detect. For example, FDG PET is limited in the evaluation of mucinous tumors, in particular, hypocellular lesions with abundant mucin.[18]

High uptake adjacent to an area of malignancy may obscure uptake at the site of malignancy, for example, at sites adjacent to the bladder or the ureter. The use of multiplanar reformats can help to avoid this error. Patients are typically asked to void before image acquisition to minimize bladder uptake.

Clinical Indications

Inflammatory bowel disease
CD and ulcerative colitis represent the majority of IBDs affecting children and adolescents in the developed world. IBD has important epidemiologic implications owing to its high incidence (10 per 100,000 children in the United States and Canada) and prevalence (100–200 per 100,000 in the United States) in the pediatric population.[19] Ulcerative colitis is a chronic condition that leads to inflammation and ulcers in the colon and rectum owing to continuous involvement of (sub)mucosal

wall tissue. CD is characterized by a chronic/relapsing course, the tendency to involve any segment of the gastrointestinal tract and by asymmetric and discontinuous transmural inflammation of the bowel wall.[20,21]

Imaging has a role in establishing the diagnosis, assessing disease extent, determining activity, and detecting and characterizing complications, including abscesses, fistulae, and strictures.[22] It can also phenotype CD into inflammatory, penetrating, and stricturing variants.[23] Although abscesses and fistulae can be confidently evaluated using several imaging modalities, strictures represent a greater challenge.[24]

Strictures are found in more than 10% of patients at diagnosis of CD, with the prevalence increasing over time. They constitute a common cause of acute clinical symptoms.[20,25,26] Strictures can be caused by acute transmural inflammation, chronic fibrosis, or a combination thereof.[25,27] Precise differentiation of inflammatory from fibrotic strictures has relevant clinical implications. Medical therapy is used to treat inflammatory strictures, whereas surgical resection or luminal dilatation is typically performed for fibrotic strictures.[20,25,28] However, this differentiation can be challenging, with endoscopic techniques often incapable of evaluating the bowel wall layers deep to the mucosa where fibrosis mainly occurs. Therefore, several clinical, laboratory, and imaging biomarkers, with variable degrees of accuracy and clinical success, have been used for this purpose.[20,25,28–30]

Hybrid imaging, including PET/CT scans and especially PET/MR imaging, has the potential to address both the basic clinical imaging needs for ulcerative colitis and patients with CD, encompassing assessment of disease extent and therapy response, as well as distinguishing inflammatory from fibrotic strictures. Despite these potential benefits, their role in clinical practice remains controversial.[24,31,32]

Inflammatory bowel disease: PET/computed tomography

^{18}F-FDG PET/CT scanning has been demonstrated to be of benefit in determining the location and severity of disease activity in many inflammatory disorders.[33,34] In particular, the maximum SUV (SUV_{max}) and partial volume-corrected mean SUV ($PVC-SUV_{mean}$) have been demonstrated to correlate significantly with Crohn's Disease Endoscopy Index subscores ($P<.05$).[35] Thus, PET has a potential role in the assessment of stricturing disease in this context. The ability of PET to detect active inflammation in strictured segments of bowel could aid in the differentiation of such regions from fibrotic strictures.

Several groups have evaluated the use of PET in CD. A study published by Skehan and colleagues[36] was performed using FDG PET in 25 pediatric patients with suspected IBD. Fifteen patients in the group had CD. Endoscopy with biopsy and small bowel follow-through were used as reference standards. This article demonstrated a sensitivity of 81% and specificity of 85%, and concluded that PET localized more inflammatory areas in the proximal large bowel than colonoscopy. In another article regarding a separate patient cohort, Skehan confirmed a high (81.5%) sensitivity for PET in identifying active inflammation. PET represents an alternative for further imaging modality in the evaluation of CD.[37] Loffler and colleagues[38] evaluated FDG-PET in 23 pediatric patients, 17 of whom had CD. This study demonstrated a sensitivity and specificity of 98% and 68% with histology as standard of reference, 92% and 65% with endoscopy as the standard of reference, respectively.

Bettenworth and colleagues[33] performed PET/CT scans in 25 patients with histologically diagnosed Crohn's colitis. Positive findings were demonstrated in 88% of extensive ulcerations, but only in 50% of superficial epithelial lesions. The group concluded that the intestinal glucose uptake is variable and pathologic segments are often not distinguishable from unaffected ones. The same group compared FDG PET/CT scanning with MR imaging-enteroclysis and transabdominal ultrasound imaging to identify a noninvasive imaging method for the detection and differentiation of inflammatory and fibrosing stenosis in CD. Endoscopy and histology were used as reference standards. The combination of transabdominal ultrasound imaging and PET/CT scanning or MR imaging-enteroclysis yielded a 100% detection rate of strictures.[28]

More recently, Russo and colleagues[39] evaluated the role of FDG PET/CT as a marker of progression of inflammatory activity and its response to anti-tumor necrosis factor therapy in 22 patients with CD. The study demonstrated a sensitivity of 88% and a specificity of 70% for PET/CT. The SUV demonstrated significant cross-sectional and longitudinal correlation with clinicopathologic markers including C-reactive protein and Harvey-Bradshaw index.

FDG-PET/CT is a reliable "paninflammatory" marker that can evaluate the whole bowel. SUV can assist in image interpretation but caution should be used owing to physiologic uptake of FDG by the bowel. However, FDG-PET cannot substitute for colonoscopy or MR imaging and should be performed in conjunction with other imaging modalities.

Inflammatory bowel disease: PET/MR imaging
PET/MR imaging offers advantages over PET/CT scanning in this context owing to the improved anatomic detail and soft tissue contrast, additional functional capabilities of MR, including DWI and apparent diffusion coefficient (ADC) maps, and the simultaneous acquisition of PET and MR.[40] The latter may allow an ideal co-registration and fusion of the PET data over the simultaneously acquired MR imaging anatomic layout of the bowel segments, overcoming the challenges imposed by bowel peristalsis that may affect the asynchronously acquired PET/CT data.

Despite the extreme paucity of literature on PET/MR imaging of CD, this new hybrid technique is promising.[8,41,42] Therefore, we have described our personal experience and reviewed the limited available PET/MR imaging literature, incorporating also stand-alone MR and PET research.

At our institutions, the first data that we evaluate from a PET/MR imaging study for CD are PET, STIR, and coronal portal venous phase contrast-enhanced images, both stand-alone and after having been co-registered and fused with PET. This process is to ascertain the quality of the acquisition, identify possible areas of active disease, evaluate disease extent and severity, and exclude false positives. Thereafter, all the other MR imaging sequences are evaluated on both a stand-alone basis and after fusion with PET.[8]

The criteria that we use to assess for active inflammation of the bowel in patients with CD have evolved from stand-alone MR imaging and PET imaging and include wall thickening (>3 mm), mural edema, prominent vasa recta, contrast enhancement, and focally increased FDG uptake, with a high SUV_{max} (>4; **Fig. 1**).[43–46] For fistulae, bowel loops are typically tethered, fixed, and distorted and demonstrate high SUV values. Increased FDG uptake is a common finding in acute inflammatory CD, in agreement with the high sensitivity reported in this setting in the PET literature.[36–38]

In the setting of inactive CD, FDG avidity is reduced, making detection more difficult on stand-alone PET.[28,47] In these cases, MR imaging demonstrates bowel wall thickening in the absence of intramural edema, reduced signal on T2-weighted images, focal, slow and progressive contrast enhancement, and lipomatous hypertrophy affecting adjacent mesenteric fat. However, the accuracy of MR imaging alone in distinguishing active from inactive CD is questionable. For example, the target sign (bowel wall thickening and stratified mural enhancement), reported to occur in 75% of fibrotic strictures, is also observed in active inflammation.[48,49] In our recently published data on the PET/MR imaging assessment of active inflammation on CD, nonincreased FDG avidity (SUV_{max} of <4) may facilitate this distinction.[50]

Strictures, regardless of the predominance of fibrosis or acute inflammation, are responsible for upstream bowel dilatation that also improves

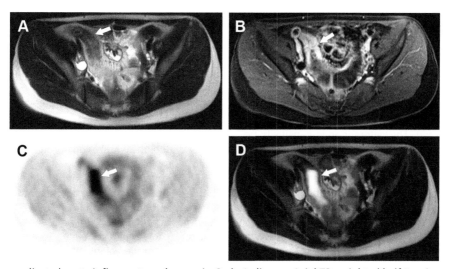

Fig. 1. Uncomplicated acute inflammatory changes in Crohn's disease. Axial T2-weighted half-Fourier acquisition single shot turbo spin echo (*A*), axial contrast-enhanced T1-weighted volume interpolated breath hold (*B*), axial PET (*C*), and fused PET/MR imaging (*D*). All the MR imaging and PET findings of active inflammation in Crohn's disease coexist in this segment of the ileum (*arrow*): bowel wall thickening with increased T2-weighted signal and intense contrast enhancement, engorgement of the adjacent vessels, and increased [18]fluorodeoxyglucose uptake. No fistulae, abscesses, or phlegmon are identified.

detection. As discussed, endoscopy or endoscopic biopsy are limited for this purpose.[29,51] Even CT enterography and MR imaging enterography, despite the ability to evaluate the entire gastrointestinal tract, and, in the case of MR imaging-enterography, to allow a multiparametric investigation (including a decreased T2-weighted signal intensity, lack of early mucosal enhancement, and slow and progressive contrast enhancement of the submucosa and muscularis) have moderate accuracy in distinguishing inflammatory from fibrotic strictures.[28–30,52,53]

In a recent study that investigated the performance of PET/MR imaging in distinguishing active versus fibrotic strictures, with surgical pathology as standard of reference, a hybrid PET/MR imaging biomarker ($ADC*SUV_{max}$) that takes into account both the FDG uptake, expressed as SUV_{max} and the diffusion of water molecules in the intercellular space (ADC), proved useful for this purpose. An $ADC*SUV_{max}$ cutoff of less than 3000 was the best discriminator between active inflammation and fibrosis with mean sensitivity of 67%, mean specificity of 73%, and mean accuracy of 71%.[8] Two other studies have demonstrated that PET/MR imaging accurately detected extraluminal disease in CD[41] and might be useful in the identification of subclinical inflammation in ulcerative colitis.[54]

In a study performed by our group, a total of 105 bowel segments were identified and evaluated among 21 patients with CD with surgical reports serving as the standard of reference. Image-based active inflammation was identified in 66 of 105 bowel segments on PET, 53 of 105 bowel segments on MR imaging, and 55 of 105 bowel segments on PET/MR imaging. On the basis of surgical reports, 59 of the 105 bowel segments were positive for active inflammation.[50]

Sensitivity for detecting active inflammation was the highest for stand-alone PET (91.5%) and 80% for MR imaging. The differences in sensitivity between stand-alone PET and stand-alone MR imaging were statistically significant ($P = .02$), although the difference in sensitivity between stand-alone PET and PET/MR imaging were not statistically significant ($P = .48$). PET/MR imaging was more sensitive in detecting active inflammation compared with MR imaging alone, but this was not statistically significant ($P = .08$).

PET/MR imaging had the highest specificity for active inflammation (93%), followed by stand-alone MR imaging (87%) and lastly stand-alone PET (74%). When compared with stand-alone PET, the higher specificities obtained with PET/MR imaging and stand-alone MR imaging were statistically significant ($P = .04$ and $P = .01$, respectively). A statistically significant difference was not identified between PET/MR imaging and MR imaging alone ($P = .37$).

PET/MR imaging exhibited the greatest diagnostic accuracy (91%), followed by stand-alone PET (84%) and stand-alone MR imaging (83%). The greater accuracy seen in PET/MR imaging in identifying active inflammation was statistically significant compared with that of stand-alone PET and stand-alone MR imaging ($P = .02$ and $P = .01$ respectively). No difference was found when comparing diagnostic accuracies between stand-alone PET and stand-alone MR imaging ($P>.5$).

As discussed, PET/CT scanning has been shown to be a useful modality for identifying bowel segments with active inflammation demonstrating good correlation in IBD patients.[34] The correlation of morphologic information from CT scans with metabolic data from PET scans have a role in predicting response of patients with CD to medical treatment and in monitoring treatment response. For example, lack of FDG avidity in abnormally enhancing bowel segments on a CT scan predicted failure of medical therapy.[55]

Similar to PET/CT scans, PET/MR imaging combines functional and morphologic data to potentially better assess the extent and location of disease than either submodality alone.[56,57] PET/MR imaging offers several advantages over PET/CT scans arising from the superior soft tissue signal-to-noise ratio and contrast-to-noise ratio of MR imaging when compared with CT scanning. MR imaging also allows a multiparametric evaluation of the bowel wall, with signal intensity on T2-weighted images correlating with signs of active inflammation in CD.[58] Furthermore, the decreased radiation burden of PET/MR imaging is especially advantageous in patients with CD who are typically young and likely to need multiple serial imaging studies.[42] The co-acquisition of PET/MR imaging allows a more accurate spatial and temporal matching of MR imaging anatomy with PET data compared with sequential acquisition in PET/CT scanning.[7] This factor is very advantageous in bowel evaluation because, owing to peristalsis, sequentially acquired PET/CT scans can lead to misregistration artifacts and difficulties in assigning anatomic correlates to areas of metabolic abnormalities highlighted by PET scanning.[59]

According to our data, PET scanning is significantly more sensitive but less specific than MR imaging in evaluating active inflammation in CD. This finding is in agreement with prior studies that have demonstrated high sensitivity (54%–100%) and lower specificity (50%–65%) of PET in evaluating active inflammation in CD.[56,57,60] The combination of the PET and MR imaging in a single technology that allows simultaneous acquisition of both modalities may overcome the intrinsic limitation of the stand-alone parent submodalities. This factor likely explains the superior performance of PET/MR imaging over stand-alone PET and stand-alone MR imaging that we observed.

Stand-alone MR imaging has false-positive rates from 7% to 21%.[61,62] Collapsed bowel loops are challenging and can be mistakenly interpreted as bowel wall thickening/enhancement/restricted loops, contributing to the false-positive rate of stand-alone MR imaging.[63] As in our recently published data, the lack of FDG uptake in areas of concern would exclude active inflammation. In contrast, stand-alone MR imaging has false-negative rates ranging from 10% to 21%, as in cases of mild inflammation or overdistended bowel loops.[61,64] However, the high sensitivity of PET for acute inflammatory changes assisted in the detection of active inflammation.[50]

In conclusion, PET/MR imaging is feasible for evaluating patients with CD and advantageous over PET/CT scanning and stand-alone MR imaging. PET/MR imaging at the expense of a reduced radiation burden compared with PET/CT scanning demonstrates better performance than stand-alone PET and stand-alone MR imaging and likely also of PET/CT scanning. PET/MR imaging

potentially has a role in the management and treatment monitoring in patients with CD (**Figs. 2** and **3**).

In the future, we foresee the use of many other radiopharmaceuticals, in addition to FDG, that have previously been successfully applied in single photon emission CT or PET/CT scanning,[65] or adapted from other chronic inflammatory diseases. These may ultimately be labeled with positron emitters (such as 18F, 68Ga, 64Cu, or 69Zr) for PET/MR imaging investigation.[66–68]

Colorectal cancer
Colorectal cancer is extremely important epidemiologically, with 139,992 new cases diagnosed in the United States in 2014 and 51,651 cancer deaths in the United States in 2014. It represents the third most common cause of cancer death worldwide.[69–71]

Overall survival is heavily influenced by stage at presentation, with a 5-year survival rate that decreased from 93% in stage I to 8% in stage IV disease.[69] Although several treatment options are available, their implementation is dictated by several factors, one of the most important being clinical stage.[72–75]

Different imaging methods are currently used for staging and restaging colorectal cancer, including CT scanning, MR imaging, PET scanning, and PET/CT scanning with FDG.[76–86] PET/CT, owing to the extremely high sensitivity to FDG uptake,

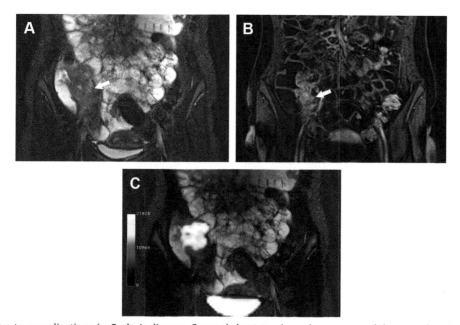

Fig. 2. Acute complications in Crohn's disease. Coronal short tau inversion recovery (*A*), coronal portal venous phase VIBE (*B*), and fused PET/MR imaging (*C*) demonstrate a phlegmon presenting as an indistinct masslike thickening of the last ileal loop and adjacent mesenteric fat (*arrow*) with associated increased [18]fluorodeoxyglucose uptake. Note the poor definition of the margins and the absence of frank areas of liquefaction.

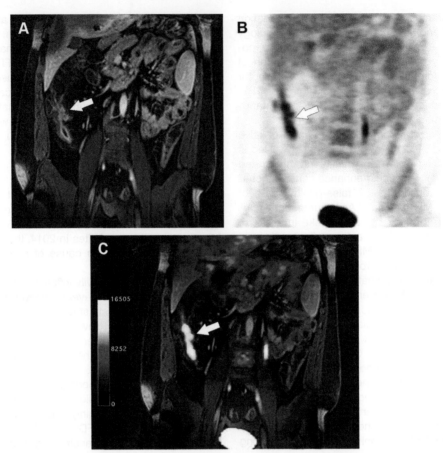

Fig. 3. Chronic complications in Crohn's disease. Coronal contrast-enhanced T1-weighted volume interpolated breath hold (*A*), coronal PET (*B*), and fused PET/MR imaging (*C*) demonstrate a fistula (*arrow*) as a complication in a Crohn's disease patient. Note distortion, tethering and fixation of the bowel loops, mucosal enhancement, adjacent lipomatous hypertrophy, and increased [18]fluorodeoxyglucose uptake.

has a superior performance for detecting distant metastases.[82,87–89] However, anatomic localization of areas of FDG uptake can be challenging with PET/CT scans, owing to the low soft tissue signal-to-noise and contrast-to-noise ratios of CT scans, as well as the asynchronous acquisition of the PET data and CT images. This factor can hamper the performance of PET/CT scans, particularly in the assessment of the T and N factors in rectal cancers, in liver lesions measuring less than 10 mm, in subcapsular liver lesions, in peritoneal metastases, and in the case of apparently nonspecific intestinal uptake of FDG.[82,87]

Conversely, MR imaging, because of its higher soft tissue signal-to-noise and contrast-to-noise ratios is preferred to CT scanning for local staging of rectal cancers (T and N factors) and for detection of smaller liver lesions.[82] For local staging, the reported sensitivity, specificity, and accuracy are 78% to 79%, 63% to 78%, and 66% to 73%, respectively, for CT scanning; 82% to 86%, 76% to 77%, and 74% to 82%, respectively, for MR imaging, and 75% to 90%, 42% to 76%, and 68% to 85%, respectively, for PET/CT scanning.[82–86] For distal staging, the reported sensitivity, specificity, and accuracy are 58% to 89%, 87% to 94.9%, and 52% to 77%, respectively, for CT scanning; 80% to 85%, 92.5% to 99%, and 82% to 98%, respectively, for MR imaging, and 66% to 86%, 67% to 97.2%, and 64% to 83%, respectively, for PET-CT scanning.[82–86]

Given these advantages of MR imaging over CT scanning and the intrinsically high sensitivity of PET scanning, the advent of hybrid PET/MR imaging scanner is expected to play a major role in rectal cancer staging.[90] In our opinion, PET/MR imaging may potentially serve as a one-stop shop assessment of both locoregional extension and distal status (**Figs. 4–6**). However, its performance is strongly influenced by the acquisition protocol.

Kang and colleagues[91] performed the largest PET/MR imaging study in patients with colorectal

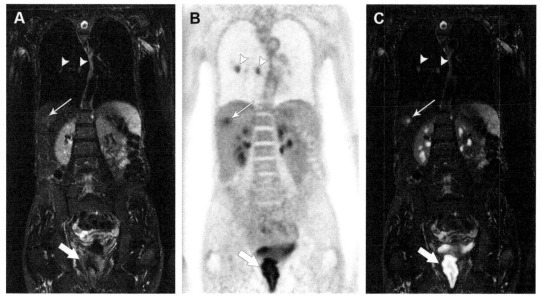

Fig. 4. Single stop shop examination. Coronal short tau inversion recovery (*A*), coronal PET (*B*), and coronal fused PET/MR imaging (*C*) demonstrate the ability to achieve local staging and search for distant metastases during the same imaging session. The rectal cancer (*solid arrow*), the hepatic (*thin arrow*), and pulmonary metastases (*arrowheads*) are clearly depicted on PET. The corresponding anatomic abnormalities are shown on the co-acquired short tau inversion recovery.

cancer (51 cases) to date, comparing PET/MR imaging with contrast-enhanced CT scanning. The authors reported potential PET/MR imaging–driven changes in treatment plans in up to 21% of cases. Specifically, they found PET/MR imaging advantageous for the detection of liver metastases, of local tumor recurrence, and to rule out malignancy in other liver lesions and in postoperative

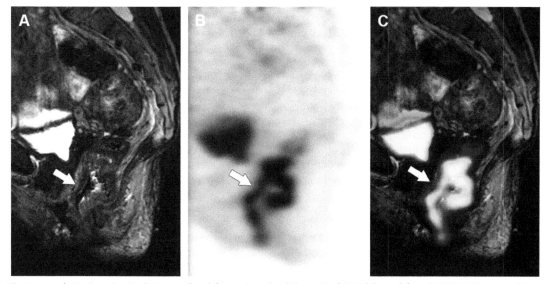

Fig. 5. Local staging. Sagittal T2-weighted fast spin echo (*A*), sagittal PET (*B*), and fused PET/MR imaging (*C*). In this case of an intensely [18]fluorodeoxyglucose-avid rectal cancer (*arrow*), note the perfect superimposition of the PET data over the co-acquired high-quality MR image. The fine details of this low rectal cancer (*arrow*), its extension into the anal canal, and the infiltration of the rectovaginal septum and of the perineum are clearly delineated owing to 2 features unique to PET/MR imaging: synchronous acquisition of PET and MR images and intrinsically high soft tissue signal to noise ratio of MR imaging.

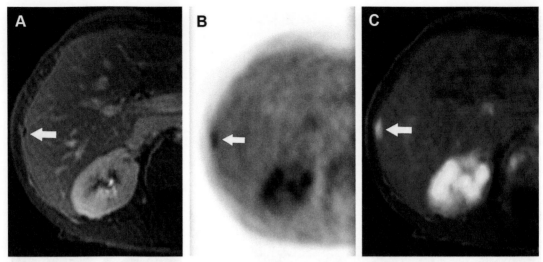

Fig. 6. Colorectal liver metastases. Axial contrast-enhanced T1-weighted volume interpolated breath hold (*A*), axial PET (*B*), and fused PET/MR imaging (*C*). PET/MR imaging is advantageous over other imaging technologies in the setting of liver metastases (*arrow*), particularly in the case of subcentimeter and subcapsular lesions, as in this case. The lesion is difficult to detect in (*A*). Localization of the focus of increased [18]fluorodeoxyglucose uptake in (*B*) would have been challenging in the absence of co-acquired PET/MR imaging and the high contrast-to-noise ratio of MR imaging. However, this is easily accomplished using PET/MR imaging (*C*).

tissues. However, these high figures may have been lower if PET/MR imaging had been matched with a state-of-the-art PET/CT protocol.

In a study performed by Brendle and colleagues[92] in 15 patients affected by metastatic colorectal cancer, the accuracy of PET/MR imaging with DWI and of PET/CT scanning were similar in evaluating for lymphadenopathy (84% each) and for nodules at the pulmonary bases (50%).

PET/MR imaging outperformed PET/CT in the assessment of hepatic metastases, with an accuracy of 74% and 56%, respectively. However, whereas PET/MR imaging with DWI achieved better overall accuracy than PET/CT scanning (69% vs 66%, respectively) the difference in performance was not statistically significant (*P* = .275). However, Brendle and colleagues[92] used a PET/MR imaging protocol that covered only the abdomen and pelvis, and did not include contrast enhanced sequences or T2-weighted high-resolution pelvic sequences.

Paspulati and colleagues[93] (2013) in a study that recruited 12 patients with colorectal cancer, demonstrated that PET/MR imaging allowed a superior assessment of the T factor in the staging of rectal cancer compared with PET/CT, and also demonstrated similar accuracy in assessing for lymphadenopathy and distant metastases. However, the authors identified that a protocol without specific bone marrow sequences could miss bone metastases, as occurred in a single patient of their cohort.

In a study by Catalano and colleagues,[94] in 26 patients affected by colorectal cancer, whole body contrast-enhanced PET/MR imaging outperformed whole-body contrast-enhanced PET/CT scanning. The PET/MR imaging protocol used by the authors covered the entire body, and in addition to the sequences reported by Brendle and colleagues, included also contrast-enhanced VIBE sequences and high-resolution T2-weighted pelvic sequences, for cases of rectal or sigmoid cancer or suspected pelvic recurrence. Although both technologies correctly and concordantly evaluated 69% of the cases, and concordantly misevaluated 1 of the 26 cases (3.8%), PET/MR imaging correctly assessed the remaining 27% of patients that were misstaged by PET/CT scanning. Specifically, PET/MR imaging identified peritoneal carcinomatosis in 1 case and lymphadenopathy in 3 that were missed by PET/CT evaluation; PET/MR imaging also excluded residual/recurrent pelvic disease in 2 cases and excluded nonregional lymphadenopathy in the remaining patient.

In our experience, which is in agreement with the limited available literature, the superior soft tissue contrast of MR imaging, the better anatomic overlay of MR imaging, and the availability of multiple MR imaging sequences, when compared with CT scanning, could enable better assessment of locoregional extension of rectosigmoid cancer, including assessment of the distance from the mesorectal fascia, involvement of adjacent anatomic structures, and evaluation of the soft tissue structures in the pelvis and perineum.[95,96] The superior anatomic depiction offered by MR imaging, compared with CT scanning, allowed for better localization of foci of FDG avidity, which in some cases led to a more accurate interpretation. This finding is in agreement with other studies that demonstrated the superior soft tissue resolution of PET/MR imaging to be advantageous compared with PET/CT scanning in better identifying perirectal implants and locoregional infiltration.[7]

In our practice, we rely on the combined assessment of all the MR imaging sequences in addition to the FDG uptake both for local and distal staging and restaging. This modality is especially useful for the assessment of small lesions in the liver and peritoneum, as well as in the evaluation of the local extension of rectal cancer.[93–99]

PET/MR imaging may underperform compared with PET/CT scanning in the evaluation for lung nodules. However, in a study by Chandarana and colleagues,[100] PET/MR imaging demonstrated a sensitivity of 70.3% for all nodules, 95.6% for FDG-avid nodules, and 88.6% for nodules 5 mm or greater in diameter. In addition, it is unclear if the lack of visibility of lung nodules less than 6 mm in dimeter may be clinically relevant.[7]

PET/CT scanning and PET/MR imaging have a clear role to play in the evaluation of inflammatory and malignant disorders of the lower gastrointestinal tract. The results of future studies evaluating novel radiotracers are eagerly awaited, which could further enhance the usefulness of these modalities.

ACKNOWLEDGMENTS

Aoife Kilcoyne was supported by the Higher Degree Bursary from the Faculty of Radiologists, Royal College of Surgeons in Ireland.

REFERENCES

1. Lee LK, Kilcoyne A, Goldberg-Stein S, et al. FDG PET-CT of genitourinary and gynecologic tumors: overcoming the challenges of evaluating the abdomen and pelvis. Semin Roentgenol 2016;51:2–11.

2. Cronin CG, Scott J, Kambadakone A, et al. Utility of positron emission tomography/CT in the evaluation of small bowel pathology. Br J Radiol 2012;85: 1211–21.

3. Delbeke D, Coleman RE, Guiberteau MJ, et al. Procedure guideline for tumor imaging with 18F-FDG PET/CT 1.0. J Nucl Med 2006;47:885–95.

4. Brix G, Lechel U, Glatting G, et al. Radiation exposure of patients undergoing whole-body dual-modality 18F-FDG PET/CT examinations. J Nucl Med 2005;46:608–13.

5. Mettler FA Jr, Huda W, Yoshizumi TT, et al. Effective doses in radiology and diagnostic nuclear medicine: a catalog. Radiology 2008;248:254–63.

6. ACR-SPR Practice parameter for performing FDG-PET/CT in oncology (Amended 2014). 2007. Available at: https://www.acr.org/~/media/71B746780F934F6D8A1BA5CCA5167EDB.pdf. Accessed October 22, 2017.

7. Catalano OA, Rosen BR, Sahani DV, et al. Clinical impact of PET/MR imaging in patients with cancer undergoing same-day PET/CT: initial experience in 134 patients–a hypothesis-generating exploratory study. Radiology 2013;269:857–69.

8. Catalano OA, Gee MS, Nicolai E, et al. Evaluation of quantitative PET/MR enterography biomarkers for discrimination of inflammatory strictures from fibrotic strictures in Crohn disease. Radiology 2016;278:792–800.

9. Atkinson W, Catana C, Abramson JS, et al. Hybrid FDG-PET/MR compared to FDG-PET/CT in adult lymphoma patients. Abdom Radiol (NY) 2016;41: 1338–48.

10. Schafer JF, Gatidis S, Schmidt H, et al. Simultaneous whole-body PET/MR imaging in comparison to PET/CT in pediatric oncology: initial results. Radiology 2014;273:220–31.

11. Blake MA, Setty BN, Cronin CG, et al. Evaluation of the effects of oral water and low-density barium sulphate suspension on bowel appearance on FDG-PET/CT. Eur Radiol 2010;20:157–64.

12. Cohade C, Osman M, Nakamoto Y, et al. Initial experience with oral contrast in PET/CT: phantom and clinical studies. J Nucl Med 2003;44:412–6.

13. Yasuda S, Takechi M, Ono M, et al. The effect of glucagon on FDG uptake in skeletal muscle. Tokai J Exp Clin Med 2012;37:11–3.

14. Blake MA, Singh A, Setty BN, et al. Pearls and pitfalls in interpretation of abdominal and pelvic PET-CT. Radiographics 2006;26:1335–53.

15. Ozulker T, Ozulker F, Mert M, et al. Clearance of the high intestinal (18)F-FDG uptake associated with metformin after stopping the drug. Eur J Nucl Med Mol Imaging 2010;37:1011–7.

16. Metser U, Miller E, Lerman H, et al. Benign nonphysiologic lesions with increased 18F-FDG uptake on PET/CT: characterization and incidence. AJR Am J Roentgenol 2007;189:1203–10.

17. Erdi YE. Limits of tumor detectability in nuclear medicine and PET. Mol Imaging Radionucl Ther 2012;21:23–8.

18. Berger KL, Nicholson SA, Dehdashti F, et al. FDG PET evaluation of mucinous neoplasms: correlation of FDG uptake with histopathologic features. AJR Am J Roentgenol 2000;174:1005–8.

19. Rosen MJ, Dhawan A, Saeed SA. Inflammatory bowel disease in children and adolescents. JAMA Pediatr 2015;169:1053–60.

20. Sleisenger MH, Feldman M, Friedman LS, et al. Sleisenger and Fordtran's gastrointestinal and liver disease: pathophysiology, diagnosis, management. 9th edition. Philadelphia: Saunders/Elsevier; 2010.

21. Ford AC, Moayyedi P, Hanauer SB. Ulcerative colitis. BMJ 2013;346:f432.

22. Anupindi SA, Grossman AB, Nimkin K, et al. Imaging in the evaluation of the young patient with inflammatory bowel disease: what the gastroenterologist needs to know. J Pediatr Gastroenterol Nutr 2014;59:429–39.

23. Baumgart DC, Sandborn WJ. Crohn's disease. Lancet 2012;380:1590–605.

24. Panes J, Bouhnik Y, Reinisch W, et al. Imaging techniques for assessment of inflammatory bowel disease: joint ECCO and ESGAR evidence-based consensus guidelines. J Crohns Colitis 2013;7:556–85.

25. Rieder F, Zimmermann EM, Remzi FH, et al. Crohn's disease complicated by strictures: a systematic review. Gut 2013;62:1072–84.

26. Speca S, Giusti I, Rieder F, et al. Cellular and molecular mechanisms of intestinal fibrosis. World J Gastroenterol 2012;18:3635–61.

27. Rieder F, Fiocchi C. Intestinal fibrosis in IBD–a dynamic, multifactorial process. Nat Rev Gastroenterol Hepatol 2009;6:228–35.

28. Lenze F, Wessling J, Bremer J, et al. Detection and differentiation of inflammatory versus fibromatous Crohn's disease strictures: prospective comparison of 18F-FDG-PET/CT, MR-enteroclysis, and transabdominal ultrasound versus endoscopic/histologic evaluation. Inflamm Bowel Dis 2012;18:2252–60.

29. Gee MS, Nimkin K, Hsu M, et al. Prospective evaluation of MR enterography as the primary imaging modality for pediatric Crohn disease assessment. AJR Am J Roentgenol 2011;197:224–31.

30. Adler J, Punglia DR, Dillman JR, et al. Computed tomography enterography findings correlate with tissue inflammation, not fibrosis in resected small bowel Crohn's disease. Inflamm Bowel Dis 2012;18:849–56.

31. Glaudemans AW, Maccioni F, Mansi L, et al. Imaging of cell trafficking in Crohn's disease. J Cell Physiol 2010;223:562–71.

32. Jamar F, Buscombe J, Chiti A, et al. EANM/SNMMI guideline for 18F-FDG use in inflammation and infection. J Nucl Med 2013;54:647–58.

33. Bettenworth D, Reuter S, Hermann S, et al. Translational 18F-FDG PET/CT imaging to monitor lesion activity in intestinal inflammation. J Nucl Med 2013;54:748–55.

34. Treglia G, Quartuccio N, Sadeghi R, et al. Diagnostic performance of Fluorine-18-Fluorodeoxyglucose positron emission tomography in patients with chronic inflammatory bowel disease: a systematic review and a meta-analysis. J Crohns Colitis 2013;7:345–54.

35. Saboury B, Salavati A, Brothers A, et al. FDG PET/CT in Crohn's disease: correlation of quantitative FDG PET/CT parameters with clinical and endoscopic surrogate markers of disease activity. Eur J Nucl Med Mol Imaging 2014;41:605–14.

36. Skehan SJ, Issenman R, Mernagh J, et al. 18F-fluorodeoxyglucose positron tomography in diagnosis of paediatric inflammatory bowel disease. Lancet 1999;354:836–7.

37. Lemberg DA, Issenman RM, Cawdron R, et al. Positron emission tomography in the investigation of pediatric inflammatory bowel disease. Inflamm Bowel Dis 2005;11:733–8.

38. Loffler M, Weckesser M, Franzius C, et al. High diagnostic value of 18F-FDG-PET in pediatric patients with chronic inflammatory bowel disease. Ann N Y Acad Sci 2006;1072:379–85.

39. Russo EA, Khan S, Janisch R, et al. Role of 18F-fluorodeoxyglucose positron emission tomography in the monitoring of inflammatory activity in Crohn's disease. Inflamm Bowel Dis 2016;22:2619–29.

40. Maccioni F, Patak MA, Signore A, et al. New frontiers of MRI in Crohn's disease: motility imaging, diffusion-weighted imaging, perfusion MRI, MR spectroscopy, molecular imaging, and hybrid imaging (PET/MRI). Abdom Imaging 2012;37:974–82.

41. Pellino G, Nicolai E, Catalano OA, et al. PET/MR versus PET/CT imaging: impact on the clinical management of small-bowel Crohn's disease. J Crohns Colitis 2016;10:277–85.

42. Beiderwellen K, Kinner S, Gomez B, et al. Hybrid imaging of the bowel using PET/MR enterography: feasibility and first results. Eur J Radiol 2016;85:414–21.

43. Toriihara A, Yoshida K, Umehara I, et al. Normal variants of bowel FDG uptake in dual-time-point PET/CT imaging. Ann Nucl Med 2011;25:173–8.

44. Allen BC, Leyendecker JR. MR enterography for assessment and management of small bowel Crohn disease. Radiol Clin North Am 2014;52:799–810.

45. Dillman JR, Trout AT, Smith EA. MR enterography: how to deliver added value. Pediatr Radiol 2016;46:829–37.

46. Grand DJ, Guglielmo FF, Al-Hawary MM. MR enterography in Crohn's disease: current consensus on optimal imaging technique and future advances from the SAR Crohn's disease-focused panel. Abdom Imaging 2015;40:953–64.

47. Jacene HA, Ginsburg P, Kwon J, et al. Prediction of the need for surgical intervention in obstructive Crohn's disease by 18F-FDG PET/CT. J Nucl Med 2009;50:1751–9.

48. Steward MJ, Punwani S, Proctor I, et al. Non-perforating small bowel Crohn's disease assessed by MRI enterography: derivation and histopathological validation of an MR-based activity index. Eur J Radiol 2012;81:2080–8.

49. Al-Hawary MM, Zimmermann EM, Hussain HK. MR imaging of the small bowel in Crohn disease. Magn Reson Imaging Clin N Am 2014;22:13–22.

50. Catalano OA, Wu V, Mahmood U, et al. Diagnostic performance of PET/MR in the evaluation of active inflammation in Crohn disease. Am J Nucl Med Mol Imaging 2018;8(1):62–9.

51. Burke JP, Mulsow JJ, O'Keane C, et al. Fibrogenesis in Crohn's disease. Am J Gastroenterol 2007; 102:439–48.

52. Lee SS, Kim AY, Yang SK, et al. Crohn disease of the small bowel: comparison of CT enterography, MR enterography, and small-bowel follow-through as diagnostic techniques. Radiology 2009;251: 751–61.

53. Siddiki HA, Fidler JL, Fletcher JG, et al. Prospective comparison of state-of-the-art MR enterography and CT enterography in small-bowel Crohn's disease. AJR Am J Roentgenol 2009;193:113–21.

54. Shih IL, Wei SC, Yen RF, et al. PET/MRI for evaluating subclinical inflammation of ulcerative colitis. J Magn Reson Imaging 2017;47:737–45.

55. Ahmadi A, Li Q, Muller K, et al. Diagnostic value of noninvasive combined fluorine-18 labeled fluoro-2-deoxy-D-glucose positron emission tomography and computed tomography enterography in active Crohn's disease. Inflamm Bowel Dis 2010; 16:974–81.

56. Louis E, Ancion G, Colard A, et al. Noninvasive assessment of Crohn's disease intestinal lesions with 18F-FDG PET/CT. J Nucl Med 2007;48:1053–9.

57. Shyn PB, Mortele KJ, Britz-Cunningham SH, et al. Low-dose 18F-FDG PET/CT enterography: improving on CT enterography assessment of patients with Crohn disease. J Nucl Med 2010;51: 1841–8.

58. Rimola J, Rodríguez S, García-Bosch O, et al. Magnetic resonance for assessment of disease activity and severity in ileocolonic Crohn's disease. Gut 2009;58:1113–20.

59. Roy P, Lee JK, Sheikh A, et al. Quantitative comparison of misregistration in abdominal and pelvic organs between PET/MRI and PET/CT: effect of mode of acquisition and type of sequence on different organs. AJR Am J Roentgenol 2015;205: 1295–305.

60. Neurath M, Vehling D, Schunk K, et al. Noninvasive assessment of Crohn's disease activity: a comparison of 18F-fluorodeoxyglucose positron emission tomography, hydromagnetic resonance imaging, and granulocyte scintigraphy with labeled antibodies. Am J Gastroenterol 2002;97:1978.

61. Kim K-J, Lee Y, Park SH, et al. Diffusion-weighted MR enterography for evaluating Crohn's disease: how does it add diagnostically to conventional MR enterography? Inflamm Bowel Dis 2015;21: 101–9.

62. Seo N, Park SH, Kim K-J, et al. MR enterography for the evaluation of small-bowel inflammation in Crohn disease by using diffusion-weighted imaging without intravenous contrast material: a prospective noninferiority study. Radiology 2015;278: 762–72.

63. Neubauer H, Pabst T, Dick A, et al. Small-bowel MRI in children and young adults with Crohn disease: retrospective head-to-head comparison of contrast-enhanced and diffusion-weighted MRI. Pediatr Radiol 2013;43:103–14.

64. Ziech ML, Hummel TZ, Smets AM, et al. Accuracy of abdominal ultrasound and MRI for detection of Crohn disease and ulcerative colitis in children. Pediatr Radiol 2014;44:1370–8.

65. D'Alessandria C, Malviya G, Viscido A, et al. Use of a 99mTc labeled anti-TNFalpha monoclonal antibody in Crohn's disease: in vitro and in vivo studies. Q J Nucl Med Mol Imaging 2007;51:334–42.

66. Nie X, Laforest R, Elvington A, et al. PET/MRI of hypoxic atherosclerosis using 64Cu-ATSM in a rabbit model. J Nucl Med 2016;57:2006–11.

67. Pedersen SF, Sandholt BV, Keller SH, et al. 64Cu-DOTATATE PET/MRI for detection of activated macrophages in carotid atherosclerotic plaques: studies in patients undergoing endarterectomy. Arterioscler Thromb Vasc Biol 2015;35:1696–703.

68. Bucerius J, Barthel H, Tiepolt S, et al. Feasibility of in vivo 18F-florbetaben PET/MR imaging of human carotid amyloid-beta. Eur J Nucl Med Mol Imaging 2017;44:1119–28.

69. Howlader N, Noone AM, Krapcho M, et al, editors. SEER Cancer Statistics review. Bethesda (MD): National Cancer Institute; 2014.

70. U.S. Cancer Statistics Working Group. United States Cancer Statistics Incidence and Mortality Web-based Report Atlanta GA Department of Health and Human Services Centers for Disease Control and Prevention and National Cancer Institute 2015. p. 1999–2012. Available at: https://nccd.cdc.gov/USCS/.

71. Research UK. Cancer. Available at: http://www.cancerresearchuk.org/health-professional/cancer-statistics/statistics-by-cancer-type/bowel-cancer/incidence - heading-Seven, Accessed February, 2016.

72. Abdalla EK, Vauthey JN, Ellis LM, et al. Recurrence and outcomes following hepatic resection, radiofrequency ablation, and combined resection/ablation for colorectal liver metastases. Ann Surg 2004;239:818–25.

73. Kanas G, Taylor A, Primrose J, et al. Survival after liver resection in metastatic colorectal cancer: review and meta-analysis of prognostic factors. Clin Epidemiol 2012;4:283–301.

74. Haug U, Engel S, Verheyen F, et al. Estimating colorectal cancer treatment costs: approach

exemplified by health insurance data from Germany. PLoS One 2014;9:e88407.

75. Nagtegaal ID, Quirke P. What is the role for the circumferential margin in the modern treatment of rectal cancer? J Clin Oncol 2008;26:303–12.

76. Bipat S, Glas A, Slors F, et al. Rectal cancer: local staging and assessment of lymph node involvement with endoluminal US, CT, and MR imaging–a meta-analysis. Radiology 2004;232:773–83.

77. Fletcher J, Djulbegovic B, Soares H, et al. Recommendations on the use of 18F-FDG PET in oncology. J Nucl Med 2008;49:480–508.

78. Brush J, Boyd K, Chappell F, et al. The value of FDG positron emission tomography/computerised tomography (PET/CT) in pre-operative staging of colorectal cancer: a systematic review and economic evaluation. Health Technol Assess 2011;15: 1–192.

79. Kwok H, Bisset IP, Hill GL. Preoperative staging of rectal cancer. Int J Colorectal Dis 2000;15:9–20.

80. Expert Panel on Gastrointestinal Imaging, Fowler KJ, Kaur H, et al. ACR appropriateness criteria® pretreatment staging of colorectal cancer. J Am Coll Radiol 2017;14(5S):S234–44.

81. Kinkel K, Lu Y, Both M, et al. Detection of hepatic metastases from cancers of the gastrointestinal tract by using noninvasive imaging methods (US, CT, MR imaging, PET): a meta-analysis. Radiology 2002;224:748–56.

82. Niekel M, Bipat S, Stoker J. Diagnostic imaging of colorectal liver metastases with CT, MR imaging, FDG PET, and/or FDG PET/CT: a meta-analysis of prospective studies including patients who have not previously undergone treatment. Radiology 2010;257:674–84.

83. Veil-Haibach P, Kuehle CA, Beyer T, et al. Diagnostic accuracy of colorectal cancer staging with whole-body PET/CT colonography. JAMA 2006;296:2590–600.

84. Cohade C, Osman M, Leal J, et al. Direct comparison of (18)F-FDG PET and PET/CT in patients with colorectal carcinoma. J Nucl Med 2003;44:1797–803.

85. Rappeport E, Loft A, Berthelsen A, et al. Contrast-enhanced FDG-PET/CT vs. SPIO-enhanced MRI vs. FDG-PET vs. CT in patients with liver metastases from colorectal cancer: a prospective study with intraoperative confirmation. Acta Radiol 2007;48: 369–78.

86. Low R, McCue M, Barone R, et al. MR staging of primary colorectal carcinoma: comparison with surgical and histopathologic findings. Abdom Imaging 2003;28:784–93.

87. Even-Sapir E, Parag Y, Lerman H, et al. Detection of recurrence in patients with rectal cancer: PET/CT after abdominoperineal or anterior resection. Radiology 2004;232:815–22.

88. Hany TF, Steinert HC, Goerres GW, et al. Accuracy: improvement with initial results. Radiology 2002; 225:575–81.

89. Nie Y, Li Q, Li F, et al. CT information to improve diagnostic accuracy for lung nodules: a semiautomatic computer-aided method. J Nucl Med 2006; 47:1075–80.

90. Al-Nabhani K, Syed R, Michopoulou S, et al. Qualitative and quantitative comparison of PET/CT and PET/MR imaging in clinical practice. J Nucl Med 2013;55:88–94.

91. Kang B, Lee J, Song Y, et al. Added value of integrated whole-body PET/MRI for evaluation of colorectal cancer: comparison with contrast-enhanced MDCT. AJR Am J Roentgenol 2016;206:W10–20.

92. Brendle C, Schwenzer NF, Rempp H, et al. Assessment of metastatic colorectal cancer with hybrid imaging: comparison of reading performance using different combinations of anatomical and functional imaging techniques in PET/MRI and PET/CT in a short case series. Eur J Nucl Med Mol Imaging 2016;43:123–32.

93. Paspulati RM, Partovi S, Herrmann KA, et al. Comparison of hybrid FDG PET/MRI compared with PET/CT in colorectal cancer staging and restaging: a pilot study. Abdom Imaging 2015;40(6):1415–25.

94. Catalano OA, Coutinho AM, Sahani DV, et al. Colorectal cancer staging: comparison of whole-body PET/CT and PET/MR. Abdom Radiol (NY) 2017; 42:1141–51.

95. Antoch G, Vogt FM, Freudenberg LS, et al. Whole-body dual-modality PET/CT and whole-body MRI for tumor staging in oncology. JAMA 2003;290: 3199–206.

96. von Schulthess GK, Schlemmer HP. A look ahead: PET/MR versus PET/CT. Eur J Nucl Med Mol Imaging 2009;36:S3–9.

97. Lee S, Seo H, Kang K, et al. Clinical performance of whole-body 18F-FDG PET/Dixon-VIBE, T1-weighted, and T2-weighted in colorectal cancer. Clin Nucl Med 2015;40:e392.

98. Boss A, Bisdas S, Kolb A, et al. MRI of intracranial masses: initial experiences and comparison to PET/CT. J Nucl Med 2010;51:1198–205.

99. Delso G, Jakoby B, Ladebeck R, et al. Performance measurements of the Siemens mMR integrated whole-body PET/MR scanner. J Nucl Med 2011;52:1914–22.

100. Chandarana H, Heacock L, Rakheja R, et al. Pulmonary nodules in patients with primary malignancy: comparison of hybrid PET/MR and PET/CT imaging. Radiology 2013;268:874–81.

Imaging of the Postoperative Colon

Eugene Huo, MD[a],*, Laura Eisenmenger, MD[b], Stefanie Weinstein, MD[a]

KEYWORDS

- Colorectal surgery • Colectomy • Postoperative complications • Colon cancer • Rectal cancer
- Colon

KEY POINTS

- The appearance of the abdomen and pelvis after colon resection can vary significantly depending on the choice of surgery.
- Imaging abnormalities can be normal, and even expected, in a postoperative patient.
- Clinical data such as laboratory abnormalities and multiple prior examinations are often required to differentiate recurrent/residual malignancy from postoperative changes.

INTRODUCTION

Colorectal surgery is commonly performed for a wide range of pathologies. The choice of surgical procedure and technical approach is often determined by the extent of disease and surgeon experience and preference.[1,2] The use of fluoroscopic evaluation of the colon has declined significantly in recent years, with newer technologies such as computed tomography (CT) colonography gaining traction with radiologists and referring physicians. Most recently, the US Preventative Services Task Force (USPSTF) recommendations no longer include double-contrast barium enema (DCBE) as a method of screening, while American College of Radiology (ACR) appropriateness criteria rating for DCBE are a 6 out of 9 (may be appropriate) compared with a 9 (usually appropriate) for CT colonography.[3] CT has become a primary imaging modality, often performed in the setting of clinical symptoms that may reflect perforation, intra-abdominal abscess, or other postoperative complications.[4–11] However, CT has been shown to have a low sensitivity for the evaluation of anastomotic leaks in postoperative patients, while fluoroscopy

has continued to demonstrate superior accuracy.[12–14] Despite the overall changes in referral and utilization, fluoroscopic evaluation is still used in the postoperative setting, specifically for the evaluation of postoperative anatomy and integrity of the anastomosis.[15,16]

This article will not be a comprehensive discussion regarding the details of colorectal surgical procedures, but will highlight some of the important imaging features and pitfalls in evaluating patients after they have undergone colorectal surgical procedures. The procedures that will be discussed include segmental colectomy, abdominoperineal resection (APR), anterior resection, Hartmann procedure, and ileal pouch-anal anastomosis (IPAA).

SEGMENTAL COLECTOMY

Segmental colon resections include ileocecal, right, transverse, and left colectomies, and are based on the location of the diseased segments typically from either inflammatory bowel disease, or colonic malignancies, unresectable polyps, inflammatory diverticular disease without complications, volvulus, or bleeding.[1,11,17] When there is a

Disclosure Statement: No disclosures.
[a] Department of Radiology, San Francisco VA Medical Center, 4150 Clement Street (114), San Francisco, CA 94121, USA; [b] Department of Radiology and Biomedical Imaging, University of California, San Francisco, 513 Parnassus Avenue, Room S-261, Box 0628, San Francisco, CA 94143, USA
* Corresponding author.
E-mail address: Eugene.huo@ucsf.edu

Radiol Clin N Am 56 (2018) 835–845
https://doi.org/10.1016/j.rcl.2018.04.006

malignant neoplasm, wider margins are typically performed as well as mesenteric, omental, and lymphatic drainage nodal resections.

Common complications include anastomotic leak (2%–3%), wound complications, postoperative hemorrhage, ileus, and recurrence of neoplasm, and less commonly ureteral injury. Trocar site complications such as hernias can also be seen. A stomal or parastomal hernia with herniation of bowel or fat at the site of the stoma can be seen after stoma creation (**Fig. 1**). Bowel herniation without accompanying fat stranding, fluid accumulation, or thickening of bowel wall to suggest strangulation is typically not concerning.[18] On imaging, expected postresection findings include absence of excised bowel segments, anastomotic clips or sutures, and typically displacement of viscera into now unoccupied postoperative spaces.[2]

In the early postoperative period, clinical suspicion for leak may warrant radiographic evaluation, for which water-soluble contrast enema has demonstrated greater sensitivity than CT imaging.[12,19] Past studies have demonstrated a reduction in adverse events with routine leak testing[20] and a link between anastomotic leakage and poor long-term outcomes.[21–23] Subsequently, fluoroscopic studies may be indicated for strictures, obstruction and functional status, or to assess anatomy. Fluoroscopic studies may be limited by overlapping loops of contrast-opacified bowel, whereas CT allows better assessment of extraluminal fluid collections and planning for drainage procedures. In some cases, CT or magnetic resonance (MR) enterography may be preferred, particularly with inflammatory bowel disease (IBD) patients to evaluate the extent of small and large bowel involvement and associated complications.[24,25]

ABDOMINOPERINEAL RESECTION

An APR involves complete rectosigmoid, anal, and perineal resection with creation of a permanent end colostomy, typically in the left lower abdomen. An APR is typically performed for low-lying rectal or anal malignancies or anorectal complications of IBD.[26,27] Postoperative imaging involves recognition of drains and/or packing material used to close the perineal defect, which can be confusing if not appropriately diagnosed. In patients undergoing preoperative radiation treatment, radical pelvic surgery, or who have large cutaneous defects, myocutaneous flaps or mesh can be used to augment the reconstruction (**Fig. 2**).[28,29] This may involve rectus, gracilis, or gluteal muscle flaps, which are felt to reduce the incidence of healing complications including abscess or perineal herniation. Denervation can cause these flaps to demonstrate on MR scan initial increased T2 signal followed by fatty infiltration and subsequent increased T1 signal. Denervation atrophy can also result in thinning of the muscle flap on subsequent examinations.[30,31]

APRs are less well-tolerated and have more complications compared with other sphincter-sparing procedures.[27,32] On CT, the uterus, seminal vesicles, and prostate are typically posteriorly displaced into the presacral space (**Figs. 3 and 4**).[9] There is often a presacral soft tissue mass, which can resemble recurrent tumor, but should be stable to decreased in size over time.[33–35] The presacral changes can range from minimal to more substantial, but residual scarring can persist indefinitely. A persistently normal carcinoembryonic antigen (CEA) level is

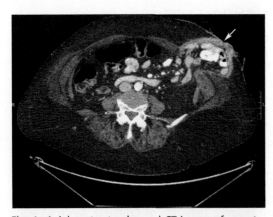

Fig. 1. Axial contrast-enhanced CT image of parastomal hernia (*arrow*) with opacified bowel and mesenteric vessels. No inflammatory changes or fluid are seen surrounding the involved bowel and the patient was asymptomatic.

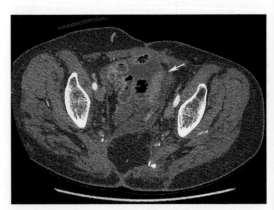

Fig. 2. APR with myocutaneous flap. Rectus muscle flap and associated feeding artery seen along the left hemipelvis (*arrow*).

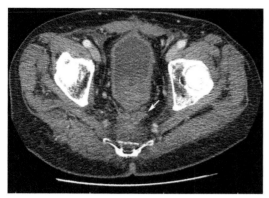

Fig. 3. Axial CT status post APR demonstrating expected elongation of the bladder in the AP direction, along with posterior displacement of the seminal vesicles (*arrow*).

an additional reassuring sign of the lack of recurrent tumor.[9] Fibroids or abscesses that fill the presacral space can be pitfalls. Postoperative fluid collections and new air may suggest infection (**Fig. 5**). Tumor recurrence (**Fig. 6**) after APR can be difficult to assess and distinguish from expected postoperative presacral soft tissue changes (**Fig. 7**). The key to recognizing tumor recurrence is that the tissue may be thickened or bulging and tumor like. New hydronephrosis also should be viewed with caution as a sign of either recurrence or ureteral injury and has a poor prognosis.[36] Positron emission tomography (PET)/CT can play a role in distinguishing recurrent disease from fibrosis but is not yet recommended for widespread routine surveillance (**Figs. 8** and **9**).[37–39] A baseline examination 2 to 4 months after surgery can be helpful for assessment of stability of soft tissue, but this is not routinely obtained. A common pitfall is the mistaken identification of asymmetric displaced seminal vesicles as lymphadenopathy.[40]

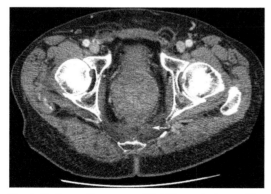

Fig. 4. Postoperative presacral fluid (*arrow*), along with a more posterior location of the prostate within the pelvis.

ANTERIOR RESECTION

Anterior resection, also known as an abdominal proctosigmoidectomy, involves resection of the rectosigmoid and repeat anastomosis of the descending colon and proximal rectum.[41] As a sphincter-sparing procedure without a perineal dissection, the bowel remains in continuity, and patients have a better functional outcome. The indication is typically for rectal cancer not involving the anal sphincter complex.

Preoperative MRI is used in local staging and surgical planning, and has become the modality of choice for evaluation and staging of rectal cancer.[42] The location of the anastomosis of the descending colon and proximal can vary, with high AR involving tumors above the peritoneal reflection and low AR tumors below the reflection. Because there is considerably less periprocedural morbidity with a preserved sphincter, fewer APRs are being performed. More patients may become candidates for an AR over an APR because of adequate margins obtained with appropriate adjuvant therapy and reduced local recurrence. Small-scale studies have demonstrated similar oncologic outcomes but with improved quality of life with neoadjuvant therapy/sphincter preservation compared with APR.[43]

Again, imaging modalities employed in the postoperative period consist of water-soluble contrast enemas or CT to identify leaks (**Fig. 10**). A Foley is used rather than the hard-tipped enema catheter, and is advanced across the anastomosis before instillation of contrast to avoid trauma to the low anastomosis.[44] If an enema is performed, postevacuation lateral or oblique views can help differentiate postoperative anatomy such as blind ending limbs versus small leaks (**Fig. 11**). CT can also detect leaks but has the additional benefit of better detecting postoperative abscess and fluid collections. Although fluoroscopic imaging of the bowel with rectal administration of water based contrast can be used to identify exact location of a leak, CT is also sensitive, particularly if rectal contrast reaches the level of the leak.[4] Perianastomatic loculated fluid containing air is a most suggestive sign of the presence of a leak.[45] CT can then be used to guide drainage. Reasons for missing an anastomatic leak include insufficient extraluminal air and fluid that may take time to accumulate in the immediate postoperative period, and a rectal contrast catheter that may inadvertently occlude the leak during the study with balloon or rectal collapse.

To a lesser extent, compared with an APR, there may still be soft tissue and/or stranding adjacent to and posterior to the anastomosis and a widened presacral space with increased fat (**Fig. 12**).

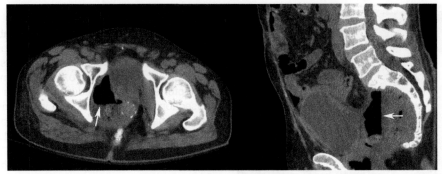

Fig. 5. Axial and coronal images of a patient with a history of LAR. Air-fluid levels (*arrows*) in a presacral fluid collection secondary to anastomotic leak. Cortical irregularity and erosions of the anterior sacrum was also noted, secondary to osteomyelitis.

Normal postoperative presacral fluid should also decrease over time. Extraperitoneal air or fluid around iliac vessels will resolve unless there is also increased bowel distention that might lead to increased air, and typically does not persist beyond 6 months.[4] Increased soft tissue or air may be more concerning for infection or recurrence. The double rectum sign was described to suggest anastomotic dehiscence with extravasation of contrast and air posterior to and mimicking the true rectum.[4] Be aware that a substantial portion of leaks may be occult and chronic and therefore may be clinically insignificant. Therefore, it is not always necessary to treat all leaks. Subclinical leaks are predicted to occur in about 5% to 10% of cases[46] and may have a higher incidence of spontaneous healing compared with clinical leaks.[47] Increasing air can occur if there is increasing bowel lumen distention or pressure occurring in the setting of ileus or obstruction. Because the inferior mesenteric artery (IMA) supply is harvested during the procedure, these patients rely on superior mesenteric artery (SMA)-IMA communications such as the marginal artery of Drummond. In the event of an underdeveloped or occluded collateral pathway, one can see non-enhancing bowel segments consistent with ischemic bowel in the correlating territory (**Fig. 13**).

HARTMANN PROCEDURE

This procedure includes a distal colectomy or sigmoidectomy with a diverting colostomy. A blind ending rectal remnant, or pouch, is left in situ. The pouch may be sutured or stapled in anticipation of an elective anastomosis at a later time. The Hartmann procedure is typically seen in patients at high risk of complications from a primary anastomosis, but who require emergent partial colectomy. Typical clinical situations include management of obstructing, perforated, or bleeding neoplasm, complicated diverticulitis with distal colonic leak, or other causes of colitis requiring emergent resection.

Imaging modalities for these patients include water-soluble contrast media enema to assess the stump or pouch to look for leak and pouch integrity.

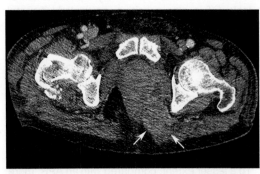

Fig. 6. Axial CT image of a patient with a history of remote APR. A soft tissue mass in the left pelvis abuts and invades the left obturator internus laterally and the gluteus maximus posteriorly (*arrows*).

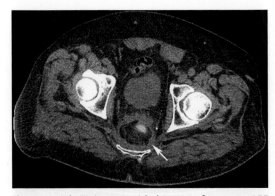

Fig. 7. Axial CT image with history of remote APR demonstrating normal presacral soft tissue changes (*arrow*).

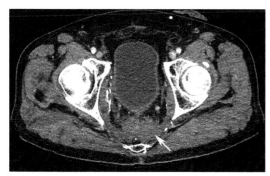

Fig. 8. 5 years after APR with rounded pre-sacral soft tissue density (*arrow*). Concerning findings would include interval growth and a rising or elevated CEA level.

Although the clinical impact of fluoroscopic evaluation in asymptomatic patients is unclear, a benefit was seen in symptomatic patients, patients with a history of prior leaks or complications such as IBD, or in cases where a different surgeon will be performing the takedown.[48] In addition, when a secondary takedown is being considered, fluoroscopic evaluation may be performed to look at the stump and upstream from the end colostomy proximally, to exclude strictures, and better detail pouch anatomy. The pouch can vary in length, from rectum only, up to the transverse colon, and can have mucus, polyps, or diverticula within it (Fig. 14). If left in the peritoneal cavity, it is considered a stump or pouch. Alternatively, it can be brought up to the abdominal wall as a mucus fistula. Other complications include wound infection, fistula, and parastomal hernia. The pouch can become distended with a large fecolith (Fig. 15), with larger pouches developing more secretions and concretions. Diversion colitis, which is a nonspecific colitis in a defunctionalized portion of the colon, can also occur, and these patients can have a variable presentation including being completely asymptomatic.[49,50] The colitis occurs because of bacterial overgrowth or deficiency.

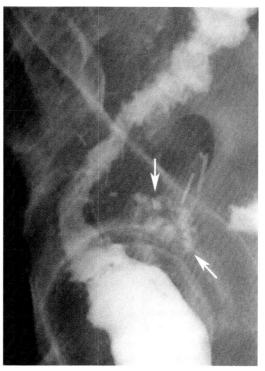

Fig. 10. Lateral image from water-soluble contrast enema with a heterogeneous collection of extraluminal contrast (*arrows*) extending anteriorly at the level of the anastamosis.

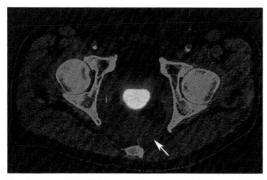

Fig. 9. Fused PET/CT image demonstrating lack of FDG uptake in the presacral mass (*arrow*), supporting a benign postoperative etiology.

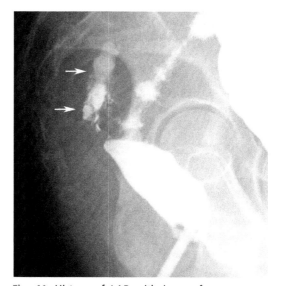

Fig. 11. History of LAR with image from a water-soluble contrast enema demonstrating a fluid and air collection (*arrows*) posterior to the anastamosis. Without postvoid images, differentiation between a leak versus a blind-ending limb from a side-to-end reconstruction is difficult.

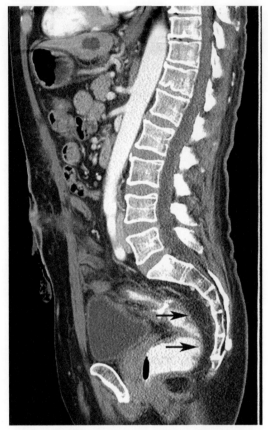

Fig. 12. Sagittal CT image of a patient with history of remote LAR demonstrating increased presacral space (*arrows*) from normal postoperative changes.

It typically resolves with closure of the colostomy and reconstitution of the fecal stream.[51]

ILEAL POUCH-ANAL ANASTOMOSIS

A restorative proctocolectomy involves a total proctocolectomy and creation of an ileal pouch

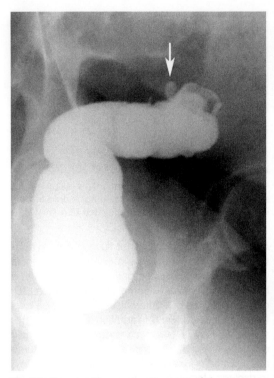

Fig. 14. Preoperative contrast enema of the Hartman pouch demonstrating diverticuli (*arrow*) along the proximal margin.

and ileo-anal anastomosis. The pouch configuration can be a J, S, or W shape (Fig. 16). This procedure is primarily performed for ulcerative colitis, family adenomatous polyps, or other colon cancers, but is contraindicated in Crohn patients with small bowel involvement. This can be performed in a single-stage procedure or initial proximal temporary loop ileostomy followed by a takedown. The disadvantage of a single-stage procedure is an increased risk of sepsis from a leak.[26]

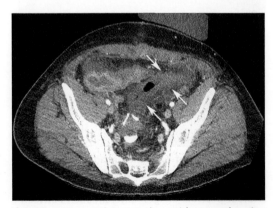

Fig. 13. Low anterior resection with nonenhancing segment of bowel (*arrows*) compatible with ischemia.

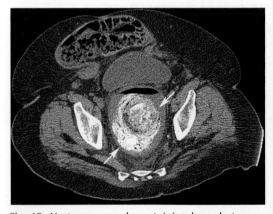

Fig. 15. Hartmann pouch containing large heterogeneously dense mass (*arrows*) corresponding to pouch fecalith.

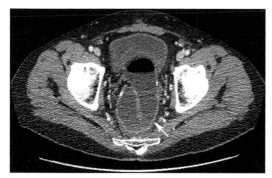

Fig. 16. Axial CT image at the level of the ileal pouch-anal anastomosis (IPAA) with a J pouch (*arrow*) configuration.

Typically, fluoroscopic pouchography has been performed after the initial stage ileal pouch-anal anastomosis (IPAA) creation and before closure of the ileostomy. Rectal administration of the water-soluble contrast allows evaluation of the integrity of the ileal pouch. Postevacuation films are needed to detect subtle leaks or strictures.[52] Images may show diffuse wall thickening and irregularity of the ileal pouch on fluoroscopy or CT and surrounding inflammatory changes of pouchitis (**Fig. 17**). Contrast-enhanced CT is favored for patients with clinical suspicion for infection or other complications.

On CT, the pouch can be seen opacified with contrast. The unique identifying linear side-to-side anastomosis with a vertical row of staples and terminal blind end staple line can be seen with a pouch-anal anastomosis.[53] Mild stranding in the peripouch fat and wall thickening of the pouch can be seen on CT in the normal postoperative period or may relate to chronic inflammation. A diagnosis of pouchitis should not be given until at least 6 to 8 weeks after surgery to allow resolution of the normal postoperative changes and edema. Typically, it is an endoscopic diagnosis.

Without treatment, chronic inflammation may lead to pouch failure. Other complications include leaks and fistula. The pouch-anal anastomosis is most commonly at risk, but also at risk is the ileo-ileo staple line or the pouch itself. Because there can be overlap between Crohn and UC, some patients who have frequent complications may actually have a form frust of Crohn disease (**Fig. 18**). These patients may require higher rates of pouch excision or a diversion. CT can also be used to define complex perianal or perineal fistulas involving the pouch. Later on, strictures can develop, secondary to anastomotic fibrosis or ischemia from stretching of the ileal mesentery during pouch creation. These can be seen as abrupt transitions near the pouch, and can be treated with dilatation.

COLORECTAL CANCER SURVEILLANCE AFTER SURGERY

High rates of recurrent or metachronous disease occur after resection. Despite a potentially curative surgical procedure, it is estimated that 29% to 40% of patients will experience recurrence of tumor.[54–56] Over 90% of recurrences occurred within 5 years of surgery, and the majority occurred within the first 3 years.[57] Different recommendations exist on the appropriate follow-up method and interval, utilizing history and physical examination, laboratory markers including CEA, and colonoscopy. CT and CEA follow-up can reduce mortality to 9% to 13%.[58] However, CEA testing by itself has been shown to be ineffective to detect recurrence.[59] Most guidelines agree on the need for optical colonoscopy at 1 year following resection, but there are differing intervals for subsequent endoscopic evaluation.

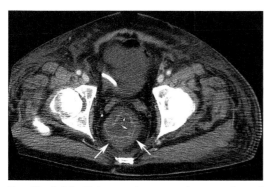

Fig. 17. Axial CT image demonstrating pouch wall thickening and surrounding inflammatory changes (*arrows*) from pouchitis.

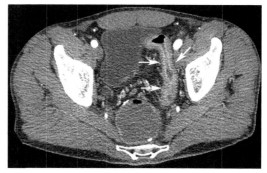

Fig. 18. History of IPAA for Crohn disease, with new abdominal pain. Axial CT image demonstrates unremarkable appearance of pouch; however bowel thickening and mucosal hyperenhancement of the small bowel more proximally (*arrows*) are consistent with recurrent IBD.

Based on American Society of Clinical Oncology (ASCO) endorsement in 2013 of the Cancer Care Ontario (CCO) guidelines,[60] ASCO recommends an annual CT of the chest and abdomen for 3 years after therapy in patients who are at higher risk for recurrence and who would be candidates for further therapy. This was not rigidly defined, and was based on evidence of survival benefit from detection of liver metastases. A pelvic CT was recommended for rectal cancer surveillance, especially in patients who were not treated with radiotherapy. Patients considered at high risk for recurrent rectal cancer should also be considered for sigmoidoscopy at more frequent intervals.

National Comprehensive Cancer Network (NCCN) and American Society of Colon and Rectal Surgeons (ASCRS) guidelines on surveillance after colon cancer resection include a yearly CT scan for 5 years.[61,62]

A meta-analysis of follow-up by more intensive and more frequent monitoring of patients who had undergone potentially curative resection of CRC showed earlier detection of recurrence by a median of 10 months, but demonstrated no clear survival benefit for colon cancers.[63] Subsequent studies[64] including a Cochrane meta-analysis[65] have demonstrated no definite benefit for intensive monitoring after resection of colon cancer. However, patients with rectal cancer have shown an improvement in survival from more intensive monitoring.[66,67]

Recommendations of the USMSTF on colorectal cancer include that patients receive a first surveillance optical colonoscopy 1 year after surgery, then at 3 years, and then at 5 years. The use of CT colonography in postoperative surveillance has been proposed to simultaneously detect metachronous lesions, local recurrence, and distant metastases.[68] Experience is needed in differentiating normal postoperative findings from true recurrent disease, in addition to standardization of protocols and reporting terminology. In 1 meta-analysis, CTC has compared favorably to optical colonoscopy, identifying 95% of patients with recurrence at the anastomosis, compared with 88% for optical colonoscopy.[69] The optimal timing for a CTC and how to incorporate it in conjunction with other tests have not been determined. Detection of recurrence may be limited for detecting flat or small lesions and nonadenomatous lesions.[68,70,71]

Current surveillance guidelines do not have a role for PET/CT; however, this is an evolving area of research. Studies have shown PET can detect additional sites of disease in 48% of patients suspected to have recurrence and led to a change in management in 66% of these patients.[72] PET/CT is being investigated for the ability to identify occult disease and distant sites of disease,[73] in addition to problem-solving in patients with indeterminate results on conventional imaging.[74] In a study of 62 patients who had undergone APR or AR, PET/CT was able to distinguish between benign and malignant presacral abnormalities with 100% sensitivity and 96% specificity. PET/CT has demonstrated an ability to increase progression-free survival in patients with proven recurrence[75] and has been used to predict response of hepatic metastasis to treatment and overall survival. Despite these successes, the role of PET/CT in routine follow-up has yet to be determined.[76–78]

MRI is another modality that has an unclear role in follow-up of postsurgical patients. Although indispensable for the staging of rectal cancer[42] and evaluation of potential hepatic metastatic disease,[79,80] the ability of MRI to identify recurrence is not as certain in the postoperative state, especially when neoadjuvant chemoradiation is utilized.[81] Postoperative or radiation-induced fibrosis can often cause incorrect estimation of disease,[82] while postoperative edema can often obscure residual viable disease.

SUMMARY

Although the standard of care methods of evaluating the postoperative colon has evolved, many of the concepts have remained the same. An understanding of the surgical changes involved and the physiologic consequences of each part of the procedure is essential to identifying normal postoperative changes on follow-up imaging. Differentiating between expected postoperative changes versus abnormalities indicating complications or early signs of recurrence allows the radiologist to provide valuable information to the clinical team and allows for appropriate treatment and patient management.

REFERENCES

1. Scardapane A, Brindicci D, Fracella MR, et al. Post colon surgery complications: imaging findings. Eur J Radiol 2005;53(3):397–409.
2. Zissin R, Gayer G. Postoperative anatomic and pathologic findings at CT following colonic resection. Semin Ultrasound CT MR 2004;25(3):222–38.
3. Yee J, Kim DH, Rosen MP, et al. ACR appropriateness criteria colorectal cancer screening. J Am Coll Radiol 2014;11(6):543–51.
4. DuBrow RA, David CL, Curley SA. Anastomotic leaks after low anterior resection for rectal

carcinoma: evaluation with CT and barium enema. AJR Am J Roentgenol 1995;165(3):567–71.

5. Ghahremani GG, Gore RM. CT diagnosis of postoperative abdominal complications. Radiol Clin North Am 1989;27(4):787–804.

6. Gore RM, Berlin JW, Yaghmai V, et al. CT diagnosis of postoperative abdominal complications. Semin Ultrasound CT MRI 2004;25(3):207–21.

7. Guillem JG, Cohen AM. Current issues in colorectal cancer surgery. Semin Oncol 1999;26(5):505–13.

8. Horton KM, Abrams RA, Fishman EK. Spiral CT of colon cancer: imaging features and role in management. Radiographics 2000;20(2):419–30.

9. Kelvin FM, Korobkin M, Heaston DK, et al. The pelvis after surgery for rectal carcinoma: serial CT observations with emphasis on nonneoplastic features. Am J Roentgenology 1983;141(5):959–64.

10. Reznek RH, White FE, Young JWR, et al. The appearances on computed tomography after abdomino-perineal resection for carcinoma of the rectum: a comparison between the normal appearances and those of recurrence. Br J Radiol 1983; 56(664):237–40.

11. Schwartz SI, Brunicardi FC. Schwartz's principles of surgery. New York: McGraw-Hill, Medical Pub. Division; 2010.

12. Nicksa GA, Dring RV, Johnson KH, et al. Anastomotic leaks: what is the best diagnostic imaging study? Dis Colon Rectum 2007;50(2):197–203.

13. Seo SI, Lee JL, Park SH, et al. Assessment by using a water-soluble contrast enema study of radiologic leakage in lower rectal cancer patients with sphincter-saving surgery. Ann Coloproctol 2015; 31(4):131–7.

14. Kornmann VN, van Ramshorst B, Smits AB, et al. Beware of false-negative CT scan for anastomotic leakage after colonic surgery. Int J Colorectal Dis 2014;29(4):445–51.

15. Levine MS, Rubesin SE, Laufer I. Barium studies in modern radiology: do they have a role? Radiology 2009;250(1):18–22.

16. Moreno CC, Hemingway J, Johnson AC, et al. Changing abdominal imaging utilization patterns: perspectives from medicare beneficiaries over two decades. J Am Coll Radiol 2016;13(8):894–903.

17. Ashley S, Cance W, Chen H. ACS surgery. Ontario: Decker Intellectual Properties; 2014.

18. Ghahremani GG, Jimenez MA, Rosenfeld M, et al. CT diagnosis of occult incisional hernias. Am J Roentgenology 1987;148(1):139–42.

19. Shorthouse AJ, Bartram CI, Eyers AA, et al. The water soluble contrast enema after rectal anastomosis. Br J Surg 1982;69(12):714–7.

20. Kwon S, Morris A, Billingham R, et al. Routine leak testing in colorectal surgery in the surgical care and outcomes assessment program. Arch Surg 2012;147(4):345–51.

21. Law WL, Choi HK, Lee YM, et al. Anastomotic leakage is associated with poor long-term outcome in patients after curative colorectal resection for malignancy. J Gastrointest Surg 2007;11(1):8–15.

22. Mirnezami A, Mirnezami R, Chandrakumaran K, et al. Increased local recurrence and reduced survival from colorectal cancer following anastomotic leak: systematic review and meta-analysis. Ann Surg 2011;253(5):890–9.

23. Marra F, Steffen T, Kalak N, et al. Anastomotic leakage as a risk factor for the long-term outcome after curative resection of colon cancer. Eur J Surg Oncol 2009;35(10):1060–4.

24. Quon JS, Quon PR, Lim CS, et al. Magnetic resonance enterography in post-operative inflammatory bowel disease. Abdom Imaging 2015;40(5):1034–49.

25. Eliakim R, Magro F. Imaging techniques in IBD and their role in follow-up and surveillance. Nat Rev Gastroenterol Hepatol 2014;11(12):722–36.

26. Monson JR, Weiser MR. Sabiston textbook of surgery, 18th ed. The biological basis of modern surgical practice. Dis Colon Rectum 2008;51(7):1154.

27. Murrell ZA, Dixon MR, Vargas H, et al. Contemporary indications for and early outcomes of abdominoperineal resection. Am Surg 2005;71(10):837–40.

28. Touran T, Frost DB, O'Connell TX. Sacral resection. Operative technique and outcome. Arch Surg 1990;125(7):911–3.

29. Wydra D, Emerich J, Sawicki S, et al. Major complications following exenteration in cases of pelvic malignancy: a 10-year experience. World J Gastroenterol 2006;12(7):1115–9.

30. Griffin N, Rabouhans J, Grant LA, et al. Pelvi-perineal flap reconstruction: normal imaging appearances and post-operative complications on cross-sectional imaging. Insights into imaging 2011;2(3): 215–23.

31. Sagebiel TL, Faria SC, Aparna B, et al. Pelvic reconstruction with omental and VRAM flaps: anatomy, surgical technique, normal postoperative findings, and complications. Radiographics 2011;31(7):2005–19.

32. Ogilvie J, Ricciardi R. Complications of perineal surgery. Clin Colon Rectal Surg 2009;22(01):51–9.

33. Husband JE, Hodson NJ, Parsons CA. The use of computed tomography in recurrent rectal tumors. Radiology 1980;134(3):677–82.

34. Lee JK, Stanley RJ, Sagel SS, et al. CT appearance of the pelvis after abdomino-perineal resection for rectal carcinoma. Radiology 1981;141(3):737–41.

35. Moss AA, Thoeni RF, Schnyder P, et al. Value of computed tomography in the detection and staging of recurrent rectal carcinomas. J Comput Assist Tomogr 1981;5(6):870–4.

36. Brown G, Drury AE, Cunningham D, et al. CT detection of hydronephrosis in resected colorectal cancer: a predictor of recurrent disease. Clin Radiol 2003; 58(2):137–42.

37. Even-Sapir E, Parag Y, Lerman H, et al. Detection of recurrence in patients with rectal cancer: PET/CT after abdominoperineal or anterior resection. Radiology 2004;232(3):815–22.

38. Goldberg S, Klas JV. Total mesorectal excision in the treatment of rectal cancer: a view from the USA. Semin Surg Oncol 1998;15(2):87–90.

39. Titu LV, Nicholson AA, Hartley JE, et al. Routine follow-up by magnetic resonance imaging does not improve detection of resectable local recurrences from colorectal cancer. Ann Surg 2006;243(3):348–52.

40. Ibarrola de Andrés C, Castellano Megías VM, Perez Barrios A, et al. Seminal vesicle epithelium as a potential pitfall in the cytodiagnosis of presacral masses. Acta Cytol 2000;44(3):399–402.

41. Weinstein S, Osei-Bonsu S, Aslam R, et al. Multidetector CT of the postoperative colon: review of normal appearances and common complications. Radiographics 2013;33(2):515–32.

42. Jhaveri KS, Hosseini-Nik H. MRI of rectal cancer: an overview and update on recent advances. Am J Roentgenology 2015;205(1):W42–55.

43. Gawad W, Fakhr I, Lotayef M, et al. Sphincter saving and abdomino-perineal resections following neoadjuvant chemoradiation in locally advanced low rectal cancer. J Egypt Natl Canc Inst 2015;27(1):19–24.

44. Akyol AM, McGregor JR, Galloway DJ, et al. Early postoperative contrast radiology in the assessment of colorectal anastomotic integrity. Int J Colorectal Dis 1992;7(3):141–3.

45. Power N, Atri M, Ryan S, et al. CT assessment of anastomotic bowel leak. Clin Radiol 2007;62(1):37–42.

46. Bielecki K, Gajda A. The causes and prevention of anastomotic leak after colorectal surgery. Klin Onkol 1999;12(Suppl 1999):25–30.

47. Lim M, Akhtar S, Sasapu K, et al. Clinical and subclinical leaks after low colorectal anastomosis: a clinical and radiologic study. Dis Colon Rectum 2006;49(10):1611–9.

48. Ballian N, Zarebczan B, Munoz A, et al. Routine evaluation of the distal colon remnant before Hartmann's reversal is not necessary in asymptomatic patients. J Gastrointest Surg 2009;13(12):2260–7.

49. Glotzer DJ, Glick ME, Goldman H. Proctitis and colitis following diversion of the fecal stream. Gastroenterology 1981;80(3):438–41.

50. Ma CK, Gottlieb C, Haas PA. Diversion colitis: a clinicopathologic study of 21 cases. Hum Pathol 1990; 21(4):429–36.

51. Whelan RL, Abramson D, Kim DS, et al. Diversion colitis. Surg Endosc 1994;8(1):19–24.

52. Crema MD, Richarme D, Azizi L, et al. Pouchography, CT, and MRI features of ileal J pouch-anal anastomosis. AJR Am J Roentgenol 2006;187(6):W594–603.

53. Seggerman RE, Chen MY, Waters GS, et al. Radiology of ileal pouch–anal anastomosis surgery. Am J Roentgenology 2003;180(4):999–1002.

54. Tjandra JJ, Chan MK. Follow-up after curative resection of colorectal cancer: a meta-analysis. Dis colon rectum 2007;50(11):1783–99.

55. O'Connell MJ, Campbell ME, Goldberg RM, et al. Survival following recurrence in stage II and III colon cancer: findings from the ACCENT data set. J Clin Oncol 2008;26(14):2336–41.

56. Gan S, Wilson K, Hollington P. Surveillance of patients following surgery with curative intent for colorectal cancer. World J Gastroenterol 2007;13(28): 3816–23.

57. Sadahiro S, Suzuki T, Ishikawa K, et al. Recurrence patterns after curative resection of colorectal cancer in patients followed for a minimum of ten years. Hepatogastroenterology 2003;50(53):1362–6.

58. Bhatti I, Patel M, Dennison AR, et al. Utility of postoperative CEA for surveillance of recurrence after resection of primary colorectal cancer. Int J Surg 2015;16(Part A):123–8.

59. Nicholson BD, Shinkins B, Pathiraja I, et al. Blood CEA levels for detecting recurrent colorectal cancer. Cochrane Database Syst Rev 2015;(12): CD011134.

60. Meyerhardt JA, Mangu PB, Flynn PJ, et al. Follow-up care, surveillance protocol, and secondary prevention measures for survivors of colorectal cancer: American Society of Clinical Oncology clinical practice guideline endorsement. J Clin Oncol 2013; 31(35):4465–70.

61. National Comprehensive Cancer Network. Colon cancer (Version 2.2017). 2017. Available at: https://www.nccn.org/professionals/physician_gls/pdf/colon.pdf. Accessed October 30, 2017.

62. Steele SR, Chang GJ, Hendren S, et al. Practice guideline for the surveillance of patients after curative treatment of colon and rectal cancer. Dis colon rectum 2015;58(8):713–25.

63. Mokhles S, Macbeth F, Farewell V, et al. Meta-analysis of colorectal cancer follow-up after potentially curative resection. Br J Surg 2016;103(10):1259–68.

64. Mant D, Gray A, Pugh S, et al. A randomised controlled trial to assess the cost-effectiveness of intensive versus no scheduled follow-up in patients who have undergone resection for colorectal cancer with curative intent. Health Technol Assess 2017; 21(32):1–86.

65. Jeffery M, Hickey BE, Hider PN, et al. Follow-up strategies for patients treated for non-metastatic colorectal cancer. The Cochrane database Syst Rev 2016;(11):CD002200.

66. Pietra N, Sarli L, Costi R, et al. Role of follow-up in management of local recurrences of colorectal cancer: a prospective, randomized study. Dis colon rectum 1998;41(9):1127–33.

67. Rodriguez-Moranta F, Salo J, Arcusa A, et al. Postoperative surveillance in patients with colorectal cancer who have undergone curative resection: a

prospective, multicenter, randomized, controlled trial. J Clin Oncol 2006;24(3):386–93.

68. Kim HJ, Park SH, Pickhardt PJ, et al. CT colonography for combined colonic and extracolonic surveillance after curative resection of colorectal cancer. Radiology 2010;257(3):697–704.

69. Porte F, Uppara M, Malietzis G, et al. CT colonography for surveillance of patients with colorectal cancer: Systematic review and meta-analysis of diagnostic efficacy. Eur Radiol 2017;27(1):51–60.

70. Hong N, Park SH. CT colonography in the diagnosis and management of colorectal cancer: Emphasis on pre- and post-surgical evaluation. World J Gastroenterol 2014;20(8):2014–22.

71. Almond LM, Snelling S, Badiani S, et al. CT colonography after colorectal cancer resection: a one-stop assessment of metachronous mucosal lesions, local recurrence, and distant metastases. Radiology 2011;260(1):302–3.

72. Scott AM, Gunawardana DH, Kelley B, et al. PET changes management and improves prognostic stratification in patients with recurrent colorectal cancer: results of a multicenter prospective study. J Nucl Med 2008;49(9):1451–7.

73. Yoon HJ, Lee JJ, Kim YK, et al. FDG-PET/CT is superior to enhanced CT in detecting recurrent subcentimeter lesions in the abdominopelvic cavity in colorectal cancer. Nucl Med Mol Imaging 2011; 45(2):132–8.

74. Donswijk ML, Hess S, Mulders T, et al. [18F]Fluorodeoxyglucose PET/computed tomography in gastrointestinal malignancies. PET Clin 2014;9(4):421–41. v-vi.

75. Tural D, Selcukbiricik F, Sager S, et al. PET-CT changes the management and improves outcome in patients with recurrent colorectal cancer. J Cancer Res Ther 2014;10(1):121–6.

76. Lastoria S, Piccirillo MC, Caraco C, et al. Early PET/CT scan is more effective than RECIST in predicting outcome of patients with liver metastases from colorectal cancer treated with preoperative chemotherapy plus bevacizumab. J Nucl Med 2013; 54(12):2062–9.

77. Xia Q, Liu J, Wu C, et al. Prognostic significance of (18)FDG PET/CT in colorectal cancer patients with liver metastases: a meta-analysis. Cancer Imaging 2015;15:19.

78. Paspulati RM, Partovi S, Herrmann KA, et al. Comparison of hybrid FDG PET/MRI compared with PET/CT in colorectal cancer staging and restaging: a pilot study. Abdom Imaging 2015;40(6):1415–25.

79. Niekel MC, Bipat S, Stoker J. Diagnostic imaging of colorectal liver metastases with CT, MR imaging, FDG PET, and/or FDG PET/CT: a meta-analysis of prospective studies including patients who have not previously undergone treatment. Radiology 2010;257(3):674–84.

80. Bipat S, Leeuwen MSV, Comans EFI, et al. Colorectal liver metastases: CT, MR imaging, and PET for diagnosis—meta-analysis. Radiology 2005; 237(1):123–31.

81. Kim DJ, Kim JH, Lim JS, et al. Restaging of rectal cancer with MR imaging after concurrent chemotherapy and radiation therapy. Radiographics 2010;30(2):503–16.

82. Dresen RC, Beets GL, Rutten HJT, et al. Locally advanced rectal cancer: MR imaging for restaging after neoadjuvant radiation therapy with concomitant chemotherapy part I. Are we able to predict tumor confined to the rectal wall? Radiology 2009;252(1): 71–80.

Moving?

Make sure your subscription moves with you!

To notify us of your new address, find your **Clinics Account Number** (located on your mailing label above your name), and contact customer service at:

Email: journalscustomerservice-usa@elsevier.com

800-654-2452 (subscribers in the U.S. & Canada)
314-447-8871 (subscribers outside of the U.S. & Canada)

Fax number: 314-447-8029

Elsevier Health Sciences Division
Subscription Customer Service
3251 Riverport Lane
Maryland Heights, MO 63043

*To ensure uninterrupted delivery of your subscription, please notify us at least 4 weeks in advance of move.

Printed and bound by CPI Group (UK) Ltd, Croydon, CR0 4YY

08/05/2025

01864727-0002